Prevention in Psychi

Edited by
E. S. PAYKEL
R. JENKINS

Prevention in Psychiatry

GASKELL

©The Royal College of Psychiatrists 1994

Gaskell is an imprint of the Royal College of Psychiatrists,
17 Belgrave Square, London SW1

All rights reserved. No part of this book may be reprinted or reproduced or utilised in any form or by any electronic, mechanical, or other means, now known or hereafter invented, including photocopying and recording, or in any information storage or retrieval system, without permission in writing from the publishers.

British Library Cataloguing-in-Publication Data

A catalogue record for this book is available from the British Library

ISBN 0-902241-72-9

Distributed in North America
by American Psychiatric Press, Inc.
ISBN 0-88048-634-1

The views presented in this book do not necessarily reflect those of the Royal College of Psychiatrists, and the publishers are not responsible for any error of omission or fact.

The Royal College of Psychiatrists is a registered charity (no. 228636).

Cover design by Julia Burnside
Phototypeset by Dobbie Typesetting Limited, Tavistock, Devon
Printed by Henry Ling Ltd, The Dorset Press, Dorchester, Dorset

Contents

Contributors   vii

Part I. General issues

1   Introduction   *E. S. Paykel*   3
2   Principles of prevention   *Rachel Jenkins*   11
3   Social factors, social interventions and prevention
     Jan Scott and Julian Leff   25
4   Genetics   *Peter McGuffin*   32
5   Biological causes   *Eve C. Johnstone*   40
6   Drug treatment in tertiary prevention   *Eve C. Johnstone*   46

Part II. Prevention of specific disorders

7   Affective disorders   *Jan Scott and E. S. Paykel*   53
8   Suicide   *Keith Hawton*   67
9   Schizophrenia   *Eve C. Johnstone and Julian Leff*   80
10   Anxiety disorders   *Peter Tyrer*   88
11   Eating disorders   *J. Hubert Lacey*   96
12   Drug and alcohol-related problems
     Andrew Johns and Bruce Ritson   103

Part III. Prevention in psychiatric specialities

13   Child psychiatry   *Issy Kolvin*   115
14   Mental handicap   *Kenneth Day*   130
15   Old age psychiatry   *David Jolley*   148
16   Forensic psychiatry   *Pamela Taylor*   157

Part IV. Prevention in medical settings

17   General hospitals   *Keith Lloyd and Simon Wessely*   177
18   Somatisation   *Christopher Bass*   188
19   Primary care   *Keith Lloyd and Rachel Jenkins*   198

Contributors

Christopher Bass, Consultant in Liaison Psychiatry, John Radcliffe Hospital, Oxford OX3 9DU
Kenneth Day, Consultant Psychiatrist and Medical Director, Northgate & Prudhoe NHS Trust, Morpeth, Northumberland NE61 3BP, and Senior Lecturer, Department of Psychiatry, University of Newcastle upon Tyne, UK
Keith Hawton, Consultant Psychiatrist and Senior Clinical Lecturer, University Department of Psychiatry, Warneford Hospital, Oxford OX3 7JX
Rachel Jenkins, Principal Medical Officer, Department of Health, 133 Waterloo Road, London SE1 6UG and Honorary Senior Lecturer, Institute of Psychiatry, De Crespigny Park, London
Andrew Johns, Senior Lecturer, Division of Psychiatry of Addictive Behaviour, St George's Hospital Medical School, London SW17 ORE
Eve Johnstone, Professor of Psychiatry, University Department of Psychiatry, The Kennedy Tower, Royal Edinburgh Hospital, Morningside Park, Edinburgh EH10 5HF
David Jolley, Consultant Old Age Psychiatrist, Honorary Reader Old Age Psychiatry, Healey House, Withington Hospital, Manchester 20
Issy Kolvin, Professor, The Tavistock Centre, Child and Family Department, 120 Belsize Lane, London NW3 5BA; Royal Free Hospital School of Medicine, London
J. Hubert Lacey, Head, Division of General Psychiatry, Department of Mental Health Sciences, St George's Hospital Medical School, Cranmer Terrace, London SW17 ORE
Julian Leff, Director, MRC Social & Community Psychiatry Unit, Institute of Psychiatry, Denmark Hill, London SE5 8AF
Keith Lloyd, Senior Lecturer in Mental Health, University of Exeter, Postgraduate Medical School, Barrack Road, Exeter EX2 5DW
Peter McGuffin, Professor of Psychological Medicine, University of Wales College of Medicine, Heath Park, Cardiff CF4 4XN
E. S. Paykel, Professor of Psychiatry, University of Cambridge, Addenbrooke's Hospital, Cambridge CB2 2QQ
Bruce Ritson, Consultant Psychiatrist, Royal Edinburgh Hospital, Morningside Place, Edinburgh EH10 5HF
Jan Scott, Professor of Psychiatry, University Department of Psychiatry, Royal Victoria Infirmary, Queen Victoria Road, Newcastle upon Tyne NE1 4LP

Pamela Taylor, Head of Medical Services, Special Hospitals Service Authority, 375 Kensington High Street, London W14 8QH

Peter Tyrer, Professor of Community Psychiatry, St Mary's Hospital Medical School, Academic Unit of Psychiatry, St Charles' Hospital, London W10 6DZ

Simon Wessely, Senior Lecturer, Department of Psychological Medicine, King's College Hospital Medical School, Denmark Hill, London

I. General issues

1 Introduction

E. S. PAYKEL

Many of the early advances in medicine, contributing to the increases in life expectancy that occurred in the 19th century, were due to developments in prevention. These particularly involved the infectious diseases, with identification of the causes and prevention of some of them, such as control of the sources of infection for cholera, enhancement of host immunity in vaccination for smallpox; and general improvements in host resistance as nutrition improved. Later, in the 20th century, the emphasis shifted to treatment, with major advances across the field of medicine.

More recently the importance of prevention has again been recognised. Epidemiological studies have pointed to major contributing factors to cancer, chest disease and heart disease, such as smoking, diet and lack of exercise. Considerable investment has been made in public health programmes to modify these. Screening programmes have been set up to detect disorder while it is early and treatable, such as those for cervical and breast cancer. In Britain, the National Health Service has undergone a recent redirection to lay more emphasis on such approaches. The Government White Paper, *Health of the Nation* (1992), has set out targets for this approach, including, within mental health, reductions both in morbidity and in mortality from suicide.

Psychiatric disorders are an important group of public health problems. Prevalences of psychiatric disorders are around 5% for depressive and anxiety disorders respectively, 0.5% for schizophrenia, 5% for dementia in people under 65 and 20% in those over 80 (Bebbington *et al*, 1981; Myers *et al*, 1984; Jorm *et al*, 1987). Lifetime risks for depression may be over 20% (Bebbington *et al*, 1989; Rorsman *et al*, 1990). Mental illness accounts in Britain for about 14% of certificated sickness absence, 14% of NHS in-patient costs and 25% of NHS pharmaceutical costs (*Health of the Nation*, 1992). About 3 per thousand of the population suffer from severe mental handicap (Fryers, 1984). Around 25% of general practice consultations have a psychiatric element (Shepherd *et al*, 1966). Psychiatric disorder causes considerable personal disability and distress in families. It has an increased mortality, notably from suicide but also from other causes; follow-up studies show increased death rates from physical illness in schizophrenia and depression (Tsuang *et al*, 1980).

Psychiatry has tended to be slower in preventive developments and the approaches have been more tentative. Early optimism in the mental hygiene movement in the 1920s and 1930s, focusing around individual work with children, was not fulfilled. The community mental health programme of the Kennedy era in the USA incorporated proposals for prevention, but was oversold and was not translated into continuing funding.

There have been some important publications since 1960. A child psychiatrist, Caplan (1964) suggested a model based on response to crises, which has been influential. He also applied the framework of primary, secondary and tertiary prevention. In recent years there have been reports from the World Health Organization, WHO European office (1988, 1991), a useful book by Newton (1988), American reports concentrating particularly on research (Steinberg & Silverman, 1987; American Psychiatric Association, 1990), and an important report in Britain on Alcohol and Public Health (Faculty of Public Health, 1991). Within mental handicap there have been more consistent preventive efforts and considerable advances.

Views expressed have varied considerably, between very cautious scepticism and over-confident optimism. At one extreme Richard Doll, doyen of British epidemiologists, stated in his Harveian oration on prevention to the Royal College of Physicians (Doll, 1983):

> "A programme for intervention is, however, unlikely to be effective unless the illnesses can be defined and attributed to single factors or groups of factors that act synergistically and are amenable to intervention. . . . it will, I suspect, be many years before we can design a programme for the prevention of mental illness, at either the individual or the social level that will be more cost-effective than a programme that provides for the treatment and support of affected individuals."

At the other extreme, statements have sometimes implied that most of the problems have been solved, and that a massive diversion of resources away from treatment and care towards preventive approaches was justified. Yet it is not easy to point to many proven achievements which might persuade the hardheaded decision maker with a tight limit on total expenditure, that the resources would be best expended on prevention of psychiatric disorders rather than, say, heart disease or early detection of cancer, or that such efforts would cut down the need for psychiatric treatment facilities.

It is noteworthy that a good deal of the published work on psychiatric prevention depends on non-psychiatrists. There have been some notable exceptions, including that of Caplan. In Britain, Jenkins (1990) has formulated useful targets for prevention and outcome indicators in relation to the National Health Service. Nevertheless psychiatrists have been at risk of leaving a vacuum in preventive formulations.

The Royal College of Psychiatrists Committee

In response to these issues the Royal College of Psychiatrists decided early in 1991 to establish a Special Committee on the Place of Prevention in Psychiatry.

The broad aim of the committee was to attempt a balanced appraisal of the present place of prevention in psychiatry, attempting to steer between unjustified optimism, and the scepticism about prevention which all too readily affects those whose main activity is treating disorder. The committee met for two years and published a report (Royal College of Psychiatrists, 1993).

As part of its activities the committee commissioned working papers from experts on various topics, both from within its membership and from outside it. Many of these provided authoritative statements and reviews on areas which had not been well summarised in the literature, and which could not be presented in detail in a committee report. They have therefore been revised and brought together here.

The book is organised in four sections. First general issues are examined, including principles, and implications of knowledge of the broad kinds of causes for prevention. The second section deals with prevention of specific psychiatric disorders. The third deals with prevention viewed from some psychiatric specialities, or regarding special groups of people, including childhood, old age, mental handicap (learning disability) and forensic psychiatry (the interface of psychiatric problems and the law). In the fourth section authors examine prevention in some special medical settings: general hospitals, general practice, and the problems of somatisation which are important in both.

Framework and problems

Attempts to apply prevention in psychiatry have encountered a number of difficulties. For primary prevention a prerequisite is an adequate base of knowledge of causes. In respect of psychiatric disorders this is only partly available, but there is now a substantial body of knowledge, particularly concerning social aspects.

A key issue is that most psychiatric causation is multifactorial. Single causes, such as adverse early home environments or recent life stresses may contribute to many disorders. A single disorder commonly appears to have many contributing causes. For instance, causes of depression range from genes and effects of some amine-depleting drugs, to psychosocial factors such as bereavement, interpersonal losses, and threats to self-esteem. Therefore a single preventive measure may not link to a specific disorder, but to many in varying degree. This need not be an argument against prevention: the same applies to the effects of smoking.

From the point of view of secondary prevention, the boundaries between pre-disorder and disorder are vague, since both can only be detected by the presence of certain symptoms, and the same symptoms, at a more severe level, define disorder. This is really a semantic issue and it applies also in other areas where screening has been used. A more substantive question is whether detecting and treating early disorder will prevent the development of major disorders and of prolonged disorders, and is a cost-effective method of doing so. It might be the case that early and mild disorders most often have a good spontaneous outcome. These are questions for empirical testing. The evidence available suggests that milder and neurotic disorders do not generally proceed to psychoses but are often prolonged, thus secondary prevention can be helpful.

From the standpoint of tertiary prevention, the major question is whether this is to be regarded as prevention rather than treatment. However, much psychiatric disorder is recurrent; effective measures to eliminate recurrence can have major effects in reducing prevalence and do not necessarily involve treatment of, or presence of, any active symptoms. Likewise psychiatric disorder may lead to major disability. Overall the classical preventive framework is applicable to psychiatry.

A particular set of problems arises in relation to positive mental health. It is not easy to define this concept without finishing up in something which is really outside the health domain: happiness. More empirically, in a similar way to with mild disorder, the question again arises as to whether positive aspects of mental well-being protect against major disorder. Some aspects of a healthy lifestyle, such as avoidance of dependence-inducing drugs, fostering of a supportive social network, development of an adaptive coping style for minor adversities, are relatively non-controversial and do have much *prima facie* evidence in their favour.

Beyond these, in the arena of policy, the general public has rightly become distrustful of the claims of psychiatrists to advise on wide aspects of how people should live, and of the reality of the knowledge base which would entitle them to do so. Psychiatrists have also, in the light of experience, become cautious in making such pronouncements. In general, this volume does not deal with direct issues of positive mental health, as we do not consider that sufficient empirically tested knowledge is yet available. Chapters do adopt relevant aspects of the health promotion approach, and also health education.

Conclusions

The general tone of this volume is one of cautious optimism. There have only been a few spectacular successes, of which the most striking are in the genetic causes of severe learning disability, where developments in biochemistry, genetics and screening have already produced dramatic results; the current revolution in molecular genetics is leading to a further acceleration, and even the possibility of reversing the causes by gene replacement. Almost as impressive are the contributions of psychotropic medications towards reducing relapse, recurrence and disability in functional psychiatric disorders. There are other more modest successes, particularly in relation to psychosocial factors in functional psychiatric disorders.

A pleasing conclusion is that the general principles of prevention as formulated in other health areas apply equally to psychiatry despite, as yet, incomplete knowledge about the aetiology of many disorders. As psychiatric disorders may have multiple causal pathways, direct approaches to prevention of causes are likely to have diffused effects across several disorders, but such efforts are nevertheless worthwhile.

Primary prevention

Regarding primary prevention the greatest successes have in fact been in the application of genetic and biochemical methods in mental handicap. Worthwhile advances have been achieved in some problems which represent end point types of behaviour, in part consequences of psychiatric disorder and in part involving many other personal and societal causes, such as suicidal behaviour, and

HIV-related consequences of drug misuse. These can respond to improvements in psychiatric services for care of the primary disorders. Two further problems, alcohol and drug misuse, are not yet well prevented but would be amenable to determined preventive measures on a societal level. Genetic counselling for psychiatric disorders needs to be more widely available. Its place is currently limited but is likely to grow. There are additional needs for primary prevention in developing countries, particularly in relation to organic disorders.

Beyond these specifics, social causative factors have implications for primary prevention. Here an important general conclusion emerges: it is better to think small than to think big. In psychiatry targeted preventive medicines are likely to be more profitable than universal measures. It is easier to modify the social microenvironment of the family than the macroenvironment of society as a whole. Similarly it is easier to tackle precipitating factors where the link with onset of disorder is closer, rather than predisposing factors. Coping responses are more amenable to intervention than is removal of social stresses themselves, many of which are bound up with the inevitable consequences of the life-cycle. What is not at present feasible in primary prevention is to change dramatically cultures or societal structures, except for the most deprived. Nor is it possible to avoid interpersonal life events, or, as yet, to prevent functional disorders by tackling fundamental biological causes and mechanisms.

What do present themselves as feasible and timely are a variety of targeted pilot projects which can be properly evaluated, to determine effectiveness and cost–benefit ratios. These pilot projects should precede any widespread introduction and major diversion of resources. Pending these, the case is not yet conclusively made that primary prevention in functional psychiatric disorders can succeed on a wide scale, so replacing some of the need for treatment services. Such pilot projects should include long-term evaluation of outcome. Their expense is justified. Examples include: further studies of benefits of crisis intervention in stressful events; provision of social support and community networks for people at high-risk such as young mothers, the bereaved, socially isolated, the elderly, those with physical or sensory disabilities, painful or life-threatening conditions; early intervention after catastrophic events; educational programmes for staff in settings where eating disorders are prevalent; intervention in post-natal depression to prevent effects on infants, work with the children of psychiatrically ill parents and children in other vulnerable situations.

Secondary prevention

The situation is similar but the opportunities greater in secondary prevention. The use of screening techniques is highly feasible with many of the common disorders in psychiatry, particularly depression, anxiety and problem drinking. It also lends itself well to the circumstances of general practice. When combined with interviewing to establish presence of disorders which exceed thresholds for clinical criteria, it is straightforward and merits wider adoption. When it involves detection of subthreshold disorders, it requires evaluation in controlled designs, to determine whether detection and intervention in early disorders is justified in terms of benefit and cost. Available evidence based on the use of the General Health Questionnaire suggests that it is effective.

Tertiary prevention

For tertiary prevention, the situation is different; it is already well established in psychiatry. It involves not only prevention of disability but prevention of recurrence. The value of prophylactic maintenance drug treatment is well proven in affective disorders and schizophrenia, and there is good evidence for the effects of family intervention in high expressed emotion schizophrenic families. The place of behavioural and cognitive approaches in anxiety and depression is growing. Service-related local case registers can be useful for identifying and monitoring vulnerable groups.

Prevention opportunities

Among the specific disorders, the possibilities for primary and secondary prevention differ. Currently they are higher for depression than for schizophrenia, potentially high but less well tested for eating disorders. Post-traumatic stress disorder offers a productive arena for early intervention. Suicidal behaviour, because it is often a consequence of psychiatric disorder, presents particular opportunities for the psychiatrist. Substance misuse is a good example of an area where much is in theory possible; it would require a commitment from society, policy makers and the media to take tough decisions, such as in respect of alcohol pricing policy and tobacco agricultural incentives. Prevention in childhood presents one of the greatest challenges to empirical long-term testing – can intervention in childhood avoid adult disorder or is this aim at present not achievable?

A multidisciplinary approach

Although the contributions to this volume are all by psychiatrists, this reflects its origin rather than any claims to ownership. Preventive activities, contributions to the theoretical debate and empirical studies extend widely to other disciplines and the authors of this volume are very clear that this is the case. In all fields of medicine preventive activities involve a wider framework than simply those who undertake treatment, and include workers in the fields of public health, education, public policy and the political arena. In psychiatry, prevention also involves those in the social and psychological disciplines. Psychiatrists can make useful contributions in care and aftercare of patients so as to avoid subsequent consequences such as disability, recurrence and suicide, in the management of mentally disordered offenders and potential offenders, and in the education of others. The other members of the multidisciplinary psychiatric team, including psychologists, psychiatric nurses and community psychiatric nurses are also of crucial importance in applying preventive strategies.

General practitioners and other members of the primary health care team are particularly well placed to contribute to psychiatric prevention, because of their responsibilities for specific populations and families, and their roles in early presentation of disorders, in regular assessment of the elderly, and in delivering continuity of care over long periods. Their contributions to prevention can include early detection, early treatment, prevention of relapse, identification and prevention of persistent somatisation in early somatisers, and amelioration of the consequences for family members of having a physically or psychiatrically ill relative. The Defeat Depression campaign jointly organised by the Royal College of Psychiatrists and the Royal College of General Practitioners is currently focusing on some of these aspects in relation to depression (Paykel & Priest, 1992).

Other health and social work personnel should also contribute, including social workers, health visitors and midwives involved in ante-natal and post-natal work, and community nurses working with the elderly. General hospital medical and nursing staff can make considerable contributions in relation to somatisation and suicide. There is a large potential contribution to be made by the voluntary sector, for example by bereavement counselling, advice centres, the Samaritans, support groups for the vulnerable, and workers with ethnic minorities.

Many of the tasks are educational. There is a need for education of medical students, postgraduate education of psychiatrists, general practitioners, other doctors and other health workers, other kinds of staff members in appropriate settings (such as dance schools in respect of eating disorders, teachers), and the general public. Some of these aspects are within professional education; some are aspects of health education to the general public. Education of the public is needed about mental disorder, availability of local treatment facilities, sensible attitudes to alcohol and drugs, and facts to lessen stigma. In respect of some other educational activities aimed at developing more mentally healthy life styles, coping mechanisms, and positive mental health, caution and evaluation as to real benefits are required. An important aspect on which there has already been considerable and commendable effort is that of safe sexual behaviour in the face of the HIV epidemic. The best methods for altering such behaviour still need to be determined.

An overall need referred to repeatedly in the chapters is for research. It is axiomatic that successful prevention depends on good knowledge of causes, but its introduction should also be dependent on careful evaluation of feasibility, short and long-term effectiveness, acceptability and costs.

However, evaluation of preventive projects is not easy and studies have sometimes been relatively unsophisticated. The difficulties include lack of evaluation expertise; lack of consensus on definitions, particularly relating to the target groups, the specification of interventions and the target measures; design and statistical problems arising from implementing programmes in a field setting rather than a laboratory (Cook & Campbell, 1979). Many potential causative factors act in childhood but the disorders to be prevented may occur in adulthood, so that long-term studies are required. These bring additional problems including changes in staff and problems in funding, making it difficult to evaluate programmes over a number of years, together with other events, political, economic or environmental, which may intervene unexpectedly, disrupting data collection and analysis.

In much of the above, it is apparent that tough realism is required. Prevention in psychiatry does not currently justify large scale investment or diversion of resources from treatment. What it does justify is cautious and limited investment, with as much money spent on evaluation of benefits, and countervailing costs, as on the preventive intervention itself.

It is unlikely that preventive approaches currently available will lessen the need for treatment services, except in a few specific aspects such as some mental handicap syndromes. The contribution of prevention is likely to grow progressively in the future as knowledge of causes increases, and with evaluative studies such as those recommended above.

References

AMERICAN PSYCHIATRIC ASSOCIATION (1990) Report of the APA Task Force on Prevention Research. *American Journal of Psychiatry*, **147**, 1701–1704.
BEBBINGTON, P., HURRY, J., TENNANT, C., *et al* (1981) Epidemiology of mental disorders in Camberwell. *Psychological Medicine*, **11**, 561–579.
BEBBINGTON, P., KATZ, R., MCGUFFIN, P., *et al* (1989) The risk of minor depression before age 65: results from a community survey. *Psychological Medicine*, **19**, 393–400.
CAPLAN, G. (1964) *Principles of Preventive Psychiatry*. London: Tavistock.
COOK, T. D. & CAMPBELL, D. T. (1979) *Quasi-experimentation: Design and Analysis Issues for Field Settings*. Chicago: Rand McNally.
DOLL, R. (1983) Prospects for prevention. *British Medical Journal*, **286**, 445–453.
FACULTY OF PUBLIC HEALTH (1991) *Alcohol and the Public Health*. London: Macmillan.
FRYERS, T. (1984) Severe intellectual impairment in the developing world. In *The Epidemiology of Severe Intellectual Impairment: The Dynamics and Prevalence*, pp. 190–202. London: Academic Press.
JENKINS, R. (1990) Towards a system of outcome indicators for mental health care. *British Journal of Psychiatry*, **157**, 500–514.
JORM, A. F., KORTEN, A. E. & HENDERSON, A. S. (1987) The prevalence of dementia: a quantitative integration of the literature. *Acta Psychiatrica Scandinavica*, **76**, 465–479.
MYERS, J., WEISSMAN, M. M., TISCHLER, G. L., *et al* (1984) Six-month prevalence of psychiatric disorders in three communities: 1980–1982. *Archives of General Psychiatry*, **41**, 959–967.
NEWTON, J. (1988) *Preventing Mental Illness*. London: Routledge.
PAYKEL, E. S. & PRIEST, R. G. (1992) Recognition and management of depression in general practice: consensus statement. *British Journal of Psychiatry*, **3051**, 1198–1202.
RORSMAN, B. A., GRASBECK, A., HAGNELL, O., *et al* (1990) A prospective study of first-incidence depression. The Lundby Study 1957–72. *British Journal of Psychiatry*, **156**, 336–342.
ROYAL COLLEGE OF PSYCHIATRISTS (1993) *Prevention in Psychiatry*. London: Royal College of Psychiatrists.
SHEPHERD, M., COOPER, M., BROWN, A. C., *et al* (1966) *Psychiatric Illness in General Practice*. Oxford: Oxford University Press.
STEINBERG, J. A. & SILVERMAN, M. D. (1987) *Preventing Mental Disorders – A Research Perspective*. US Department of Health and Human Services – Public Health Service: Alcohol, Drug Abuse and Mental Health Administration.
THE HEALTH OF THE NATION (1992) A strategy for health in England. London: HMSO.
TSUANG, M. T., WOOLSON, R. F. & FLEMING, J. A. (1980) Causes of death in schizophrenia and manic depression. *British Journal of Psychiatry*, **136**, 239–242.
WORLD HEALTH ORGANIZATION (1988) *Prevention of Mental, Psychosocial and Neurological Disorders in the European Region*. Geneva: WHO Regional Office for Europe.
——— (1991) *Implications for the Field of Mental Health of the European Targets for Attaining Health for All*. Geneva: WHO Regional Office for Europe.

2 Principles of prevention

RACHEL JENKINS

This chapter aims to introduce the conceptual framework of prevention, to discuss its applicability to mental illness, and to explore recent theoretical developments underpinning strategies of primary prevention. It then goes on to discuss the general policy issues of whether there is an adequate knowledge base, what are appropriate targets for prevention, factors to consider in setting objectives, the boundaries of mental health prevention activities, and what is known of professional attitudes towards preventive interventions. It concludes with a review of research and evaluation issues in prevention.

Conceptual and theoretical issues

Traditional public health definitions

Most people are by now familiar with the traditional public health definitions of prevention (Caplan, 1964), which are as follows:

Primary prevention is directed at reducing the incidence (rate of occurrence of new cases) in the community. Primary prevention efforts are those directed at reducing the incidence (rate of occurrence of new cases) in the community. Primary prevention efforts are directed at people who are essentially normal, but believed to be 'at risk' from the development of a particular disorder.

Secondary prevention involves efforts to reduce the prevalence of a disorder by reducing its duration. Thus secondary prevention programmes are directed at people who show early signs of disorder, and the goal is to shorten the duration of the disorder by early and prompt treatment.

Tertiary prevention is designed to reduce the severity and disability associated with a particular disorder.

Application of these definitions to mental health

It has been argued that, while this model of prevention is quite useful where specific diseases or other causal factors are easily identifiable, it is less helpful in the field of mental health where precise definitions and specific disease entities with known aetiologies are the exception rather than the rule. However, these arguments would only seem to hold up in relation to primary prevention;

they do not militate any more against secondary and tertiary prevention than in physical medicine.

Many psychiatrists consider primary prevention of mental illness a hollow term, and they have not forgotten the failed dreams of prevention promised in the community psychiatry movement of the 1970s. However, other disciplines and some psychiatrists have continued to be interested in the possibilities and have slowly developed both a framework for health promotion and primary prevention, as well as the research methodologies required. Toews & El-Guebaly (1989) have called strongly for psychiatrists to contribute to this debate, lest insufficient attention is paid to the realities of treating the mentally ill.

The debate about secondary and tertiary prevention has focused, not on their definition or boundaries which have remained relatively unchallenged and uncontroversial, but rather on whether they qualify as 'prevention' proper at all, rather than simply aspects of good clinical practice (e.g. Bower, 1987; Newton, 1988). (Indeed this viewpoint illustrates how little doubt there is of the effectiveness of secondary and tertiary prevention.) My opinion is that they do qualify as prevention simply because they do prevent something. Secondary prevention shortens the duration of illness, and hence prevents chronic morbidity and even mortality, as well as preventing some of the knock-on consequences of depression to other people, e.g. to children and spouses; while tertiary prevention minimises handicap and disability and thus prevents many of the associated sequelae of chronic illness.

In contrast, the debate, both theoretical and practical, about primary prevention is considerable and somewhat complex, and is most readily understood from a historical perspective. Caplan's presentation of the definition of primary prevention was based on the public health model of eradication of disease, where each disease was assumed to have a single biological cause and where no accompanying psychological or social factors were considered (Caplan, 1964). However, in psychiatry, the hereditability of various disorders is relatively low, and many other factors influence the development of conditions such as schizophrenia. Therefore more recent concepts of prevention have stressed the *multifactorial approach* to the aetiology of disease and hence to preventive strategies (Bloom, 1981). Such a multifactorial aetiology usually includes both psychological and social components.

The second major development in the concept of prevention has been the notion of targeting. In order to clarify the issues surrounding targeting it is necessary here to introduce three further definitions (Gordon, 1983).

Universal prevention measures are those which are regarded as desirable for everyone, and the decision to implement them is taken if their benefits clearly outweigh the costs and risks of implementing them (e.g. seat belts, encouragement of safe drinking, reduction of cigarette smoking, nutrition and exercise).

Selective prevention measures are deemed to be appropriate when an individual is a member of a subgroup of the population (e.g. age, sex, occupation) whose risk of becoming ill is above normal. Examples are good antenatal and perinatal care and preventive activities in pregnant women; health interventions in young unsupported teenage mothers and socially isolated elderly.

'Indicated' measures for groups at sufficiently high risk, for an illness like schizophrenia in which a genetic susceptibility is strongly suspected, and for

groups who have experienced severe, clearly defined emotional stress (e.g. children exposed to disasters or to violence).

Goldston (1977a, b) and others have argued that primary prevention encompasses those activities which are directed towards specifically identified vulnerable high risk groups in the community who have not been labelled psychiatrically ill and for whom measures can be undertaken to avoid the onset of emotional disturbance and/or enhance their level of positive mental health. Thus, prevention, by this definition, is directed at specific targets rather than at the whole population. Thus it would include indicated and possibly selective measures, but certainly not universal measures.

On the other hand, authors such as Newton (1988) have argued from the implicit standpoint that primary prevention does include universal, selective and indicated measures, but that the only strategies worth doing are those which are highly targeted.

Relationship of mental health promotion to primary prevention

A related issue is that the concept of primary prevention has been used interchangeably with health promotion. Toews & El-Guebaly (1989) assert that primary prevention is directed towards populations at risk while promotion involves the population at large. This would suggest that health promotion refers to universal strategies while primary prevention refers to selective and indicated measures (Fig. 2.1, model 1).

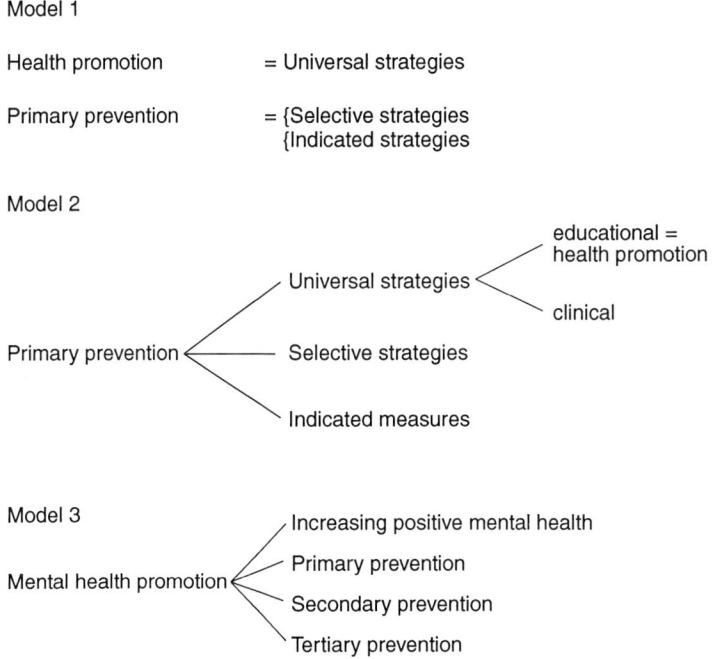

Fig. 2.1. Relationship of mental health promotion to primary prevention

Goldston (1977b) goes still further, and asserts that mental health promotion programmes are "primarily educational rather than clinical in conception, their ultimate goal being to increase people's capacities for dealing with crises and for taking steps to improve their own lives". So far, it would seem that we could regard health promotion as a subset of universal strategies (i.e. the educational rather than the clinical strategies), which is itself a subset of primary prevention (Fig. 2.1, model 2). However, mental health promotion literature generally assumes that mental health is a positive state which is not synonymous with the absence of illness, and furthermore that mental health promotion activities may include those who are ill as well as those who are well and those who are at risk. Thus, we have reached the alternative situation where, from a mental health promotion standpoint, primary prevention is a subset of mental health promotion (Fig. 2.1, model 3).

It is therefore clear that there is some conceptual muddiness in the field. As Toews & El-Guebaly (1989) argue

> "the conceptual diffuseness suggests the need for crisper definitions; and the semantics involved are determined by ideologies regarding the causes of mental illness, professional advocacy and social agendas."

My opinion is that the definitions of primary, secondary and tertiary prevention are in fact as useful in delineating opportunities for preventive action in mental illness as in physical illness and, furthermore, that the division of primary prevention into universal, selective, and indicated strategies is an extremely helpful aid to considering the value and effectiveness of primary preventive strategies. The reminder that preventive strategies may be educational as well as clinical in focus is also useful. I find the term health promotion redundant, and potentially confusing, and would favour model 4 (Table 2.1). The terms which have not yet been discussed, namely proactive and reactive, microlevel and macrolevel, will be dealt with in the next section.

TABLE 2.1
Proposed classification of prevention strategies

Primary prevention (Aims to stop illness from occurring)
   Macrolevel and microlevel strategies
   Educational and clinical strategies
   Proactive strategies (aims to remove/reduce stressors)
   Reactive strategies (aim to improve supports)
   Universal, selective and indicated strategies

Secondary prevention (Aims to detect and treat existing illness as soon as possible)

Tertiary prevention (Aims to reduce chronic disability and avoid long-term handicap)

Recent conceptual developments in primary prevention

Predisposing and precipitating factors

As our conceptual understanding of the difference between *predisposing factors* (e.g. loss of mother in childhood, genetic loading) and *precipitating factors* (e.g. stressful life events) has developed, more practical opportunities have arisen for prevention in the domain of precipitating factors rather than predisposing factors. In practice, this has meant a shift of interest from 'high risk populations' to 'high risk situations' and events. There are two possible reasons for this: the greater difficulty in identifying high risk populations in clinical practice than of identifying those in high risk situations; and that the prevention payoff or return is probably greater if one concentrates on the high risk situations, since these are more likely to be otherwise closely followed by illness in the short term, than if one concentrates on the high risk populations who may not have developed illness in any case for many years to come (Price *et al*, 1989).

Lack of specificity of causes

It is now well recognised that in mental illness, rather than a specific cause being associated with a specific illness (e.g. vitamin deficiency: pellagra), a variety of stressful events may lead in a variety of people to a variety of illness outcomes. Again this situation is not unique to mental illness. In physical illness as well, stressful events and environments may lead to a variety of diseases, for example myocardial infarction, vitiligo and skin diseases.

Caplan (1981) summed it up:

> "Years ago we used to think that particular sets of such events in association with certain personality patterns would cause specific bodily or mental illnesses. Nowadays, many of us believe that individuals exposed to such circumstances may suffer an increase in nonspecific vulnerability to a wide range of bodily and mental illnesses."

Preventing the risk factor and improving the coping response: a distinction

Catalano & Dooley (1980) have distinguished, within primary prevention, between preventing the occurrence of the risk factor and improving the coping response triggered by stressors. The first strategy assumes that it is possible to control or prevent the occurrence of the causal agent while the second strategy assumes that the agent, if unavoidable, can be resisted. They cite the public health examples of eliminating breeding grounds of malaria-carrying mosquitoes as preventing occurrence of the risk factor, and vaccinating for polio and smallpox as improving the coping response triggered by stressors, and they have termed the first approach '*proactive primary prevention*' and the second '*reactive primary prevention*'. Reactive primary prevention can occur before or after the stressor, but is aimed at preparing the individual to react effectively to the stressor. In contrast proactive primary prevention attempts to avoid the stressor altogether.

Micro v. macro proactive primary prevention

There are different levels of intervention, especially in relation to proactive primary prevention, which can be classified on a continuum ranging from micro to macro (Bronfenbrenner, 1977), which Catalano & Dooley (1980) have condensed into two broad categories of the *macroenvironment* (social and large organisational conditions) and the *microenvironment* (family and individual characteristics).

At the *microlevel*, proactive prevention might take the form of education about parenting to reduce the occurrence of damaging parenting, child abuse and divorce. At the *macrolevel*, proactive prevention might involve transport policies and planning to prevent excessive automobile lead exhausts and airport noise from occurring near school playgrounds.

In general, people have been optimistic about microlevel prevention at the biological and family levels, but have avoided thinking about macrolevel prevention. This has arisen because conditions such as unemployment, social discrimination, poverty and so forth are not always regarded as within the purview of mental health, and psychiatry has tried to learn from the lessons of the 1960s and '70s when some psychiatrists went far beyond their areas of expertise to treat the community as the patient. Also, such considerations may sometimes involve sufficiently controversial social values that it is deemed politically wise to avoid them.

Thus the general view seems often to be that microlevel proactive and reactive primary prevention approaches are helpful, while macrolevel proactive prevention is regarded as beyond the province of the mental health worker.

But Catalano & Dooley (1980) argue that macrolevel proactive primary prevention should be more carefully considered. They believe that opportunities for macrolevel primary prevention are often ignored because mental health disciplines are used to taking the individual as the unit of analysis, and have little experience with or methodological equipment for aggregate level analysis.

Strategies based on life event and social support theory

Researchers have not only developed scales which attempt to assign stress weights to various life events (Holmes & Rahe, 1967) but have also examined individual differences in the perception of and the response to similar events (Masuda & Holmes, 1974). In addition, other researchers have begun to try to identify situations (Cassel, 1976; Cobb, 1976) and personal variables (Kobasa, 1979) which may influence an individual's ability to cope with similar levels of stress. Bloom (1985) has thoroughly reviewed the research concerned with factors that appear to attenuate the effects of stressful life events. Important factors include the availability of social support or a helping social network for people undergoing life stressors, and social competence or coping ability and style. Both factors lend themselves to the development of preventive strategies.

There have been two main approaches to identifying the target population for preventive activities. Firstly the identification of all those who are *multiply* stressed. This is helpful at an individual level but difficult at population level. Secondly, the identification of those who have experienced a *particular* life event.

It draws on crisis theory which states that interventions keyed to central life points can reduce the incidence of emotional disturbance (Goldston, 1977a, b).

In an attempt to help the development of preventive strategies from the perspective of stressful life events, Bloom (1979) has outlined the following paradigm:

(a) Identify a stressful life event that appears to have undesirable psychological consequences in a significant proportion of the population. Develop procedures for reliably identifying people who have undergone or who are undergoing that stressful experience.
(b) By traditional epidemiological and laboratory methods, study the consequences of that event and develop hypotheses related to how one might go about reducing or eliminating the negative consequences of the event.
(c) Mount and evaluate experimental preventive intervention programmes based on these hypotheses.

Potentially targetable stressful life events include both predictable transition points or 'normal' crises which are potentially periods of lengthened stress, for example starting school, moving school at 11, job entry, retirement, are all 'normal' life events; and unpredictable high frequency events or crises, for example unemployment or physical illness or injury.

The second and third steps of Bloom's list are less easily dealt with because not all individuals respond to an event in the same way or to the same extent. Some individuals cope well, while others experience considerable difficulties. Therefore, in order to understand the differential impact of life events, and hence to design effective prevention strategies, we have to find out more about the modes of action of different kinds of social support (e.g. instrumental appraisal, emotional, informational) (Cobb, 1976; House, 1981), and coping abilities.

Besides avoiding specific stresses and improving coping capacities, it is also possible to alter environmental settings. People are often at risk due not only to their individual characteristics but also the situation they are in. Price (1979) suggested that environmental settings can be specifically selected, changed or created in prevention strategies. For example, helping people find opportunities for recreation, education or self-help groups would qualify as selecting the environmental setting. Changing the environmental setting might be achieved by consulting or intervening with the family or the organisation. Creating a setting occurs when a new structure is created, for example, a walk-in mental health centre. While most individuals engage in setting selection naturally, its possibilities in prevention strategies have often been overlooked.

Research has elucidated three broad mechanisms by which social support may affect mental health: by a direct effect on well-being regardless of whether the individual is under stress; indirectly by reducing exposure to social adversity (for example, individuals with deficient social networks may be more likely to experience stressful events, and to use less effective coping strategies) and interactively by buffering the individual from the maladaptive effects of stress (Mitchell *et al*, 1982). Moos & Mitchell (1982) suggested that the different types of support include social companionship, emotional support, cognitive guidance and education, and material aid and services; Jenkins *et al* (1981) pointed out that all social domains may be either stressful or supportive or both.

Support needs to be related to the coping task required for a particular stress. Moos (1982) suggests that an individual with a chronic physical illness may benefit more from companionship and assistance with maintaining regular routines than from 'emotionally supportive' discussions that focus on aspects of the sickness.

Jason (1980), writing about children, describes four distinct types of primary prevention strategies in children.

Preventing vulnerable populations from succumbing to disorders (Poser & Hartman, 1979). High risk target groups might include children with one or two schizophrenic parents (Garmezy, 1971); children of alcoholics and drug addicts; or those experiencing the death of a parent; and children with physical handicaps. A potential iatrogenic hazard in this approach involves inadvertently labelling or stigmatising normal functioning children as being marginally adjusted.

Preventing the onset of carefully defined specific disorders (Plunkett & Gordon, 1960). For example, poisoning from lead-based paints, infections such as syphilis, genetic diseases such as PKU, nutritional diseases (e.g. pellagra), school phobias, or addictive behaviour patterns. The value of this approach is a direct function of the extent to which these disorders are associated with short-term as well as long-term psychological and physical conditions.

Promoting and enhancing adaptivity and healthy functioning is emphasised, rather than preventing illness. Building or strengthening social skills typify this orientation, which focuses on goals no-one could disagree with, and precludes unintentional stigmatisation.

Easing the impact of traumatic milestones, and transitional events in three areas – school, family life and work.

Developing natural support systems

Facilitating the development of natural support systems in the community relies on the evidence that social supports act as a buffer protecting individuals from the effects of external stressors (Cassel, 1973; Caplan, 1974; Bloom, 1979). These strategies may be further categorised:

(a) *Supporting existing systems*. Providing consultative services to natural support systems is illustrated by Collins & Pancoast (1976) who developed collaborative ties with natural neighbours and helpers who provide support to individuals and groups at risk. Their strategy involved identifying high risk neighbourhoods, conducting a preliminary assessment of the area, identifying natural neighbours, and establishing a consultative relationship with them, and assisting natural helpers in carrying out helping roles by giving consultation and support (Note: This could be done in Britain via general practice).

(b) *Creating a new but natural support system*. As exemplified by Silverman (1969), who set up self-help groups for widows.

(c) *Educating carers*. The knowledge and skills of professional and non-professional carers can be improved so that they will be more effective in the future (Caplan, 1970).

(d) *Organisational consultation*. This aims to create more responsive organisations. This is based on the premise that schools, police, law system, social services and other key organisations have a profound effect on attitudes and behaviour, and are not neutral in their influence (Maclennan *et al*, 1975).

(e) *Development of alliances*. Coalition building aims to develop community networks to bring together the relevant agencies, and also to increase the community's involvement in health issues, e.g. on children's welfare, on rape or domestic violence. The community may then start to develop on advocacy role as well, arguing for more resources, lobbying for support and so forth.

(f) *Mental health education*. This can be aimed at several different levels. Mental health education seeks to inform the general public about mental health problems and about available treatment and health promoting resources. Research indicates that local residents often have minimal knowledge about mental health services offered in their vicinity. It is particularly important to reduce stigma, and here, school and the media have an important role; it aims to develop important competencies within normal and at risk groups, in order to improve the capacity to cope both with predictable life transitions and with less predictable stresses. The premise is that disorders can be avoided by strengthening an individual's or group's capacity to handle environmental stress or life issues (Cowen, 1977); it can be used to increase the knowledge and skills of both patients and their relatives; and can be specifically targeted by providing important information to people in a community who are in key positions to affect lives of others – formal and informal, such as clergy, teachers, employers and doctors. Lastly, it is important to influence public policies which affect the mental health and well-being of individuals and groups in the community. Keeping policy makers informed about mental health issues and sensitive to the effects of service programmes on human lives, and developing position papers on key policy issues, are among the strategies open to health promotion professionals who wish to influence the public policy process.

General policy issues in mental health prevention

Is there an adequate knowledge base?

This is a question to be considered in detail in following chapters, and is clearly a vital one where scarce resources are to be allocated.

Pardes *et al* (1989) highlight some of the research cornerstones of preventive efforts. Briefly they argue that these rest on:

(a) *The refinement of psychiatric diagnosis*. Greater specificity and validity of diagnostic criteria make epidemiological studies much more informative, while enabling psychiatrists to tailor treatment to diagnosis more appropriately and to carry out more specific studies of homogeneous groups of illnesses.
(b) *Epidemiology*. Epidemiological studies enable the elucidation of environmental and sociodemographic risk factors. The increasing use of longitudinal designs, linkage with health service use data, and replication of design and method in multiple sites will generate valuable information for the evaluation of preventive interventions.

(c) *Genetics*. Molecular genetic technology is advancing the understanding of the genotypes of illnesses, including Alzheimer's disease, Huntington's disease, bipolar affective disorders and schizophrenia. Genetic counselling may become a significant element in primary prevention, although the ethical and emotional implications need to be clearly addressed (Wexler, 1985).

(d) *Neurobiology and biotechnology*. New non-invasive methods of visualising the brain are allowing us to increase our understanding of cerebral function and dysfunction in relation to particular psychiatric illness, and may in the long run aid in the identification of prophylactic measures.

However, to some prevention advocates, it appears that a double standard is being applied in relation to the adequacy of the knowledge base for action. More evidence on effectiveness seems to be required before prevention programmes are supported than is the case for treatment activities. Generally there is greater public demand to do something when a person is ill or suffering than to undertake primary preventive efforts. Prevention is accepted in principle, but when hard resource allocations are made, the decision usually goes for treatment services rather than primary preventive programmes.

Appropriate targets for prevention/promotion activities

Some have argued that the priority targets for preventive work should be the major mental illnesses (schizophrenia and manic depressive disorders). However, there is little evidence for the effectiveness of primary prevention here other than the limited scope for genetic counselling, although plenty on secondary and tertiary prevention strategies. Some have also suggested non-psychotic depression where there are many possibilities for primary and secondary prevention (Jenkins *et al*, 1992). Taking a longitudinal perspective, Eisenberg & Parron (1979) suggested preventing developmental attrition, "a sequential and cumulative failure to attain levels of cognitive and affective development sufficient for personal and social competence". On the other hand, others have argued the need to move away from the focus on specific illness, and instead promote and reinforce the strengths of community systems. There is no consensus on which of the above targets is most important. Different assumptions underlie the various approaches, and call for different strategies.

In choosing objectives for prevention it is important to consider (a) the social cost or burden of illness involved in the particular problem or condition including death, disability, days off work, impaired functioning or extent of suffering; (b) the current knowledge about the aetiology of the condition, and how persuasive is the evidence that interventions are effective; (c) what is the feasibility of the proposed programme in terms of political acceptance, nature of public attitudes, balance between risk and gain factors, and then availability of funds; (d) how appropriate it is for mental health personnel to take the lead in developing or organising the activity, for example, in improving availability of public housing or in ensuring improved prenatal care for teenage mothers. Should mental health personnel only focus on those areas that are specifically within their own competence?

We are generally agreed that it is usually acceptable for prevention activities to modify individual or family behaviour. How far do we agree that prevention activities should seek to bring about broader changes in society? There is considerable evidence that rates of mental disorders are related to social class and to other measures of economic deprivation. Should prevention programmes then seek to bring about greater equity in society generally, income redistribution, reduce poverty, racism or sexism?

Eisenberg & Parron (1979) have argued that "Mental health professionals bear a special responsibility to bring to public attention the urgency of concerted social action".

There are probably opportunities for previously unexplored collaboration between mental health programmes and other programmes, for example on diet, exercise, relaxation and health education. The Look After Your Heart campaign is a possible avenue for improved collaboration with mental health programmes. Some mental health centres have consultation and education activities in schools, police, day care centres, and work places.

Professional attitudes towards preventive interventions

Because opportunities for prevention in psychiatry are less immediately obvious than in physical medicine, they are often overlooked by the psychiatrist who may feel frustrated or disenchanted with the philosophy of prevention, feeling it has little to offer psychiatry. A recent American survey (Linn *et al*, 1988) showed that while psychiatrists have generally positive attitudes towards the idea of prevention, they are uncertain about the ethics and knowledge basis of specific preventive activities, and they also perceive serious barriers to implementation including resources, educational and time factors (see also Yager *et al*, 1989).

Research and evaluation

Strategies need to be evaluated, but the unspecific nature of objectives often makes this difficult. Improving coping skills or providing support systems to bereaved individuals sets a methodological challenge in deriving a specific set of measurable outcomes. The evaluation of prevention strategies involves all the difficulties associated with evaluation of psychotherapy, and some of the effects are likely to be measurable only over very long periods of time.

The level of evaluation of prevention programmes is often primitive due to lack of evaluation expertise, and of widely accepted models for evaluation; lack of consensus on definitions particularly relating to the target groups, the specification of the interventions and the outcome measures; changes in staff and lack of funding making it difficult to monitor and evaluate programmes over a number of years; design and statistical problems arising from implementing programmes in a field setting rather than in a laboratory (Cook & Campbell, 1979); together with events, either political, economic, or environmental which may intervene unexpectedly, disrupting data collection and analysis. It is of course important to have a representative design that it is possible to generalise from.

Most evaluation tends to rely on process measures and client satisfaction scales, but there is no good reason not to use before and after tests and control groups as in classic research methodology. In planning the research design, it is important to adopt multifactorial models of causation. Research in prevention must tease apart the separate effects of individual risk factors in order to discover the elements that need to be included in a prevention package. In order to maximise the likelihood of showing population-wide reduction in incidence, prevention programmes will need to address a group of contributing risk factors simultaneously.

TABLE 2.2
Specification of target groups, interventions and expected outcome

General questions	Examples of available data
Prevention target	
What is the evidence for the suspected vulnerability of the specific target group?	Prevalence rates, and associated factors in particular populations such as age, sex, race, family history, economic status, geographic location – obtained from epidemiological surveys
What is the evidence for the risk potential of the specific target situation?	Prevalence rates and associated factors in particular settings or events e.g. work or school environments, or events such as separations, loss, hospitalisation, or school or work transitions – obtained from epidemiological surveys.
Interventions	
What specific procedures are to be used to increase the coping capacity of population?	Education, skill training, stress management, social problem-solving training – manuals, workshops
What specific procedures are to be used to reduce the risk producing features of the environment?	Selecting the setting: matching person to an appropriate setting e.g. school, day centre, self-help group
	Changing the setting: consulting with existing social institutions e.g. schools, churches
	Creating the setting: establishing new settings such as interest and support groups
Expected outcomes	
What is the evidence that the programme elements were implemented?	Attendance records, dropout rates, behaviour observation samples, survey feedback, rearrange service delivery interviews
What is the evidence that goals were met?	Coping capacity – criterion tests of new skills, knowledge, abilities or behaviour of setting participants
	Setting selection, change or creation – Documentation of change in attitude knowledge or behaviour of setting participants
What is the evidence for programme popularity, cost, and impact on other systems?	Surveys, services load data, cost per unit of service delivery, change in service load of other agencies
What is the evidence that long-term prevention goals were met?	Longitudinal evidence, follow up studies, or epidemiological surveys indicating a reduction in specific negative outcomes for which the interventions were originally designed

(From *Prevention in Mental Health: Research, Policy and Practice*. (1980), Vol. 1, p. 306 (eds R. H. Price, R. F. Ketterer, B. C. Bader & J. Monahon). Reprinted by permission of Sage Publications, Inc.).

Vulnerability factors may operate in childhood, and disorders occur in adulthood. Most prevention programmes will have difficulty demonstrating an impact on long-term goals, due to this time factor, and the difficulty of controlling other variables for so long. This also causes practical problems of obtaining sufficient funding and of staff turnover.

So how can researchers hope to demonstrate the effectiveness of prevention programmes? This may be attempted by specifying some immediate goals which are linked to the long-term goals. For example, increased social competence has been seen as a worthwhile goal in its own right, but we still need to prove that it makes individuals less vulnerable to disorder.

Prevention strategies may be evaluated against a number of different criteria. Effectiveness is to do with whether the strategy worked in the short term; preventive potential describes the contribution in the long term to a preventive goal of high priority, which is likely to have a large mental health impact. For example, a strategy to improve the social skills of children may have more eventual impact than one for mature adults. This is very difficult to measure and is subject to value judgements; the cost of the strategy can be assessed in terms of finances and people, and side-effects of the intervention; acceptability is partly a function of consistency with prevailing social values.

Guidelines for development and evaluation of prevention strategies

It is important to specify the target (either a population at risk or risk situations) the strategy or intervention, and the expected outcome, both short-term and long-term. Many programmes have not clearly specified all these components, which are detailed in Table 2.2. The importance of considering the varying mechanisms of social support is also emphasised.

References

BLOOM, B. L. (1979) Prevention of mental disorders: recent advances in theory and practice. *Community Mental Health Journal*, **15**, 179–191.
—— (1981) The logic and urgency of primary prevention, *Hospital Community Psychiatry*, **32**, 839–843.
—— (1985) *Life Event Theory and Research: Implications for Primary Prevention*. (DHSS (ADM) 85-1385) Washington, DC: DHSS.
BOWER, E. M. (1987) Prevention: A word whose time has come. *American Journal of Orthopsychiatry*, **57**, 4–5.
BRONFENBRENNER, U. (1977) Toward an experimental ecology of human development. *American Psychologist*, **32**, 513–531.
CAPLAN, G. (1964) *Principles of Preventive Psychiatry*. New York: Basic Books.
—— (1970) *The Theory and Practice of Mental Health Consultation*. New York: Basic Books.
—— (1974) *Support Systems and Community Mental Health*. New York: Behavioural Publications.
—— (1981) Mastery of stress: psychological aspects. *American Journal of Psychiatry*, **138**, 413–420.
CASSEL, J. (1973) The relation of the urban environment to health: implications for prevention. *Mount Sinai Journal of Medicine*, **40**, 539–550.
—— (1976) The contributions of the social environment to host resistance. *American Journal of Epidemiology*, **104**, 107–123.
CATALANO, R. & DOOLEY, D. (1980) Economic change in primary prevention. In *Prevention in Mental Health – Research, Policy and Practice* (eds R. H. Price, R. J. Ketterer, B. C. Bader & J. Monahan), pp. 21–40. London: Sage Publications.
COBB, S. (1976) Social support as a moderator of life stress. *Psychosomatic Medicine*, **38**, 300–314.

COLLINS, A. H. & PANCOAST, O. L. (1976) *Natural Helping Network*. New York: National Association of Social Workers.
COOK, T. D. & CAMPBELL, D. T. (1979) *Quasi-experimentation: Design and Analysis Issues for Field Settings*. Chicago: Rand McNally.
COWEN, E. L. (1977) Baby steps toward primary prevention. *American Journal of Community Psychology*, **5**, 1–22.
EISENBERG, L. & PARRON, D. (1979) Strategies for the prevention of mental disorders. In *Healthy People, the Surgeon General's Report on Health Promotion and Disease Prevention*. Background Papers, DHEW (PHS), Publication No. 79.55071A. Washington, DC: US Government Printing Office.
GARMEZY, N. (1971) Vulnerability research and the issue of primary prevention. *American Journal of Orthopsychiatry*, **41**, 101–116.
GOLDSTON, S. E. (1977a) An overview of primary prevention programming. In *Primary Prevention: An Idea Whose Time has Come* (eds D. C. Klein & S. E. Goldston). Washington, DC: US Government Printing Office.
––––– (1977b) Defining primary prevention. In *Primary Prevention of Psychopathology, Vol. 1* (eds G. W. Albee & J. M. Joffe). Hanover, NH: University Press of New England.
GORDON, R. S. (1983) An operational classification of disease prevention. *Public Health Reports*, **98**, 107–109.
HOLMES, T. H. & RAHE, R. (1967) The social readjustment rating scale. *Journal of Psychosomatic Research*, **11**, 213–218.
HOUSE, J. S. (1981) *Work, Stress and Social Support*. Reading, MA: Addison-Wesley.
JASON, L. A. (1980) Prevention in the schools: behaviour approaches. In *Prevention in Mental Health – Research, Policy and Practice* (eds R. H. Price, R. F. Ketterer, B. C. Bader & J. Monahan), pp. 109–134. London: Sage Publications.
JENKINS, R. (1981) The background, design and use of a short interview to assess social stress and support in research and clinical settings. *Social Science and Medicine*, **15E**, 195–203.
–––––, NEWTON, J. & YOUNG, R. (1992) *The Prevention of Depression and Anxiety – the Role of the Practice Team*. London: HMSO.
KOBASA, S. C. (1979) Personality and resistance to illness. *American Journal of Community Psychology*, **7**, 413–423.
LINN, S., YAGER, J. & LEAKE, B. (1988) Psychiatrists' attitudes toward preventive intervention in routine clinical practice. *Hospital and Community Psychiatry*, **39**, 637–642.
MACLENNAN, B. W., QUINN, R. D. & SHROEDER, D. (1975) The scope of community mental health consultation. In *The Practice of Mental Health Consultation* (eds F. V. Mannine, B. W. Maclennan & M. F. Shore). Washington, DC: Mental Health Study Center, Division of Mental Health Service Programs. NIMH, 3–24.
MASUDA, M. & HOLMES, T. H. (1978) Life events: perceptions and frequencies. *Journal of Psychosomatic Medicine*, **40**, 236–261.
MITCHELL, R. E., BILLINGS, A. G. & MOSS, R. H. (1982) Social support and well being: implications for prevention programmes. *Journal of Primary Prevention*, **3**, 77–98.
MOOS, R. H. (1982) Coping with acute health crises. In *Handbook of Health Care Clinical Psychology* (eds T. Millon, C. Green & R. Meagher). New York: Plenum.
––––– & MITCHELL, R. E. (1982) Social network resources and adaptation: a conceptual framework. In *Basic Processes in Helping Relationships* (ed. T. A. Wills). New York: Academic Press.
NEWTON, J. (1988) *Preventing Mental Illness*. London: Routledge & Kegan Paul.
PARDES, H., SILVERMAN, M. & WEST, A. (1989) Prevention and the field of mental health: a psychiatric perspective. *Annual Review of Public Health*, **10**, 403–422.
PLUNKETT, R. J. & GORDON, J. E. (1960) *Epidemiology and Mental Illness*. New York: Basic Books.
POSER, E. G. & HARTMAN, L. M. (1979) Issues in behavioural prevention: empirical findings. *Advances in Behaviour Research and Therapy*, **2**, 1–25.
PRICE, R. H. (1979) The social ecology of treatment gain. In *Maximising Treatment Gains: Transfer Enhancement in Psychotherapy* (eds A. P. Goldstein & F. J. Kaufer). New York: Academic Press.
–––––, BADER, B. C. & KETTERER, R. F. (1980) Prevention in community mental health. The state of the art. In *Prevention in Mental Health – Research, Policy and Practice* (eds R. H. Price, R. F. Ketterer, B. C. Bader & J. Monahan), pp. 9–20. London: Sage Publications.
SILVERMAN, P. R. (1969) The widow to widow program. *Mental Hygiene*, **53**, 333–337.
TOEWS, J. & EL-GUEBALY, N. (1989) A call for primary prevention: reality or utopia. *Canadian Journal of Psychiatry*, **34**, 928–933.
WEXLER, N. S. (1985) Genetic jeopardy and the new clairvoyance. In *Progress in Medical Genetics* (eds A. G. Bearn, A. G. Motulsky & B. Childs), pp. 277–304. New York: Praeger.
YAGER, J., LINN, L. S., LEAKE, B., et al (1989) Attitudes toward mental illness prevention in routine paediatric practice. *American Journal of Diseases of Children*, **143**, 1087–1090.

3 Social factors, social interventions and prevention

JAN SCOTT and JULIAN LEFF

Campbell (1981) suggested that social psychiatry is characterised by "its emphasis on environmental influences and the impact of the social group on the individual". The ideology of social psychiatry also promotes the view that a significant proportion of mental morbidity in the community is preventable by social means (Jablensky, 1990). It is widely acknowledged that social factors are important both in determining risk of onset of mental illness and in influencing prognosis (Leighton, 1989). Global interventions based on the notion of changing society are theoretically possible but lie in the sphere of politics rather than medicine. Social approaches appropriate to psychiatry are more specific and utilise strategies centred around individuals and their interaction with the social system (Leighton, 1989). Preventive interventions can be focused at the primary (reduction of incidence), secondary (early detection and treatment) or tertiary (reduction of consequent disabilities) level. Cooper (1989) points out that given our current stage of knowledge, a balanced preventive programme will give higher priority to secondary and tertiary measures directed at diagnosed cases of mental illness. However, within the spectrum of social interventions it is possible that secondary prevention for one individual may offer primary prevention to another individual (who is linked to the first by a meaningful relationship).

In order to avoid overlap with the detailed reviews provided, this chapter briefly describes the social factors that may identify groups at high risk of mental disorder. It then gives a broad overview of the social strategies available and provides examples of the types of intervention that may be possible at different levels of the social system.

The need to identify high risk groups

A central requirement for social prevention strategies is a detailed knowledge of the epidemiology of the disorder being investigated. By comparing the frequency of a disorder in different groups it is possible to develop hypotheses as to when, why and under what circumstances particular individuals present with a specific type of problem (Morris, 1974). This knowledge can be used in two ways: it allows the identification of high risk groups (important in primary prevention) and, by comparing known cases with population levels of morbidity, it allows comment on help-seeking behaviour and accessibility of services (important in secondary prevention).

Almost any social factor can be regarded as affecting an individual's 'risk' status. Socio-economic or employment status may act as a source of stress or support in an individual's life. Age, gender, ethnicity, marital status, family background and the presence or absence of social support (particularly an intimate or confidante) may also be associated with the development or maintenance of a variety of mental disorders. External factors such as recent life events or ongoing difficulties are also implicated. In order to use this information to constructively guide preventive strategies it is helpful to categorise the factors into:

(a) predisposing – those which increase individual vulnerability to onset of a disorder at some future date, e.g. childhood deprivation
(b) precipitating – those determining timing of onset, e.g. recent life events (particularly events involving threatened or actual loss)
(c) maintaining – those factors which prolong a disorder, e.g. chronic social stress, lack of a supportive relationship.

Research supporting the role of predisposing, precipitating and maintaining factors, while extensive, is mainly correlational. It is not yet possible to define pathogenic factors. However, some variables (e.g. sociodemographic characteristics) function more as associated factors whereas others (such as life events and social support variables) are more likely to have a causal role.

No model of mental illness is robust enough to allow clear definition of 'high risk' groups. This fundamental problem will always impede progress on prevention in psychiatry. In order to achieve the maximum impact possible, primary prevention strategies should be targeted at specific groups where either the social factors are amenable to change or where the response to the factors can be altered before pathological changes occur. For example, interventions might be aimed at young women at home with children who are regarded as at high risk of depression. Alternatively, interventions could be 'event-centred'. Those exposed to an extreme environmental stress such as a major disaster may be at risk of developing post-traumatic stress disorder (PTSD). Inter-agency interventions can be beneficial to both professionals and 'victims' involved in the incident. Even within these selected samples clinical and cost effectiveness will be difficult to achieve. Not all those exposed to an event or experience will develop disorder.

Categories of social interventions

Social interventions can be divided into two broad categories (Henderson, 1988):

Behavioural change – efforts are directed at improving the individual's coping repertoire and social skills. While these changes can be brought about by the use of specific therapies, social interventions are not usually aimed at the individual in isolation but at the individual within their social system.

Environmental manipulation – this involves alteration of the individual's social environment, changing the behaviour of others and reducing the level of social stress. Examples are helping individuals to develop a more adaptive life style, family interventions, or enhancing social support.

Few of the above interventions should be regarded as an approach to use in isolation. A bio-psycho-social strategy is likely to be required in most circumstances although the relative emphasis on different interventions will obviously vary depending on the disorder being treated.

Levels of social intervention

While a vast array of social and ecological factors have been proposed as risk factors for mental disorder, it is perhaps more useful to systematically outline levels within the social order where interventions could be made.

Level one: the individual

How an individual acts and reacts both determines and is determined by their personality resources or vulnerabilities. The personal make-up of the individual may enhance their resilience in the face of adversity (Rutter, 1985). Interpersonal behaviour will partly determine the extent of primary group and social networks. However, while interventions at this level can undoubtedly be preventive, individual therapies will not be addressed here.

Level two: the primary group

Cooley (1909) defines this as consisting of those people in the social world with whom there is both interaction and commitment. This group usually comprises the family and significant others. A variety of social interventions are possible at this level.

Maintaining an intact family

Isolated individuals are frequently over-represented in epidemiological studies of all diagnostic subgroups. In order to maintain a mentally ill individual within the family, support must be offered to reduce the burden of care. Social interventions at this level would involve early intervention services (e.g. through careful follow-up or assertive outreach programmes) to ensure that episodes of illness are treated quickly and families are engaged in education/communication programmes. The latter might involve education about the disorder to increase understanding or more specific interventions to improve marital or family functioning. Programmes to reduce expressed emotion or to improve the quality of marital relationships can significantly reduce relapse in schizophrenia (Vaughan & Leff, 1976; Leff *et al*, 1985) and depression respectively (Hooley *et al*, 1986; O'Leary & Beach, 1990).

The family and the 'identified patient'

There are many examples of the symptomatic individual being the identified patient within a dysfunctional family. Such a situation may particularly apply to children presenting with disturbance. Children who have been physically abused might come to the attention of school or other agencies because of behaviour change or disturbance. A social intervention aimed at the parents including attempts to improve their parenting skills may be as relevant as an intervention focused on the child. These interventions can also be seen as damage limitation exercises as they may interrupt cycles of deprivation. Children who have experienced poor parenting may themselves fail to function adequately in this role in the future without intervention at this stage.

This type of intervention might be further extended to proactively target 'at risk' families. The Homestart scheme was a community-based support programme primarily aimed at helping high-risk children, through the use of volunteers to visit the family home and develop a relationship with the parents (Van der Eyken, 1982). Invariably the relationships focused on the mother, but theoretically it could in future extend to fathers as well. The aim was to enhance parenting skills in disadvantaged families (i.e. those whose circumstances made them particularly vulnerable) through modelling positive parenting behaviours and engaging parents and their children with available community resources. Families were referred by health visitors, social workers or other professionals and 226 families were matched with a 'homestart' volunteer. Fifty families had children on the 'at risk' register, or otherwise identified as vulnerable. Over four years of operation it was reported that 92% of families showed attitudinal shifts, improved quality of relationships with parents and children, and improved self-esteem in the parents (Newton, 1988).

Level three: the social network

The term network refers to those with whom there is some degree of social interaction (Henderson, 1988). It tends to be looser but numerically larger than the primary group. Several studies have identified the importance of social networks in buffering the self-esteem of the vulnerable individual in the face of adversity. The work of Brown and colleagues (Brown, 1986) has identified the role of social support as a protective factor in women at risk of depression. Developing a confiding peer relationship as described by the Newpin project (Pound *et al*, 1985) can be beneficial to women and secondarily may enhance their parenting skills. This project also showed the benefit of recruiting volunteers from similar (often deprived) backgrounds to the clients.

An alternative social support model for those with mental illness might aim at introducing befrienders. The aim of these schemes is to recruit volunteers to visit isolated and lonely patients and to engage them in activities such as attending leisure centres. Kingdon *et al* (1989) suggest the scheme can be successful in reducing the distress that accompanies loneliness and patients who refuse day care may be willing to accept befrienders. Furthermore, volunteers are more appropriate than professionals in this role as they often form part of the client's community and can help them integrate into it. Befriending projects also have benefits for the community in general. Mental health professionals are involved in training the befrienders and therefore have an opportunity to disseminate important knowledge about mental disorders. The befrienders offer the same professionals a point of interaction with the community to enable them to gain information about local concerns regarding service provision and the care of the mentally ill. Befrienders have also been recruited from religious organisations, which can also provide a support function for mentally ill people.

Level four: culture

Ethnic origin and subculture influence individual patterns of behaviour and living. Henderson (1988) points out that ideas of what is valued by people, and the extent to which an individual experiences themselves as part of a larger social organisation are critically important. Interventions at this level might involve making services more accessible to different ethnic or social groups. However, making a service geographically accessible to a local community will not automatically ensure its appropriate use. Social strategies for intervention at this level will involve raising the awareness of professionals of the need to make the services acceptable to those from different cultural backgrounds and attempting to acccess different cultural groups to inform them about the services currently on offer and to gain advice from them on their requirements. The strategy should involve inquiring into the beliefs about psychiatric disorders and treatment held by members of the ethnic groups concerned. Another helpful strategy is to liaise with leaders of the local ethnic communities. These interventions largely operate on a community level but are ultimately focused on trying to promote attitudinal shifts in individuals.

Level five: society

Social forces appear to operate beyond the interpersonal level (Henderson, 1988). Macrosocial factors such as the general environment in which people exist (e.g. socio-economic status) and the social and physical strains imposed on individuals within a particular group are all relevant here. Interventions at this level are invariably political rather than clinical and are beyond the reach of psychiatry. However, influencing fiscal policy and legislation by disseminating information and research data can be considered as preventive strategies. Publicising the adverse effects on mental health of poor housing, unemployment and poverty may act to reinforce those promoting change in these areas. An obvious intervention at this level involves the need to educate society at large about the adverse effects of excess alcohol intake and to promote and encourage appropriate action, including at governmental level, to prevent the continued expansion of this problem. Education aimed at improving mental health is probably most effective if it is incorporated into the school curriculum. In addition to information about the effects and dangers of alcohol and drugs, an education programme could include advice on parenting, and facts about the nature of psychiatric illness intended to dispel myths and misconceptions about the subject. This could lead to people seeking appropriate help earlier in future, and possibly to a greater acceptance of psychiatrically ill people by the community.

Conclusions

Primary prevention probably represents the only 'true' preventive strategy as secondary and tertiary approaches systematise good clinical practice (detection of conspicuous and hidden morbidity, early intervention, and effective aftercare).

To be clinically and cost effective social primary preventive strategies are currently targeted at 'high risk' groups. Unfortunately, risk factors are not clearly determined and a large part of the variance for onset and course of disorder remains unaccounted for. This issue is particularly pertinent when trying to identify childhood factors that may predispose to onset of mental disorder in later life. The complexity of establishing a causal relationship between experiences occurring at such a temporal distance clearly undermines the prospects for primary prevention.

Explanatory models of the role of precipitating and maintaining factors show greater coherence and may provide opportunities for secondary and tertiary interventions. However, the proposed models underline the multifactorial aetiology of mental illness. While life events appear to have a role in the onset of many disorders, it is clear that many people experiencing such events do not suffer adversely. Social interventions will be most potent for the individual if used in combination with psychological and biological approaches.

Apart from the considerable body of literature available on expressed emotion, few of the interventions documented here have been subject to systematic exploration. The 'macrolevel' interventions would be difficult to evaluate reliably but should be promoted on the basis that they represent good clinical practice (e.g. opening up a dialogue with members of ethnic minorities). The individual, family and social network levels of intervention offer a number of opportunities for promoting improvement in interpersonal relationships and personal functioning (such as improving self-esteem). There are also possibilities for evaluating these interventions. Even here it will be difficult to demonstrate efficacy either because of low base rates of mental disorder or because few of the interventions are operationally defined with sufficient reliability to allow replication. Overall, it would appear that the area of social interventions requires more detailed investigation and further development.

References

BROWN, G. (1988) Depression: a radical social approach. In *Depression: An Integrative Approach* (eds K. Herbst & E. S. Paykel), pp. 21–44. Oxford: Heinemann Medical.
CAMPBELL, R. (1981) *Psychiatric Dictionary*. 5th Edn. Oxford: Oxford University Press.
COOLEY, C. (1909) *Social Organisation: A Study of the Larger Mind*. New York: Scribner.
COOPER, B. (1989) Strategies of prevention. In *Epidemiology and the Prevention of Mental Disorders* (eds B. Cooper & T. Helgason), pp. 3–16. London: Routledge.
VAN DER EYKEN, W. (1982) *Homestart: A Four Year Evaluation*. Leicester: Homestart Consultancy.
HENDERSON, A. (1988) *An Introduction to Social Psychiatry*, pp. 73–156. Oxford: Oxford Medical Publications.
HOOLEY, J., ORLEY, J. & TEASDALE, J. (1986) Levels of expressed emotion and relapse in depressed patients. *British Journal of Psychiatry*, **148**, 642–647.
JABLENSKY, A. (1990) Public health aspects of social psychiatry. In *The Public Health Impact of Mental Disorder* (eds D. Goldberg & D. Tantum), pp. 5–13. London: Wisepress.
KINGDON, D. (1989) Befriending: cost effective community care. *Psychiatric Bulletin*, **13**, 350–351.
LEFF, J., KUIPERS, L., BERKOWITZ, R., et al (1985) A controlled trial of social intervention in the families of schizophrenic patients. *British Journal of Psychiatry*, **149**, 594–600.
LEIGHTON, A. (1989) Global and specific approaches to prevention. In *Epidemiology and the Prevention of Mental Disorders* (eds B. Cooper & T. Helgason), pp. 17–29. London: Routledge.
MORRIS, J. (1974) Four cheers for prevention. In *Uses of Epidemiology*. 3rd Edn (Ed. J. Morris), pp. 270–283. Edinburgh: Churchill Livingstone.
NEWTON, J. (1988) *Preventing Mental Illness*, pp. 134–196. London: Routledge.

O'LEARY, K. D. & BEACH, S. R. (1990) Marital therapy: a viable treatment for depression and marital discord. *American Journal of Psychiatry*, **147**, 183–186.

POUND, A., MILLS, M. & COX, T. (1985) A pilot evaluation of Newpin. *Newsletter of the Association of Child Psychology and Psychiatry*, October, 2–4.

RUTTER, M. (1985) Resilience in the face of adversity: protective factors and resistance to psychiatric disorder. *British Journal of Psychiatry*, **147**, 719–724.

VAUGHN, C. & LEFF, J. (1976) The influence of family and social factors on the course of psychiatric illness. A comparison of schizophrenic and depressed neurotic patients. *British Journal of Psychiatry*, **129**, 125–137.

4 Genetics

PETER McGUFFIN

Is psychiatric genetics ethical?

The study of molecular genetics currently offers one of the most exciting approaches to understanding the causes and discovering cures for common diseases including cancer, heart disease and psychiatric disorder. However, the view that there is something slightly sinister about investigating the inheritance of abnormal behaviours is still surprisingly persistent in some quarters.

It is not too difficult to trace the historical roots of such views. The first of these probably stems from a reaction to the eugenics movement in the early part of the century. This arose from the optimistic notion that a knowledge of genetics would not only enable the abolition of certain diseases but might also lead to improvement of human stock in general (Carlson, 1987; Roll-Hanssen, 1988). Some believed that such improvement could be implemented on a national basis and it has been alleged that beliefs about genetic and racial influences on IQ and other behavioural characteristics played a part in the way immigration policies were carried out in the USA (Kamin, 1974). But, as is well known, much worse was to come. Eugenic arguments were commandeered by the German Third Reich in a way that blended an astonishing mixture of scientific naïvety and evil intent. Despite the fact that such policies were seen by most of the scientific community as not just morally repugnant but intellectually bone-headed, psychiatric genetics still acquired a sort of guilt by association. Perhaps not surprisingly a reactive antagonism to psychiatric genetics among politicians is still more evident in Germany than in other parts of Europe.

The second source of feeling against psychiatric genetics is more intuitive. This derives from the idea that to say a condition is genetic is to say that it is fixed, inborn, and immutable. Such conditions must be difficult or even impossible to treat, and are certainly unlikely to be susceptible to psychological interventions. Allied to this gut feeling is the objection that it is somehow demeaning to invoke genetic causes for human behaviour and that genetic theories of psychiatric disease are crude, simplistic and mechanistic.

Fortunately counter arguments are not too difficult to find. The whole thrust of modern genetics is towards defining aetiology precisely, both at a molecular level and at the level of interplay between genes and environment. At both levels, by defining causes more precisely, we should in the long term be able to acquire knowledge which allows the development of rational therapies. Physical disorders with simple Mendelian inheritance provide good examples of the benefits which might be reaped in psychiatric disorders by applying the molecular biological strategies of 'positional cloning'. Broadly, this means detecting genes of major effect, locating them precisely and then moving from marker loci to the genes themselves, and hence establishing the exact nature of the biochemical abnormality.

However, even in disorders where the application of molecular genetic strategies seems far off, there is no reason why the finding that there are genetic influences on the disorder should rule out psychological or behavioural treatments. For example, two recent important findings have emerged from the Maudsley where it has been shown that anorexia nervosa is (i) substantially heritable (Treasure & Holland, 1991) and (ii) responsive to psychotherapy (Russell et al, 1987).

Psychiatric genetics is now a very vigorous and energetic field. It is therefore worth briefly surveying the present state of knowledge before discussing current and future strategies and the implications for prevention.

Current knowledge

For the major psychoses, manic depression and schizophrenia, genetic studies have provided the most consistent aetiological clues. The notion that there is a genetic contribution to schizophrenia has been attacked, partly on ideological grounds but for some reason the inheritance of manic depression has provoked almost no controversy. In both cases the combined evidence from family, twin and adoption studies is convincing and quantitative studies suggest that genes are responsible for the greater part of the variance in liability to these disorders. On the other hand, identical twin discordance rates of 50% in schizophrenics and 30% in manic depression provide sufficient proof (if the twins have lived through the period of risk) that environmental influences are also necessary. So far such environmental factors as have been identified are controversial and the interplay between environmental insults and genetic liability is poorly understood. Similarly the modes of transmission of schizophrenia and manic depression are unknown, and aetiological heterogeneity is likely. Although the familial distribution of typical forms of the two major psychoses is clearly distinct the degree of aetiological overlap in intermediate or 'schizoaffective' psychoses remains a matter of debate.

So called unipolar depression has been less intensively studied using genetic strategies than bipolar manic depression. Nevertheless there is virtual unanimity among investigators that unipolar depression aggregates in families. The separation from bipolar disorder is incomplete and their overlap can be as well explained by a multiple threshold model with differing levels of severity as by the hypothesis that there are two or more distinct conditions. Although some smaller and earlier studies were contradictory, recent investigations of twins suggest that unipolar depression is substantially heritable even in the absence of overt psychotic symptoms. Environmental influences, particularly various forms of social adversity, have been very carefully studied in depression. Unfortunately evidence on the interplay between genetic and environmental factors is again sparse. A recent study of the families of depressed patients shows that not only was the risk of depression increased compared with the general population but so also was the rate of reported life events (McGuffin *et al*, 1988) raising the possibility that at least part of the often reported association between life events and depression is due to the fact that both are familial. Indirect support for the familiality of reporting life events has subsequently come from twin studies (Kendler *et al*, 1991; Plomin & Rende, 1991).

The literature on neurotic and personality disorders is fragmentary. Nevertheless there is a coherent body of evidence that antisocial personality and/or criminality has a genetic component. Early studies suffered from methodological flaws and an oversimplistic interpretation of their results but more recent, scientifically sound investigations confirm a moderate degree of heritability for adult criminality, particularly petty recidivism (Cloninger & Gottesman, 1987). There is good evidence for the familial aggregation of anxiety disorders, particularly phobic disorders or anxiety with panic. Studies of anxiety symptoms in non-clinical twin samples together with such data as is available in clinical samples, strongly suggest a genetic component. Similar types of family and twin evidence suggest a genetic contribution to obsessive compulsive disorder.

Alcoholism is common and clinically very variable in Western populations and the genetic data are difficult to interpret. There is strong familiality but some evidence suggests an environmental explanation (for example similar concordance rates in male half siblings and full siblings). The twin data on alcohol dependence are conflicting with recent results suggesting either no genetic contribution or only modest heritability. On the other hand studies of alcohol use in normal twins suggest genetic influences, as do animal studies of strain differences in alcohol preference (Merikangas, 1990). The strongest evidence for a genetic contribution to clinically significant alcoholism comes from adoption studies carried out in Denmark and in Sweden. A genetic effect is convincing only in men and the proposal that there are two subtypes, one 'milieu limited' which is mild and affects both sexes, and the other 'male limited' which is more severe and associated with criminality, has been provocative (Cloninger, 1987).

Childhood disorders probably represent the largest piece of under-explored territory in psychiatric genetics. This may be partly related to the overt antagonisms which (as already noted) are still occasionally shown by child psychiatrists to the whole topic of genetics. Despite this the importance of genetic factors has been amply demonstrated in childhood autism (Rutter, 1991) and a wide variety of other conditions (Rutter *et al*, 1990). Even eating disorders such as anorexia nervosa which in the recent past were attributed to abnormal 'family dynamics' would now appear, on the basis of twin study evidence, to have a definite genetic contribution (Treasure & Holland, 1991).

The genetics of common forms of dementing disorders and disorders of late life have also been somewhat neglected until quite recently. Here the explanation has not been clinicians' antagonism to biological mechanisms but rather the sheer practical difficulties of carrying out family or twin studies and the near impossibility of performing adoption studies in elderly populations. Nevertheless a tendency for familial aggregation in Alzheimer's disease particularly of the early onset type has long been established and the association with Down's syndrome first focused attention on chromosome 21 (Wright, 1991). The subsequent localisation of the amyloid precursor protein (APP) gene on chromosome 21q and the flurry of linkage results using markers nearby, even though somewhat contradictory, make it likely that Alzheimer's type dementia will be the first complex disorder of psychiatric interest whose aetiology can be understood at a molecular level. It is now known that a minority of early onset cases are associated with a mutation in the APP gene and that most of the rest are due to a dominant gene or chromosome 14. It has also recently been shown that carrying a certain apolipoprotein E allele, Apo e4 increases the risk of late onset Alzheimer's disease (Owen *et al*, 1994). Important and clinically relevant advances have meanwhile taken place with less common, Mendelian forms of dementia, notably Huntington's disease where the gene, or chromosome 4, has now been identified.

Current research and future prospects

It will be clear from the above brief survey that most psychiatric phenotypes have complex inheritance and only a few of the rarer disorders of psychiatric interest such as Huntington's disease exhibit regular Mendelian inheritance. This has important implications for preventive strategies and genetic counselling since even in 'loaded' pedigrees where conditions such as schizophrenia appear to segregate in a Mendelian like fashion, risk predictions based on Mendelian assumptions are unreliable. Even state-of-the art statistical methods are not foolproof against culturally transmitted traits simulating Mendelism. Recently we were able to demonstrate (McGuffin & Huckle, 1990) that attendance of medical school among relatives of our medical students in Cardiff segregates as an autosomal recessive! However linkage studies offer a more certain method of detecting genes of major effect. Initial claims of dominant-like genes for schizophrenia (Sherrington *et al*, 1988) and manic depression (Egeland *et al*, 1987) were unsupported and the optimism surrounding these findings proved to be premature.

However, it would be equally premature to react to such disappointment by assuming that linkage studies offer no prospect for advance. The problems in carrying out a linkage study in a disorder such as schizophrenia include the fact that the mode of transmission is unknown. Studies therefore need to incorporate an exploratory approach to mode of inheritance and recognise that realistic models may include very low penetrance, heterogeneity and a degree of diagnostic uncertainty. Large sample sizes are required and this together with laboratory resources needed for a systematic genome search necessitate large scale collaborative studies. Such programmes are currently underway under the auspices of the European Science Foundation (ESF) and the National Institute of Mental Health (NIMH) in the United States. If these programmes progress according to plan, genes of major effect for manic depression and schizophrenia will, if they exist, be detected within the next few years.

However, if these disorders have genetic components which result purely from additive effects of many minor genes, linkage strategies are unlikely to prove successful. By analogy with succcessful molecular genetics strategies in studies of multigenic traits in plants, Plomin (1990) has advocated that a search for so-called quantitative traits loci (QTL) represents the most rational approach to the molecular genetic study of human behaviour. One such method is to aim to detect associations in populations rather than linkage within families. Association studies have the disadvantage of being very poor at detecting genes of large effect at some distance from marker loci but can detect genes of comparatively small effect at the very close range. It is theoretically feasible, although in practical terms an enormous amount of work, to scan the entire genome using an association rather than linkage strategy (Owen, 1991).

In terms of non-molecular research the methodology in family, twin and adoption studies has been greatly refined in recent years and methods of statistical analysis have been greatly advanced by the introduction of model fitting approaches. These in turn have been facilitated by the widespread availability of high speed computers. A major criticism of quantitative methods is that until recently the environment has been conceptualised either as a latent variable contributing to the correlation between relatives ('shared environment') or as everything that is left over once genetic and shared environment effects have been taken into account ('non-shared environment'). However, researchers interested in environmental effects have been almost equally guilty of ignoring genetic influences. It is only comparatively recently that attempts have been made to integrate direct observations of environmental factors in genetic studies of psychiatric disorders. So far research has yielded some unexpected results. For example, a study of depression found that the relatives of depressed patients not only had an increased risk of depression but also had high rates of reported life events. The unlikely notion that having (or reporting) life events may be partly genetic has since been confirmed by twins studies in Scandinavia and the United States (Plomin & Rende, 1991). We therefore must conclude that genes and the environmental factors relevant to disorders such as depression are (i) not independent of each other and (ii) cannot be assumed to act together in a simple additive fashion.

Implications for prevention

There is no place for a public health campaign persuading people with psychiatric disorder, or a strong family history of psychiatric disorder, not to have children. Still less is there a place for any attempts to legislate on this matter. However, an informed and responsible genetic counselling service has a small but definite current role and this is likely to increase in the future. Most genetic counsellors in current practice adopt a non-directive educational approach (Harper, 1994). Appropriate emphasis is therefore given to counsellees' personal autonomy. Again in practice much of the work of a genetic counsellor is to allay anxiety and dispel mistaken beliefs, for example that all the offspring of a parent with serious mental illness necessarily have the same 'hereditary taint' or that all disorders with a genetic component are necessarily untreatable. However, it may be legitimate to not only lower anxiety by providing information and reassurance but also to raise the individual's anxiety and the awareness of potential problems where this is appropriate. The counsellor needs to help the counsellee assess the risk as accurately as possible and understand the potential burdens. However, finally, after assessing the risk/burden ratio, the ultimate decision must be that of the counsellee.

For psychiatric disorders most of the information imparted in genetic counselling derives from *empirical* sources, i.e. estimates based on the best available research data. *Modular* information (Murphy & Chase, 1975) derives from a scientific understanding of the mode of inheritance of the disorder. This is usually lacking in psychiatry and it is important for anyone attempting genetic counselling not to confuse tentative hypotheses with proven facts. For example, I fairly recently saw a young man with a strong family history of early onset dementia. He had previously consulted a genetic counsellor elsewhere who confidently informed him that this was the pre-senile form of Alzheimer's dementia, that it had a dominant pattern of inheritance and that his risk of becoming affected was 50%. The young man was consulting me not for further genetic counselling but for treatment of the depression resulting from his previous consultation.

Murphy & Chase (1975) also refer to the use of *particular* information in genetic counselling which is a compilation of all the data that can be utilised in assessing the risks of a particular family. For example in schizophrenia the risks to relatives increase according to the numbers and classes of relatives already affected (Gottesman, 1991). Age of onset shows some tendency to 'breed true' as, to a much lesser extent, does the subtype of disorder (McGuffin *et al*, 1987).

Whatever the type of information available, and in psychiatry this is nearly always just empirical information, the role of the genetic counsellor is to educate and inform rather than to direct or advise. For example, a couple planning a family, one of whom has a schizophrenic parent, might beneficially be told that the average risk for each of their children displaying the disorder is about 3%, which although small is three times the rate in the general population. It must then be their decision rather than the counsellor's whether this risk is acceptable. Other than advising potential parents about risks to their offspring how might empirical knowledge about genetics be used in counselling individuals or families about prevention? One obvious answer is that for most psychiatric disorders it is a diathesis that is inherited and environmental stresses are necessary before the disorder becomes manifest. Often (as in schizophrenia) the nature of the relevant stresses is controversial or unknown. Alternatively, as in depression, relevant environmental insults have been defined with some certainty. However, it is of little use advising someone with a familial diathesis to depression to avoid threatening life events. On the other hand it may be quite legitimate and useful to advise an individual with a strong family history of alcoholism that he may be more than usually susceptible to moderate use becoming immoderate.

In the future, advances in molecular genetics should make for much greater accuracy in prediction. So far Huntington's disease provides the best prototype. In specialised centres predictive tests in pregnancy as well as predictive tests for individuals at genetic high risk have now been offered for several years. There has been careful research and evaluation from which important results have emerged (Morris *et al*, 1989). In addition to expected problems, such as reaction to adverse test results, many other difficulties have emerged, including unintentional risk alteration (e.g. participation in a linkage study by a relative who has not volunteered for predictive testing may reveal that the relative is at higher risk than had been thought). Although it is unlikely that genetic marker research will allow similar levels of predictive certainty for common disorders such as schizophrenia, predictive tests may soon have a place in subforms of Alzheimer's dementia and the ethical and psychological issues here are closely similar to those in Huntington's disease.

The need and demand for expert psychiatric genetic counselling is likely to increase as the accuracy and utility of such counselling increases. The rudiments of genetic counselling could usefully be covered in general professional psychiatric training. It would also be prudent to plan for the development of psychiatric genetic counselling services. These could be set up on a regional basis (probably jointly within University departments of psychiatry and medical genetics) within the next 5–10 years. Until this is achieved genetic counselling for psychiatric disorders is likely to be carried out by general psychiatrists or geneticists. Since misinformation may be more damaging to the counsellee than no information at all, the main message for both groups is to be frank and open about the inherent complexities and ambiguities in psychiatric genetic counselling and to be prepared to seek advice from colleagues with specialist knowledge even if this means a letter or long distance phone call.

Finally, the area in which most long-term benefit is likely to come using molecular genetic techniques is better understanding of aetiology leading to improved therapies. It has already been noted that a straightforward application of positional cloning strategies as in Mendelian disorders presents problems. Nevertheless the identification of genes involved in the aetiology of psychiatric disorders, whether of major or minor effect, must eventually inform therapeutic strategies and help provide a rational basis for the prevention of disability.

References

CARLSON, E. A. (1987) Eugenics and basic genetics in H. J. Muller's approach to human genetics. *History and Philosophy of the Life Sciences*, **3**, 57–78.

CLONINGER, C. R. (1987) Neurogenetic adaptive mechanisms in alcoholism. *Science*, **236**, 410–416.

—— & GOTTESMAN, I. I. (1987) Genetic and environmental factors in antisocial behaviour disorders. In *The Causes of Crime* (eds S. A. Mednick, T. E. Moffitt & S. A. Stack), pp. 92–109. Cambridge: Cambridge University Press.

EGELAND, J. A., GERHARDT, D. S., PAULS, D., et al (1987) Bipolar affective disorders linked to DNA markers on chromosome 11. *Nature*, **325**, 393–399.

GOTTESMAN, I. I. (1991) *Schizophrenia Genesis. Origins of Madness*. San Francisco: W. H. Freeman.

HARPER, P. (1994) *Practical Genetic Counselling*, 4th edn. Bristol: Wright.

KAMIN, L. J. (1974) *The Science and Politics of IQ*. Chichester: John Wiley.

KENDLER, K. S., NEALE, M. C., HEATH, A. C., et al (1991) Life events and depressive symptoms: a twin study perspective. In *The New Genetics of Mental Illness* (eds P. McGuffin & R. M. Murray), pp. 146–164. Oxford: Butterworth Heinemann.

McGUFFIN, P., FARMER, A. E. & GOTTESMAN, I. I. (1987) Is there really a split in schizophrenia? The genetic evidence. *British Journal of Psychiatry*, **150**, 581–592.

——, KATZ, R. & BEBBINGTON, P. (1988) The Camberwell Collaborative Study. III. Depression and adversity in the relatives of depressed probands. *British Journal of Psychiatry*, **152**, 775–782.

—— & HUCKLE, P. (1990) Simulation of Mendelism revisited: the recessive gene for attending medical school. *American Journal of Human Genetics*, **46**, 994–999.

MERIKANGAS, K. R. (1990) The genetic epidemiology of alcoholism. *Psychological Medicine*, **20**, 11–22.

MORRIS, M. J., TYLER, A. LAZAROU, I., et al (1989) Problems in genetic prediction of Huntington's Disease. *Lancet*, **i**, 601–603.

MURPHY, E. A. & CHASE, G. A. (1975) *Principles of Genetic Counselling*. Chicago: Yearbook Publishers.

OWEN, M. J. (1992) Editorial. Will schizophrenia become a graveyard for molecular geneticists? *Psychological Medicine*, **22**, 289–293.

——, LIDDELL, M. & McGUFFIN, P. (1994) Alzheimer's disease. *British Medical Journal*, **308**, 672–673.

PLOMIN, R. (1990) The role of inheritance in behaviour. *Science*, **248**, 183-188.
―― & RENDE, R. (1991) Human behavioural genetics. *Annual Review of Psychology*, **42**.
ROLL-HANSEN, N. (1988) The progress of eugenics: growth of knowledge and change in ideology. *History of Science*, **26**, 295-331.
RUSSELL, G. F. M., SZMUKLER, G. I., DARE, C., *et al* (1987) An evaluation of family therapy in anorexia nervosa and bulimia nervosa. *Archives of General Psychiatry*, **44**, 1047-1056.
RUTTER, M. (1991) Autism as a genetic disorder. In *The New Genetics of Mental Illness* (eds P. McGuffin & R. M. Murray), pp. 225-244. Oxford: Butterworth Heinemann.
――, MACDONALD, H., LE COUTEUR, A., *et al* (1990) Genetic factors in child psychiatric disorders – II. Empirical findings. *Journal of Child Psychology and Psychiatry*, **31**, 39-83.
SHERRINGTON, T., BRYNJOLFFSON, J., PETURSSON, H., *et al* (1988) Localization of a susceptibility locus for schizophrenia on chromosome 5. *Nature*, **336**, 164-167.
TIENARI, P. (1963) Psychiatric illness in identical twins. *Acta Psychiatrica Scandinavica* (suppl.) **171**.
TREASURE, J. L. & HOLLAND, A. J. (1991) Genes and the aetiology of eating disorders. In *The New Genetics of Mental Illness* (eds P. McGuffin & R. M. Murray), pp. 198-211. Oxford: Butterworth Heinemann.
WRIGHT, A. F. (1991) The genetics of the common forms of dementia. In *The New Genetics of Mental Illness* (eds P. McGuffin & R. M. Murray), pp. 259-273. Oxford: Butterworth Heinemann.

5 Biological causes

EVE C. JOHNSTONE

Only a few psychiatric disorders have a proven biological cause and preventive measures are not applicable in all of those which have. Organic disorders by definition have a biological basis, but preventive measures are applicable to relatively few of those. The fact that some once common organic psychiatric disorders such as neurosyphilis and pellagra have now become extremely rare is the result of past successes in preventive medicine based on understanding of the aetiology of the conditions. Delirious states may result from a wide range of biological causes. Most dementing illnesses are the result of demonstrable pathology. Sometimes, as in multi-infarct dementia, the biological cause is known. However, in this example, the underlying pathology of arteriosclerosis is of relatively ill-understood multifactorial aetiology. Another common cause of dementia is senile dementia of the Alzheimer's type (SDAT). Again the pathology has been clearly described but, although genetic factors are known to be important at least in early onset varieties (Goate *et al*, 1991), other possibilities such as damage related to the presence of aluminium (Perry, 1986) have been considered. Numerous biological causes of an environmental and genetic nature are known to be associated with mental handicap and are reviewed in Chapter 14.

The evidence for biological causes in the so-called 'functional' psychoses and in neurotic illness is less strong, although certainly as far as psychotic illnesses are concerned there can now be little doubt that biological causes are important. In this chapter biological causes will be classified by mechanisms and not by individual causes. The reader is referred to the previous chapter for a review of genetic mechanisms and the potential for preventive action.

Disorders of function of the CNS

Neurotransmission

Largely on the basis of psychopharmacological findings, hypotheses relating serious psychiatric disorder to neurotransmission have been derived in the last 20 years and have received much support: noradrenaline and 5-hydroxytryptamine for affective disorders (Schildkraut, 1965; Lapin & Oxenkrug, 1969); dopamine for schizophrenia (Snyder *et al*, 1974). Considerable research effort has been expended upon the study of these classic neurotransmitters, but much remains to be discovered. Evidence has accumulated to show that other substances, in particular peptides, are present in the nervous system and that these may possess neurotransmitter/modulator properties (Roberts et al, 1984). Hypotheses that psychiatric disorders are associated with altered availability or function of neurotransmitters at certain sites in the brain cannot be directly tested in human subjects but various indirect methods may be used.

Measurements of neurotransmitters, their precursors and metabolites in body fluids were widely conducted at one time and have produced evidence which supports, although does not prove, biological causations of psychiatric disorder (Johnstone, 1982). Neuroendocrine studies allied with histochemical and immunofluorescence techniques have established that neurotransmitters play a critical role in the modulation of anterior pituitary memories through an action on the hypothalamic hypophysiotropic neurons (Fuxe & Hokfelt, 1969). Dopamine, growth hormone, luteinising hormone, follicle stimulating hormone and adrenocorticotrophic hormone have been studied in relation to psychiatric disease (for review see Johnstone & Ferrier, 1981), and in addition to direct measures of hormone levels, functional tests like dexamethasone suppression (Carroll et al, 1981), growth hormone and prolactin responses to apomorphine, and growth hormone responses to adrenoreceptor blockers (Checkley, 1980) have also been used.

It is quite possible to analyse post-mortem brain tissue for monoamine-related substances and relevant enzymes. The nature and number of various types of receptor may be assessed using receptor labelling assays (Costall & Naylor, 1986) and immunocytochemistry may be used to examine brain tissue for peptides (Roberts et al, 1984). Post-mortem assays have greatly illuminated the biological basis of Parkinsonism (Hornykiewicz, 1963); Huntington's chorea (Bid & Iversen, 1974) and SDAT (Bowen et al, 1976), and although such clear-cut results have yet to be obtained in schizophrenia or affective illness, this area of work proceeds and it may be hoped advancing technical methods (Parnavelas & Papadopoulos, 1990) will allow the contradictions in previous work (Costall & Naylor, 1986) to be resolved.

Special techniques such as ^{33}Xenon inhalation (Obrist et al, 1975), SPET (Crawley et al, 1986) and positron emission tomography (PET) (Frackowiak, 1986) allow the possibility of measurement of cerebral blood flow, glucose and oxygen metabolism in various conditions and in various circumstances. It may be hoped that such methods will provide replicable findings which will illuminate the biological basis of various disorders.

Psychophysiological studies of various kinds, including measures of cardiovascular function, respiratory function, salivation, skin conductance and electromyography, have been used to investigate psychiatric disorders. Abnormalities have been found, but it is important to take account of the effects of environmental physical factors, such as exercise, rest and temperature. The effects of drug treatment must also be taken into account in interpreting the findings (Yannitsi et al, 1987).

Electroencephalography has been used for many years as a diagnostic and research tool. In the technique of evoked responses the output following some discrete stimulus of sound or light flashes or electric shock is recorded and separated from background activity. EEG monitoring and evoked responses have been used to investigate sleep, depression (Flor-Henry & Koles, 1980) and schizophrenia (Connolly et al, 1983). BEAM (brain electrical activity mapping) involves the analysis of EEG signals using a computer and displaying them on a VDU. It has been used in the study of schizophrenia (Morihisa et al, 1983).

Disorders of structure of the CNS

The post-mortem structure of the brain in psychiatric disorders received much attention at the turn of the century and the introduction of pneumocephalography allowed the possibility of examining the anatomy of the brain in life. There are a number of problems associated with pneumocephalography and the introduction of computed tomography (Hounsfield, 1973) greatly enhanced the possibilities of examining the structure of the brain. The first CT scan study in schizophrenia (Johnstone et al, 1976) found lateral ventricular area to be increased ($P<0.01$) in a group of chronically institutionalised schizophrenic patients in comparison with age-matched normal controls. This area of work has been well reviewed (Weinberger et al, 1983; Dewan et al, 1986) and it appears that evidence of reduction of brain substance occurs in patients with schizophrenia more often than in controls and is not due to treatment (Owens et al, 1985). This ventricular enlargement is not a necessary concomitant of schizophrenia, even in its most severe and chronic forms, nor is it sufficient for the development of the disease, as such enlargement has been noted in manic depressive illness (Rieder et al, 1983) and as a reversible phenomenon in alcoholism (Carlen et al, 1978), anorexia nervosa (Heinz et al, 1977) and possibly in patients dependent upon benzodiazepines (Lader et al, 1984).

The later development of magnetic resonance imaging (MRI) has built upon the findings of CT. It has the advantage of providing greater resolution and a high level of contrast between grey and white matter. The results of imaging studies have re-awakened interest in post-mortem studies of the structure and aetiology of the brain in functional psychosis (Kovelman & Scheibel, 1984; Benes et al, 1986; Bruton et al, 1990; Johnstone et al, 1994).

Other aspects

Biological psychiatry is concerned with the idea that psychiatric disorders are associated with demonstrable anatomical or physiological abnormality. Generally the abnormalities are envisaged as being in the CNS but other abnormalities may be relevant.

Minor physical abnormalities (Waldrop et al, 1986) may be associated with academic failure, behavioural disturbance and possibly early schizophrenia (Green et al, 1987).

Investigations relating to diet with reference to psychiatric disorder have been conducted. These include estimation of antibodies to food fractions (Dohan et al, 1972) and intestinal permeability studies (Wood et al, 1987).

Epidemiological studies may have considerable relevance to biological research. Studies of the association of psychiatric illness and physical disease (Baldwin, 1979) and of the relationship between seasonality of birth and psychiatric disease (Hare & Walter, 1978) have been conducted and may yield relevant information, although work of this kind demands very large numbers of patients, and careful control for factors such as availability of beds and patterns of care as well as diagnostic accuracy.

Acquired immunodeficiency syndrome (AIDS)-related psychiatric disorders may present in many ways (Perry & Jacobsen, 1986; Fenton, 1987). They are not yet common in most areas of the UK, but it is expected that they will become more frequent.

Preventability of psychiatric disorders of biological cause

Because our knowledge of biological causes of most psychiatric disorders is limited, the opportunities for primary prevention are restricted. Although the evidence that so-called 'functional psychoses' have a biological basis is increasing, it is not yet sufficiently strong for primary preventive measures based upon it to be suggested, other than careful genetic counselling as discussed in Chapter 5. At present there is no evidence to suggest that primary preventive measures for neurotic disorder based upon any biological considerations would be appropriate. Delirious states can occur in relation to a very wide range of physical disorders. Clearly if the health of the population could be generally improved and the management of physical illness made more effective, so that it was associated with less biochemical derangement and pyrexia, then rates of delirium might be reduced. Specific education of health professionals about detection, assessment and management of delirious states is important.

There is perhaps a little more scope as far as dementias are concerned. Genetic factors are important in Alzheimer's disease, although it is difficult to see how this could lead to preventive measures at the present time. Issues relating aluminium to Alzheimer's disease are currently too uncertain for recommendations arising from this area of information to be made. Recent epidemiological work suggests an inverse association between smoking and Alzheimer's disease (van Duijn & Hofman, 1991), but it is pointed out that smoking cannot be advocated for other health reasons. The role of smoking, diet and lifestyle in the production of arterial disease has received increasing emphasis in recent years, although of course genetic factors are also known to be important (Dargie, 1989; Rosengren *et al*, 1990; Chen *et al*, 1991). It may be hoped that reduction in the incidence of hypertension and arterial disease brought about by changes in lifestyle could reduce the frequency of arteriosclerotic dementia and that effective control of hypertension might also have a beneficial effect.

It may be hoped that the psychiatric aspects of AIDS, like the other features of the disorder, will be reduced in frequency by changing the behaviour of the population with regard to needle sharing habits in drug users and sexual practices in the population in general.

References

BALDWIN, J. A. (1979) Schizophrenia and physical disease. *Psychological Medicine*, **9**, 611–618.
BENES, F. M., DAVIDSON, J. & BIRD, E. D. (1986) Quantitative cytoarchitectural studies of the cerebral cortex of schizophrenia. *Archives of General Psychiatry*, **43**, 31–35.

BIRD, E. D. & IVERSEN, L. L. (1974) Huntington's chorea – post-mortem measurement of glutamic acid decarboxylase, choline acetyl transferase and dopamine in basal ganglia. *Brain,* **97**, 457–472.

BOWEN, D. M., SMITH, C. B., WHITE, P., *et al* (1976) Neurotransmitter-related enzymes and indices of hypoxia in senile dementia and other abiotrophies. *Brain,* **99**, 459–496.

BRUTON, C. J., CROW, T. J., FRITH, C. D., *et al* (1990) Schizophrenia and the brain: a prospective cliniconeuropathological study. *Psychological Medicine,* **20**, 285–304.

CARLEN, P. L., WROTZMAN, G. & HOLGALE, R. C. (1978) Reversible cerebral atrophy in recent abstinent chronic alcoholics measured by computed tomography scans. *Science,* **200**, 1076–1078.

CARROLL, B. J., GREDEN, J. F. & FEINBERG, M. (1981) A specific laboratory test for the diagnosis of melancholia. *Archives of General Psychiatry,* **38**, 15–22.

CHECKLEY, S. A. (1980) Neuroendocrine text of monoamine function in man: a review of basic theory and the application to the study of depressive illness. *Psychological Medicine,* **10**, 35–53.

CHEN, Z., PETO, R., COLLINS, R., *et al* (1991) Serum cholesterol concentration and coronary heart disease in a population with low cholesterol concentrations. *British Medical Journal,* **303**, 276–282.

CONNOLLY, J. F., GRUZELIER, J. H. & MANCHANDA, R. (1983) Electrocortical and perceptual asymmetries in schizophrenia. In *Laterality & Psychopathology. Developments in Psychiatry, Vol. 6* (eds P. Flor-Henry & J. Gruzelier), pp. 363–378. Amsterdam: Elsevier Science.

COSTALL, B. & NAYLOR, R. J. (1986) Neurotransmitter hypothesis of schizophrenia. In *The Psychopharmacology of Schizophrenia* (eds P. B. Bradley & S. R. Hirsch). Oxford: Oxford University Press.

CRAWLEY, J. C. W., CROW, T. J. & JOHNSTONE, E. C. (1986) Uptake of 77Br-Spiperone in the striata of schizophrenic patients and controls. *Nuclear Medicine Communications,* **7**, 599–607.

DARGIE, H. J. (1989) Scottish hearts but British habits. *British Medical Journal,* **299**, 1475–1476.

DEWAN, M. J., PANDURANGI, A. K., LEE, S. H., *et al* (1986) A comprehensive study of chronic schizophrenic patients. *Acta Psychiatrica Scandinavica,* **73**, 153–160.

DOHAN, F. C., MARTIN, L., GRASBERGER, J. C., *et al* (1972) Antibodies of wheat gliadin in psychiatric patients: possible role of emotional factors. *Biological Psychiatry,* **5**, 127–137.

VAN DUIJN, C. M. & HOFMAN, A. (1990) Relation between nicotine intake and Alzheimer's disease. *British Medical Journal,* **302**, 1491–1494.

FENTON, T. W. (1987) Aids-related psychiatric disorder. *British Journal of Psychiatry,* **151**, 579–588.

FLOR-HENRY, P. & KOLES, Z. J. (1980) EEG studies in depression, mania and neural evidence for partial shifts of laterality in the affective psychoses. *Advances in Biological Psychiatry,* **4**, 21–43.

FRACKOWIAK, R. S. J. (1986) An introduction to positron tomography and its application to clinical investigation. In *New Brain Imaging & Psychopharmacology. BAP Monograph No. 9* (ed. M. R. Trimble), pp. 25–34. Oxford: Oxford University Press.

FUXE, K. & HOKFELT, T. (1969) Catecholamines in the hypothalamus and pituitary gland. In *Frontiers in Neuroendocrinology* (eds W. F. Ganong & L. Martini). New York: Oxford University Press.

GOATE, A., CHARTIER-HARLIN, M. C., MULLAN, M., *et al* (1991) A missense mutation in the amyloid precursor protein gene segregates with familial Alzheimer's disease. *Nature,* **349**, 704–706.

GREEN, M. F., SALZ, P., SOJAR, H. V., *et al* (1987) Relationship between physical abnormalities and age of onset of schizophrenia. *American Journal of Psychiatry,* **144**, 666–667.

GUSELLA, J. F., WEXLER, N. S., CONNEALLY, P. M., *et al* (1983) A polymorphic DNA marker genetically linked to Huntington's disease. *Nature,* **306**, 234–238.

HARE, E. H. & WALTER, S. D. (1978) Seasonal variation in admissions of psychiatric patients and its relation to seasonal variation in their births. *Journal of Epidemiology and Community Health,* **32**, 47–52.

HEINZ, R., MARTINE, Z. J. & HAENGGLI, A. (1977) Reversibility of cerebral atrophy in anorexia nervosa and Cushing's syndrome. *Journal of Computer Assisted Tomography,* **1**, 415–418.

HORNYKIEWICZ, O. (1963) Topography and behaviour of noradrenaline and dopamine (3-hydroxytyramine) in the substantia nigra of normal and Parkinsonian patients. *Wiener Klinische Wochenschrift,* **75**, 309–312.

HOUNSFIELD, G. N. (1973) Computerised transverse axial scanning (tomography). Part I. Description of the system. *British Journal of Radiology,* **46**, 1106–1022.

JOHNSTONE, E. C. (1982) Affective disorder. In *Disorders of Neurohumoral Transmission* (ed. T. J. Crow). London: Academic Press.

——, CROW, T. J., FRITH, C. D., *et al* (1976) Cerebral ventricular size and cognitive impairment in chronic schizophrenia. *Lancet,* **ii**, 924–926.

—— & FERRIER, N. (1981) Neuroendocrine markers of CNS drug effects. In *Methods of Clinical Pharmacology – Central Nervous System* (eds M. H. Lader & A. Richens). London: Macmillan Press.

——, BRUTON, C. J. & CROW, T. J. (1994) Clinical correlates of post-mortem brain changes in schizophrenia: decreased brain weight and length correlate with indices of early impairment. *Journal of Neurology, Neurosurgery & Psychiatry,* **57**, 474–479.

KOVELMAN, J. A. & SCHEIBEL, A. B. (1984) A neurohistological correlate of schizophrenia. *Biological Psychiatry*, **19**, 1601–1621.

LADER, M. H., RON, M. & PETURSSON, H. (1984) Computed axial brain tomography in long-term benzodiazepine users. *Psychological Medicine*, **14**, 203–206.

LAPIN, I. P & OXENKRUG, G. F. (1969) Intensification of the central serotoninergic processes as a possible determinant of the thymoleptic effect. *Lancet*, **i**, 132–136.

MORIHISA, J. M., DUFFY, F. H. & WYATT, R. J. (1983) Brain electrical activity mapping (BEAM) in schizophrenic patients. *Archives of General Psychiatry*, **40**, 719–728.

OBRIST, W. D., THOMSON, H. K., WANG, H. S., et al (1975) Regional cerebral blood flow estimated by ^{33}Xenon inhalation. *Stroke*, **6**, 245–256.

OWENS, D. G. C., JOHNSTONE, E. C. & CROW, T. J. (1985) Lateral ventricular size in schizophrenia: relationship to the disease process and its clinical manifestations. *Psychological Medicine*, **15**, 27–41.

PARNAVELAS, J. G. & PAPADOPOULOS, G. C. (1990) Neuroanatomy: a psychiatric perspective. In *Principles & Practice of Biological Psychiatry, Vol I*. (ed. T. Dinan). London: Clinical Neuroscience Publishers.

PERRY, R. H. (1986) Recent advances in neuropathology. *British Medical Bulletin*, **42**, 34.

PERRY, S. & JACOBSEN, P. (1986) Neuropsychiatric manifestations of AIDS-spectrum disorder. *Hospital & Community Psychiatry*, **37**, 135–142.

RIEDER, R. O., MANN, L. S. & WEINBERGER, D. R. (1983) Computed tomographic scans in patients with schizophrenia, schizo-affective and bipolar affective disorder. *Archives of General Psychiatry*, **40**, 735–739.

ROBERTS, G. W., POLAK, J. M. & CROW, T. J. (1984) Peptide circuitary of limbic system. In *Psychopharmacology of the Limbic System* (eds M. R. Trimble & E. Sarifan). Oxford: Oxford University Press.

ROSENGREN, A., WILHELMSEN, L., ERIKSSON, E., et al (1990) Lipoprotein (a) and coronary heart disease: a prospective case control study in a general population of middle-aged men. *British Medical Journal*, **301**, 1248–1251.

SCHILDKRAUT, J. J. (1965) The catecholamine hypothesis – a review of the supporting evidence. *American Journal of Psychiatry*, **122**, 509–522.

SNYDER, S. H., BANERJEE, S. P., YAMAMURA, A. I., et al (1974) Drugs, neurotransmitters and schizophrenia. *Science*, **184**, 1243–1253.

WALDROP, M. F., PEDERSON, F. A. & BELL, R. Q. (1986) Minor physical abnormalities and behaviour in preschool children. *Child Development*, **39**, 391–400.

WEINBERGER, D. R., WAGNER, R. L. & WYATT, R. J. (1983) Neuropathological studies of schizophrenia: a selective review. *Schizophrenia Bulletin*, **9**, 193–212.

WOOD, N. C., HAMILTON, I. & AXON, A. T. R. (1987) Abnormal intestinal permeability an aetiological factor in chronic psychiatric disorders. *British Journal of Psychiatry*, **150**, 853–856.

YANNITSI, S., LIAKOS, A. & PAPAKOSSTAS, Y. (1987) Electrodermal responding and chlorpromazine treatment in schizophrenia. *British Journal of Psychiatry*, **150**, 850–853.

6 Drug treatment in tertiary prevention

EVE C. JOHNSTONE

Tertiary prevention is defined as referring to measures to limit disability and handicaps consequent upon impairment or disease which may not be fully treatable. In this chapter treatment to prevent relapse has been included. Drug treatment has a role in this area in the management of some psychiatric disorders but not others. It probably does not have such a role in the management of neurotic illness. Although various anxiolytics were in the past used over long periods for persisting anxiety symptoms, the intention was to treat ongoing symptoms rather than to prevent relapse or to limit handicap. The dangers of actually producing disability by such methods are now well appreciated.

As far as psychotic illness is concerned, drug treatment as a means of limiting handicap may have some part to play in the management of organic conditions, particularly dementias.

It is relatively rare for delirious states to become chronic and when they do it is generally in the context of very serious untreatable physical diseases such as intractable cardiac, respiratory or hepatic failure. Similarly, delirious states may relapse but this is usually due to recurrence of the underlying physical disorder. Although the disabilities produced by the delirium in such states may be substantial, they tend to be less pressing than the physical problems of these serious situations and it would generally be considered that the appropriate drug treatment would be that directed to the alleviation of the underlying physical problems.

It is very rare for dementias to be fully treatable and the usual course of such illnesses is one of progressive decline with increasing handicap. As these conditions are not normally characterised by remission, the prevention of relapse is not really an issue. Some neuroleptics or other drugs are used with a view to limiting associated agitation and behavioural disturbance, but the value of this, other than on a short-term basis, is not clear. Various drugs including tetrabenazine are used in Huntington's chorea, mainly with a view to lessening the movement disorder. It is possible that such measures may to some extent limit the handicap of this condition. Recent evidence indicates that tacrine (tetrahydroaminoacridine + lecithin) may produce slight benefits in patients with Alzheimer's disease in terms of some psychological assessments, although these were not seen in ratings of daily living skills (Eagger et al, 1991). It would at present be over-optimistic to say that this treatment limits disability and handicap in a condition that is far from fully treatable, but the results of Eagger *et al* (1991) do suggest that it is possible such benefits may become available in time.

As far as functional psychoses are concerned the introduction of drugs which are effective in the prevention of relapse has been given a major advance. The role of neuroleptic drugs in the prevention of schizophrenic relapse has been demonstrated beyond doubt. The benefits in this situation of both oral (Leff & Wing, 1971) and depot parenteral medication (Hirsch *et al*, 1973) have been well established, and in a review of 24 controlled studies of maintenance neuroleptic treatment in schizophrenia Davis (1975) concluded that the evidence for such efficacy is overwhelming. Neuroleptics do not, however, prevent relapse. In a study by Hogarty *et al* (1974) 48% of patients on active medication relapsed within two years; this figure was not substantially different in a later study (Hogarty *et al*, 1979) of depot prophylactic neuroleptics (i.e. in a situation where compliance was assured).

Effective prophylactic agents are also available for affective disorders. Lithium has been shown to be effective as a prophylactic agent against the recurrence of both manic and depressive episodes of affective illness and the evidence for its value in these situations is substantial (Baastrup & Schou, 1967; Coppen *et al*, 1971; Prien *et al*, 1974). Although lithium is undoubtedly effective in the prevention of recurrent episodes of affective illness, it is not, of course, totally successful. Study of the findings reviewed by Davis (1976) shows that while recurrent episodes are less common in lithium-treated patients than in those not receiving lithium, they do still occur. It has been suggested that poor response is commonest in rapid cycling manic-depressive illnesses (Stancer *et al*, 1970; Dunner & Fieve, 1974), but this may mean no more than that these patients are particularly severely affected. Recurrent attacks of depressive illness may be prevented by maintenance antidepressants as well as by maintenance lithium, but again, although the benefits are not doubted, prophylactic maintenance is not completely effective (Davis, 1976). It has, however, been clearly established that the frequency of relapses of schizophrenia and of both manic and depressive relapses of affective disorder is significantly, and indeed very substantially, reduced by appropriate maintenance medication. In other words, many attacks of these illnesses can be prevented by appropriate treatment.

The success of tertiary prevention in the sense of limiting disability consequent upon disease which is not fully treatable has been less substantial. Tertiary prevention in this sense is not a major issue with regard to the affective disorders, as the disabilities of these conditions relate to the symptoms of depressed or elevated mood. When the symptoms of mood disturbance are under control, then the patient is on the whole well and there is no question of the progressive development of an underlying state of increasingly limited function. Such limitation of function does not seem to occur in affective disorder, but it certainly occurs in schizophrenia (Johnstone *et al*, 1992), and indeed chronic deterioration of function has been held to be the hallmark of schizophrenia. It is therefore very important to consider what steps can be taken to minimise the development of the negative features of the defect state. An unresolved question is the relationship between the occurrence of acute episodes of positive symptoms and the development of the defect state. It is established that maintenance neuroleptic treatment will reduce the frequency of such acute episodes, but we do not know whether or not this will have an effect on the development of defect.

Although neuroleptics may be recommended as being likely to improve positive symptoms, no physical treatment can be recommended as affecting negative symptoms in such a way.

The effect of neuroleptics upon these symptoms is uncertain. At present controlled trials have yielded evidence that neuroleptic medications may improve, have no significant effect upon, or may exacerbate negative symptoms (Pogue-Geile & Zubin, 1988). L-dopa, amphetamines and anti-Parkinsonian medications have all been tried as treatments for negative symptoms, but consistent evidence that they are clearly effective is so far lacking (for review see Pogue-Geile & Zubin, 1988). Other unconventional drug treatments for schizophrenia include carbamazepine, which has generally been suggested for patients with very disturbed behaviour (Post *et al*, 1986). The limited nature of the evidence for the efficacy of this drug in schizophrenia is presented in a review by Donaldson *et al* (1983) in which other unconventional treatments of schizophrenia including propranolol, clonidine and benzodiazepines are also discussed, and it is concluded that none of these has out-performed conventional neuroleptics in treatment of schizophrenia. Small studies have been described using endorphins and opiate blocking agents (Mueser & Dysken, 1983), but the value of these drugs has not been demonstrated and the neuropeptide cholecystokinin has not been shown to be effective in the treatment of schizophrenia. Atypical neuroleptics such as clozapine may be of value in the management of treatment-resistant positive symptoms (Kane *et al*, 1988), but that they have anything particular to offer in terms of lessening the development of the defect state is unclear.

Some studies have suggested that lithium is of value in the disorder of schizophrenia and schizoaffective disorders (Prien, 1979). These studies concern acute treatment. A recent study has examined the value of prophylactic lithium in patients with functional psychosis (mainly schizophrenia), but over a 2-year period did not find it to be of benefit (Johnstone *et al*, 1991).

It will be evident from the above that there is ample evidence for the efficacy of various drugs, principally neuroleptic, in the treatment of positive schizophrenic symptoms and in the prophylaxis of relapse of such symptoms. That such benefits have an influence on the development of defect symptoms is unclear, and the evidence that defect symptoms themselves are affected by drug treatment is uncertain. There is, however, evidence that appropriate adjustment of the dosages of maintenance treatment and thoughtful use of additional medication can limit the reduction in wellbeing and function of these patients (Johnstone, 1990).

References

BAASTRUP, P. C. & SCHOU, M. (1967) Lithium as a prophylactic agent. *Archives of General Psychiatry*, **16**, 162–172.

COPPEN, A., NOGUERA, R. & BAILEY, J. (1971) Prophylactic lithium in affective disorders: controlled trial. *Lancet*, **ii**, 275–279.

DAVIS, J. M. (1975) Overview: maintenance therapy in psychiatry. I. Schizophrenia. *American Journal of Psychiatry*, **132**, 1237–1245.

—— (1976) Overview: maintenance therapy in psychiatry. II. Affective Disorders. *American Journal of Psychiatry*, **133**, 1–13.

DONALDSON, S. R., GELENBERG, A. G. & BALDESSARINI, R. J. (1983) The pharmacologic treatment of schizophrenia: a progress report. *Schizophrenia Bulletin*, **9**, 504–527.

DUNNER, D. L. & FIEVE, R. R. (1974) Clinical factors in lithium carbonate prophylaxis failure. *Archives of General Psychiatry*, **30**, 229–233.

EAGGER, S. A., LEVY, E. R. & SAHAKIAN, B. J. (1991) Tacrine in Alzheimer's Disease. *Lancet*, **337**, 989–992.

HIRSCH, S. R., GAIND, R., ROHDE, P. H., et al (1973) Out-patient maintenance of chronic schizophrenic patients with long acting fluphenazine: double blind placebo trial. *British Medical Journal*, **1**, 633–637.

HOGARTY, G. E., GOLDBERG, S. C., SCHOOLER, N. R., et al (1974) Drugs and sociotherapy in the aftercare of schizophrenic patients. II. Two year relapse rates. *Archives of General Psychiatry*, **31**, 603–608.

———, SCHOOLER, N. R. & ULRICH, R. (1979) Fluphenazine and social therapy in the aftercare of schizophrenia patients. *Archives of General Psychiatry*, **36**, 1283–1294.

JOHNSTONE, E. C. (1990) Chronic schizophrenia: can one do anything about persistent symptoms? In *Dilemmas in the Management of Psychiatric Patients* (eds K. Hawton & P. Cowen). Oxford: Oxford University Press.

———, CROW, T. J., OWENS, D. G. C., et al (1991) The Northwick Park 'functional' psychosis study. Phase 2: maintenance treatment. *Journal of Psychopharmacology*, **5**, 338–395.

———, FRITH, C. D., CROW, T. J., et al (1992) The Northwick Park 'functional' psychosis study: diagnosis and outcome. *Psychological Medicine*, **22**, 331–346.

KANE, J., HONIGFELD, G., SINGER, J., et al (1988) Clozapine for the treatment-resistant schizophrenic. *Archives of General Psychiatry*, **45**, 789–796.

LEFF, J. P. & WING, J. K. (1971) Trial of maintenance treatment in schizophrenia. *British Medical Journal*, **3**, 599–604.

MUESER, K. T. & DYSKEN, M. W. (1983) Narcotic antagonists in schizophrenia: a methodological review. *Schizophrenia Bulletin*, **9**, 213–225.

POGUE-GEILE, M. F. & ZUBIN, J. (1988) Negative symptomatology and schizophrenia: a conceptual and empirical review. *International Journal of Mental Health*, **16**, 3–45.

POST, R. M., RUBINOW, D. R., UHDE, T. W., et al (1986) Dopaminergic effects of carbamazepine. *Archives of General Psychiatry*, **43**, 392–396.

PRIEN, R. F. (1979) Lithium in the treatment of schizophrenia and schizoaffective disorders. *British Journal of Psychiatry*, **141**, 387–400.

———, KLETT, J. & CAFFEY, E. M. (1974) Lithium prophylaxis in recurrent affective illness. *American Journal of Psychiatry*, **131**, 198–203.

STANCER, H. C., FURLING, F. W. & GODSE, D. D. (1970) A longitudinal investigation of lithium as a prophylactic agent for recurrent depression. *Canadian Journal of Psychiatry*, **15**, 29–40.

II. Prevention of specific disorders

7 Affective disorders

JAN SCOTT and E. S. PAYKEL

Causative factors

Affective disorders span a range of psychotic and neurotic illnesses. Disorders at each end of the spectrum show considerable differences and causative factors may also be very different. The most useful distinctions appear to be:

(a) Bipolar v. unipolar disorder: bipolar disorder tends to show much higher familial rates (although about half the familial affective disorder is unipolar), to have an equal gender ratio, to have earlier onset and to be more recurrent.

(b) Within unipolar disorder, psychotic and melancholic clinical picture v. non-melancholic: this distinction is less clear cut, and it is now recognised that presence or absence of recent life stress shows little relation to symptom profile. When based solely on symptom pattern the distinction appears to have validity for genetic loading, neuroendocrine findings, and treatment outcome.

There has been progress in the understanding of the aetiological role of social processes in depression and similar advances in the field of biological psychiatry, but work on these models has tended to be pursued in isolation (Monroe, 1988). Ultimately the aim must be to produce more integrated theories as the available evidence suggests a multifactorial causation of affective disorders (Akiskal & McKinney, 1975). 'Stress-diathesis' models predominate in the literature (Scott, 1988).

Epidemiology

Affective disorders are essentially a community problem: only one per thousand of the population are admitted to hospital annually in England because of severe illness (Bebbington, 1978). However, approximately 3% are seen annually by GPs with recognised depression, with about an equal number unrecognised, and community six month prevalence is 3–5% (Smith & Weissman, 1992). The life-time rate is around 1.2 per 100 for bipolar disorders, and much higher for unipolar disorders. Except for bipolar disorder, depression is twice as common in women than in men, with particularly high rates in younger married women with children. The explanation probably involves a mixture of psychosocial and hormonal factors, and the differential acknowledgement of distress (Paykel, 1991). The disorders have a median age of onset of under 30 years and morbidity and mortality rates are high. Bipolar disorder may be a little more common in upper social classes, and milder depressions more common in working class populations subject to greater social stress.

Genetic factors

Bipolar disorder is the most familial form, with morbid risks in first degree relatives of approximately 9% for bipolar disorder and 11% for unipolar. In severe unipolar disorder the risk is 9% for unipolar disorder, and only 0.6% for bipolar (McGuffin & Katz, 1986). Twin studies show much higher concordances for MZ than DZ twins in bipolar disorder and severe unipolar disorder, but findings are equivocal for milder/neurotic depression, leaving the possibility of environmental explanations for concordances found. The mode of inheritance is not clear and is likely to involve multiple genes. Genetic linkage studies have not so far produced any strong replicated linkages, but there are several studies finding X linkage in bipolar disorder, with other negative studies, suggesting heterogeneity.

Biological causes

Although many years of biological studies have produced an increasing body of consistent findings, the extent to which these represent causes or secondary consequences of affective disorder remains unclear. The original monoamine hypotheses suggesting diminished noradrenergic or serotoninergic neurotransmission associated with depression remain plausible, and are supported by the fact that most antidepressant drugs potentiate neurotransmission in one or both systems. Serotoninergic antidepressants appear superior to noradrenergic drugs in obsessional and panic disorders, but there do not appear to be major differences in depression. Low CSF serotonin turnover appears to be a more reliable correlate of suicidal and impulsive behaviour than of depression. Other than older anti-hypertensives which are now little used, the evidence that therapeutic drugs produce depression of major clinical degree is weak (Edwards, 1989). Platelet studies have consistently shown reduced serotonin uptake in depression but the explanation is unclear. The most consistent neuroendocrine findings are hypercortisolaemia and dexamethasone non-suppression; both are clearly state markers. Blunted hormonal responses to the alpha 2 adrenoceptor agonist clonidine and the serotonin precursor tryptophan appear common during depression but again the explanations are unclear. None of these findings lead to firm aetiological conclusions yet.

Personality

Most work on personality has been in relation to vulnerability to stress (see below). Conclusions are hampered by difficulties in measuring personality independently of the effects of being depressed. There is some evidence that dependency and neuroticism may be associated with increased risk of depression (Hirschfeld & Shea, 1992).

Social factors

There is a consistent body of data implicating psychosocial stress in the onset of depressive episodes. Since this has greater implications currently for prevention it will be reviewed in more detail. One of the most robust findings is the higher morbidity rates for depression in females when compared to males (Weissman & Klerman, 1977; Robins *et al*, 1984). Social explanations focus on female roles and their status in society (Weissman & Klerman, 1977). Further support for this theory is adduced from the finding that, with regard to depressive disorders, marriage is detrimental to women but protective for men (Der & Bebbington, 1987) and there are particularly high rates in women with children. Biological differences or differences in acknowledgement of distress may also contribute to the differential gender ratio. Many community studies have suggested an inverse relationship between socio-economic status and depression (Brown & Harris, 1978; Goldberg & Huxley, 1980). Studies in more severe depressives and bipolars do not show this, suggesting the relationship is with milder depression.

While unemployment is likely to lead to lower socio-economic status, its association with depression may arise from other mechanisms. In particular the role of work in maintaining self-esteem has been noted (Bolton & Oakley, 1987).

Numerous studies have demonstrated that depressives (in comparison with the general population) experience a significant excess of life events in the six months prior to the onset of the disorder. The information on mania and life events is conflicting and there are few studies of bipolar depression. (For a detailed review see Paykel & Cooper, 1992.) Loss and separations are particularly common, although they show only weak specificity for depression. The strongest relationship is demonstrated between threatening or undesirable events and the onset of depression. An increase in independent undesirable events may also be implicated in recurrence or persistence of depression, while 'fresh start events' may be associated with recovery (Brown *et al*, 1987). There is a sixfold increase in the relative risk of becoming depressed within six months of experiencing a life event. Approximately 30% of those experiencing depression fail to report any life events prior to onset. McGuffin *et al* (1987) found that both depression and the tendency to experience adversity showed familial aggregation.

Social support may modify the impact of life stresses (Paykel & Cooper, 1992). Background adversity and variation in levels of support may predict illness (Bhugra, 1988). Inappropriate excessive social support (which reduces the sense of personal control) may be as damaging as too little support (Krause, 1987). It is also reported that many depressives show deficits in making and sustaining relationships premorbidly (Bhugra, 1989). Findings regarding social support are less clear than those for life events, and the independence of social support from the individual's personality and ability to generate relationships is also less clear.

The role of social support in depression is further complicated by differing interpretations of this concept. Brown & Harris (1978) have investigated a specific form of social support, the presence of a confidant in reducing vulnerability to depression. Recent attempts to identify the role of social support in depression have used a wider definition but suggest that perceived numerical and qualitative deficiencies in close personal relationships may predict onset and course of the illness (Bhugra, 1988). While depression itself may increase marital discord (Weissman & Paykel, 1974), a discordant marriage may significantly increase the risk of onset (Brown, 1989), relapse (Hooley et al, 1986) or chronicity (Scott, 1992a) of depression. Vaughn & Leff (1976) found that there was a relationship between relatives' high expressed emotion (EE) scores and relapses among neurotic depressives. Hooley et al (1986) confirmed this finding and demonstrated that high EE spouses tended to be rated high on the basis of critical comments rather than overinvolved attitudes. Hooley (1987) has further demonstrated an association between high EE and relapse of manic symptoms.

The most problematic area is that of early childhood environment and depression. Findings regarding early parental loss by death are inconsistent and the effect is at best a small one. There are more consistent associations with loss for other reasons, usually parental marital breakdown, but here other interpretations arise, such as effects of the parental disharmony preceding breakdown and the possibility of predisposing transmitted personality difficulties.

Several studies have investigated how the loss translates into adult vulnerability and have concluded that lack of adequate parental care in childhood may be an important intervening variable and independent causative factor (Harris et al, 1986; Bifulco et al, 1987). Inadequate parental care of a child may be caused by many factors (Monroe, 1988). For example it is proposed that high parental concern in childhood increases the risk in adulthood of neurosis in general and depression in particular (Perris et al, 1986; Parker et al, 1987). This 'affectionless overcontrol' may reduce self-esteem and self-efficacy and adversely affect the development of social competence (Henderson, 1988). At present these findings depend largely on retrospective reports by adult depressives and require replication in long-term prospective studies.

Studies suggesting that low self-esteem may interact with life events to produce depression (Brown et al, 1987) must be considered in the light of studies which may suggest that low self-esteem is itself a consequence of repeated depressive episodes (Ingham et al, 1987).

The interaction between the individual and provoking or protective factors in their environment occurs at many conceptual levels (Jenkins, 1976). Jenkins' model emphasises that those with a strong array of individual adaptive capacities are less likely to reach the pathological end-state of depression in response to stress.

Pearlin & Schooler (1978) argue that a coping repertoire consists not only of what an individual does but also of what resources are available to them. They describe general psychological and social resources (defined in terms of personal and interpersonal factors respectively) as well as specific coping responses (referring to types of behaviour, cognitions and perceptions that modify the impact of problematic social experiences). Not only do individual coping repertoires vary significantly, but the coping mechanisms used by people vary in their efficacy in responding to different stresses (Pearlin & Schooler, 1978). Also, strength in one area of the specific coping response may compensate for deficits in another: a small but interesting study demonstrated that those showing cognitive distortions were less likely to become depressed if they engaged in 'coping' behaviours (Burns et al, 1987). It can be seen that the models of individual coping put forward (Jenkins, 1976; Pearlin & Schooler, 1978) are similar, in as much as both define coping in terms of an inward perspective (e.g. personality, self-image, biological predisposition) that is balanced by an outward perspective (interactions with other people and the environment).

Prevention

Prevention will be discussed on three levels:

(a) Primary prevention, aiming to reduce the incidence of the disorder
(b) Secondary prevention, aiming at early detection and treatment of conspicuous and hidden morbidity
(c) Tertiary prevention, aiming to reduce disabilities arising as a consequence of the disorder.

Biological causes are not sufficiently clear cut and specific to be amenable currently to preventive approaches. Constitutional aspects of temperament will also be shaped into personality through interaction with the environment, with limited options for modification (Rutter, 1985). Socio-cultural factors are not readily amenable to direct change by the mental health services because they operate at a societal level. Accessibility of services and gender or cultural biases in the communication of distress can be addressed. Primary care physicians can be encouraged to improve detection rates of affective disorders and help-seeking behaviour may be promoted through public education. Interventions aimed at changing the social conditions for high prevalence groups, such as those of lower socio-economic status, in poor housing, in overcrowded conditions or unemployed are more clearly the domain of politics than psychiatry (Scott, 1992*b*), although attempts to influence fiscal and government policy are important (see chapter 3).

Interventions at the level of individuals and their immediate environment are more likely to be successful. Most work on prevention of affective disorders has focused on the role of psycho-social factors in the onset of depression (Brown & Harris, 1978) and on the influence of the disorder on the sufferer, their life style and their family (Wing, 1971; Monroe, 1988).

Primary prevention

The risk of adult depression is modified throughout life by the interaction between the individual and events occurring in childhood, adolescence and adulthood (Rutter, 1985). Recognition of those people at greatest risk of depression is important as it reduces the size of the target population for preventive intervention (Newton & Craig, 1991).

Genetic counselling

This is discussed in chapter 4. It is clear that the value of genetic counselling aimed at avoidance of birth of high risk individuals is restricted by limited knowledge as to mode of inheritance, absence of reliable genetic markers, and limited heritability. Even in bipolar disorder average morbid risks in offspring are probably not sufficiently high nor treatability so low as to justify avoidance of having children. The exceptions are occasional families with very high family histories, families with both parents affected, or mothers with postpartum severe affective disorder, where the 1:5 risk in subsequent pregnancies suggests postponement of next pregnancy until the index infant is sufficiently old not to be very vulnerable both to poor mothering and to an additional family stress. For mothers who have had two or more postpartum episodes, subsequent risks do appear to be sufficiently high to indicate avoidance of further pregnancies.

Interventions in parent–child relationships

Associations of adult depression with damage to early parent–child relationships suggest careful consideration of the possibility of early intervention. If parental care could be improved, or self-esteem of the individual at risk enhanced, it might be possible to prevent the onset of affective episodes at some future point. Few attempts to enhance self-esteem in young people have been evaluated, although Jorm (1987) describes a project focused on reducing neurotic traits in adolescents through the use of rational emotive therapy.

Attempts to enhance parental care, focusing on depressed or vulnerable mothers have been tried in both England and Australia. At present these are best seen as secondary prevention to mothers reducing depression and enhancing parental coping skills, and are discussed under that heading in due course, but they might also have a long-term primary preventive impact on children.

Any such attempts will require critical long-term evaluation, both on account of the inconclusive state of current aetiological evidence and in view of the likelihood that the aetiological effect may be over a range of disorders and behaviours, so that little impact may occur on any specific disorder.

Event centred interventions

Most life events implicated in studies of depression are unavoidable, being such inevitable consequences of the life cycle as interpersonal difficulties, departure of child, retirement, and death of spouse. In less developed societies where premature death, crippling disease and natural disaster are more common, true primary prevention may be directed towards reducing the frequency of events. In well developed countries, government policies may modify the occurrence of poverty, unemployment and poor housing. These lie within the domain of political action; their effect on the incidence of depression might be small.

An alternative approach to prevention uses the knowledge of the timing of the occurrence to signal that action should be taken. This lies on the border between primary and secondary prevention and is discussed in that section. Examples include bereavement counselling and counselling for patients undergoing surgery for carcinoma.

Secondary prevention

Essentially the secondary prevention of affective disorders encompasses early detection of the illness and early initiation of treatment.

Early detection of affective disorders depends in part on the behaviour of mental health professionals but also upon the attitude of the individual towards any symptoms which develop (Goldberg & Huxley, 1980). Recent studies suggest that fewer than 50% of those developing depressive disorders in the community seek professional help (Dew et al, 1988; Lehmann et al, 1988; Meller et al, 1989). Patients with endogenous depression were more likely to seek help (Meller et al, 1989). Other important variables in help-seeking behaviour were limitation in the ability to work (Meller et al, 1989), impaired functioning, and lack of social support (Dew et al, 1988).

In the UK most treatment for depression is by general practitioners. Overall GPs fail to recognise at least 50% of psychiatric disorders presenting (Goldberg & Huxley, 1980), and available figures suggest about the same rates for depression. Factors affecting the early recognition of affective disorders by GPs have been analysed by a number of researchers (Freeling et al, 1985). Many strategies have been proposed to overcome this problem:

(a) *Education.* In Sweden, Rorsman et al (1990) described a programme that improved detection and management of depression. Evidence from England (Gask et al, 1987; Boorman et al, 1992) suggests that an educational package aimed at improving the interviewing skills of primary care physicians produces similar results. These types of programmes have encouraged action at a national level in the USA and Britain where the professional colleges have respectively initiated the 'DART' (Depression Awareness, Recognition and Treatment) and the 'Defeat Depression' campaigns. Both campaigns aim to improve knowledge and treatment skills among professionals and also to raise public awareness about this disorder and encourage help-seeking.

(b) *Screening.* One approach to improving case finding would be the use of screening instruments such as the General Health Questionnaire (GHQ), the Beck Depression Scale, the Zung Scale or the Hospital Anxiety and Depression Questionnaire.

(c) *Psychiatric outreach.* Other approaches focus on practices that may enhance access to mental health services, either by deployment of mental health professionals in a liaison-consultation role with the primary care team or by offering direct access to mental health professionals by self-referral to a community mental health centre. Research on the general efficacy of these service models is available (Talbott et al, 1987; Tyrer et al, 1990) but the specific use of these approaches in affective illnesses is under-researched.

Early recognition would only be of value if shown to alter outcome. Johnstone & Goldberg (1976) found that notification to the GP that a patient was a psychiatric case produced a better outcome than non-notification, and it was suggested that individual psychological distress was reduced by 2.8 months if GPs were informed of a patient's high GHQ score. This finding was replicated by Zung et al (1983). Patients with high Zung depression scores were randomised to 'conspicuous' and 'hidden' groups. In the former group the GP was informed of the patients' high depression rating, while the scores of the latter group were not revealed. Outcome at four week follow-up revealed that 68% of patients who scored highly on the Zung scale and who also received treatment were significantly improved, compared to 28% whose score had been revealed to the GP but who had not received treatment. Only 18% of the control group (where the high depression scores had not been revealed) had improved.

Early intervention

Early intervention offers possibilities both of interrupting distress before it reaches the level of clinical depression, and of markedly shortening more clear cut clinical episodes. The first approach lies on the borderline between primary and secondary prevention. Some attempts have been made to initiate and evaluate such preventive interventions.

Event centred interventions. Bereavement has been the best studied situation. Parkes (1981) and Raphael (1977) have demonstrated the beneficial effects of support and counselling in reducing psychiatric morbidity in those at high risk of abnormal grief reactions to the same levels as low risk individuals.

Maguire *et al* (1980) offered counselling and practical advice to women exposed to a threatening life event, namely surgical treatment for breast cancer. Women were randomly assigned to counselling or a non-counselled control group. The prevalence of anxiety and depression was similar in both groups, but episodes were of shorter duration in the counselled group and they showed better social and psychological adjustment at 18 month follow-up after the operation. This offered some evidence of a possible primary preventive intervention, but, as Maguire *et al* (1983) pointed out, the reduced morbidity during episodes might have been a function of early recognition and prompt referral to additional specialist services by the counsellor (i.e. secondary prevention).

Interventions with vulnerable families. Two British befriending projects are described by Newton (1988). Homestart is a community-based support programme which has demonstrated enhanced child development and improved parental functioning in families identified as 'at risk' (Van der Eyken, 1982). The 'Newpin' project relates more closely to those at risk of depression (Pound *et al*, 1985). Mothers who were vulnerable to depression according to the Brown & Harris model (1978), who are isolated, or who show problems in parenting, form a contract with a volunteer supporter from a similar social background. Preliminary evaluation of the project did not use any recognised depression rating scales. However, self-evaluation by the women ($n = 12$) suggested that self-esteem, self-confidence and interpersonal relationships had improved and that the mothers related better to their children (Newton, 1988).

In New South Wales Barnett & Parker (1985) assigned highly anxious primiparous women (who had been shown by previous research to be at greater risk of neurotic and depressive disorders) post-natally to either professional support, lay support or a control group with no additional help offered. The results on the specific role of this social support were difficult to interpret, but those who received professional help showed a significant reduction in post-natal anxiety levels compared with the other groups. Those receiving lay support showed a non-significant reduction in their anxiety levels. Pregnant and post-natal women merit special targeting because of emerging evidence that post-natal depression may produce persistent disturbances in infant cognitive and emotional development. Cox *et al* (1987) undertook in Edinburgh a controlled trial of intervention by Health Visitors and Murray & Cooper in Cambridge are undertaking studies of screening and intervention on high risk groups.

These intervention studies offer support for the possibility of prevention of major affective disorders by intervention at the subclinical level. The studies are a useful starting point but more systematic research would be required before resources could be committed to this area with confidence. Given the high prevalence of subclinical and early clinical disorder early intervention might only be cost-effective if short-term outcome were markedly improved: the spontaneous short-term outcome of such early episodes is not yet clear. There would be a major benefit if early intervention had a major effect in reducing long-term consequences in morbidity and disability, as in some physical disorders such as cancer: again evidence is lacking.

Tertiary prevention

Rehabilitation

There has been a failure to investigate or attempt to eliminate the residual disabilities in patients with affective disorders, which contrasts sharply with the extensive literature on the rehabilitation of schizophrenics (Scott, 1992*b*). This may partly be because schizophrenics form the majority of the long-stay hospital population. In addition, the disabilities seen in schizophrenia tend to be global and more progressive than those found in chronic affective disorders, perhaps leading to more intensive efforts at rehabilitation.

Compared to patients with schizophrenia, vocational rehabilitation of patients with affective disorders focuses less on the role of work performance and more on its potential for restoring confidence and self-esteem and enhancing feelings of mastery (Bebbington & Kuipers, 1983). Weissman & Paykel (1974) reported that women working outside of the home showed less impairment following depression than housebound housewives. Brown & Harris (1978) also saw work as having a protective function in women at risk of depression. Re-employment may also reduce depression in socially isolated men who were made redundant (Bolton & Oakley, 1987). Again only broad guidelines on vocational training for patients with affective disorders are currently available (Bennett, 1982; Shaw & Koch, 1982).

Chronic neurotic disorders may cause significant limitations in social functioning (Henderson, 1988). These individuals and their families may benefit from the support of a community psychiatric nurse rather than merely receiving intermittent out-patient appointments (Paykel *et al*, 1992).

Depression produces secondary consequences in impaired marital and family relationships and these may respond to family intervention (Scott, 1992*a*).

Prevention of relapse and recurrence

An important aspect of tertiary prevention in affective disorder is prevention of further episodes. It has recently become clear that there is a high risk of these, at least with the more severe forms of disorder. It has become customary to distinguish between relapse, or early return of symptoms in the first six months or so after remission, which can be viewed as return of the original episode, and recurrence, or later symptom return, which can be regarded as a new episode. Both are common. Short-term follow-up studies show relapse in 30% or more of out-patients or in-patients. Earlier long-term follow-up studies of severe affective disorder showed common occurrence of further episodes, with more recurrences in bipolar than unipolar disorder. More recent studies confirm this picture, with at least 50% of those with first episodes having a further attack, higher recurrence rates for those with previous episodes, and a proportion showing mild to moderate persistent symptoms (Kiloh et al, 1988; Lee & Murray, 1988). About 15% of deaths are due to suicide and mortality rates from other causes are also increased. It is not known if similar actions apply to milder depression at general practice or hospital out-patient level.

The role of pharmacotherapy in preventing further episodes has been well studied and clear guidelines have been developed (Prien, 1992). Continuation of antidepressants for at least 4 months after complete symptom remission has been shown to halve relapse rates compared with early withdrawal, and should take place routinely. It is sometimes described as continuation therapy. There is suggestive evidence that antidepressants or lithium are of similar value after ECT.

Longer term maintenance where there have been at least two separate episodes recently has also been shown to be of value. Both antidepressants and lithium appear effective in unipolar depressives, with particularly high rates of recurrence on antidepressant withdrawal after a shorter continuation period, where there has been a good acute response and a recurrent history (Frank et al, 1990). In bipolar disorder lithium is most effective, with carbamazepine also of value and accumulating evidence for sodium valproate.

Non-pharmacological approaches are less clearly of value. Interpersonal psychotherapy was of significant but very limited value in reducing recurrence in one study (Frank et al, 1990) but did not reduce early relapse in a controlled study of continuation medication (Paykel et al, 1976). There is accumulating evidence from follow-ups of short-term controlled trials, not yet conclusive, that cognitive therapy may reduce relapse rates in milder unipolar depressives, compared with those treated acutely with antidepressants (Williams, 1989). Further studies in this promising area are required. The research on expressed emotion (EE) demonstrated that (in contrast to schizophrenia) depressives with high EE relatives were not protected by drug treatment or by reduced contact (Vaughn & Leff, 1976). However, Jacobson (1984) has reported that marital therapy alone or in combination with individual cognitive therapy can offer effective treatment of the acute episode and may prevent relapse. Other approaches which have been advocated include improving coping repertoires (not yet critically evaluated), and social skills training, which has been evaluated in acute treatment but not for long-term effects.

Although the above measures lie more within the realm of treatment they have preventive implications since they reduce prevalence rates of symptomatic disorder.

Research required

None of the measures discussed in the previous section have been shown conclusively to be of benefit in prevention of affective disorder, and some areas await further elucidation of causes and mechanisms before useful preventive measures can be devised.

There are some areas where possibilities are promising and further research studies are strongly indicated. These should focus both on benefits and on costs of any preventive approach and should wherever possible adopt rigorous controlled designs.

Primary prevention

(a) The role of genetic counselling in bipolar disorder and its practical take up will require evaluation, but not until reliable genetic markers are developed. There will then need to be careful consideration of levels of risk which justify specific advice, of practical take up, and emotional consequences.

(b) Further work employing large-scale and expensive longitudinal studies is required to identify major early environmental antecedents of affective disorder, before childhood preventive strategies can be evaluated.

Secondary prevention

This appears sufficiently promising to be an important area for evaluation in selected studies using rigorous controlled methodologies and cost–benefit assessments. Benefits will need careful evaluation where spontaneous outcome may turn out to be equally good; as will costs, given the high prevalence of milder disorder.

(a) Effects of screening in general practice and in high risk groups

(b) Effects of early intervention in screened groups, high risk groups, subjects undergoing stressful life events

(c) Effects of GP educational programmes directed towards better recognition and better management

(d) Effects of outreach psychiatric and community mental health programmes.

Tertiary prevention

(a) Effects of medication have been well demonstrated in trials. Evaluation of quality of aftercare actually received is indicated, and effects of introducing model programmes, together with development of further predictors of who requires maintenance treatment.

(b) High recurrence rates after discontinuation of antidepressants even after standard continuation therapy, in recurrent depressives, suggest the need to study potential sensitising effects of antidepressant treatment, and the importance of evaluating non-pharmacological approaches to prevention of symptom return, of which cognitive therapy appears at present the most promising.

(c) The value of programmes aimed at reducing disability and secondary interpersonal and social consequences of depression requires further evaluation after the acute episode, particularly in the more chronic and recurrent depressives.

References

AKISKAL, H. A. & MCKINNEY, W. T. (1975) Overview of recent research in depression. Integration of ten conceptual models into a comprehensive clinical frame. *Archives of General Psychiatry*, **32**, 285–305.

BARNETT, B. & PARKER, G. (1985) Professional and non-professional intervention for highly anxious primiparous mothers. *British Journal of Psychiatry*, **146**, 287–293.
BEBBINGTON, P. (1978) The epidemiology of depressive disorder. In *Culture, Medicine and Psychiatry* (ed. A. Kleinnman), pp. 297–341. Dordrecht: Reidal.
—— & KUIPERS, L. (1983) Social management of depression. *The Physician*, August, 176–179.
BENNETT, D. H. (1982) Management and rehabilitation of affective psychoses. In *Handbook of Psychiatry, Volume 3; Psychoses of Uncertain Aetiology* (eds J. K. Wing & L. Wing), pp. 173–176. Cambridge: Cambridge University Press.
BHUGRA, T. S. (1988) Social support. *Current Opinion in Psychiatry*, **1**, 206–211.
—— (1989) Social support and social networks. *Current Opinion in Psychiatry*, **2**, 278–282.
BIFULCO, A., BROWN, G. W. & HARRIS, T. O. (1987) Childhood loss of parent, lack of adequate parental care and adult depression: a replication. *Journal of Affective Disorders*, **12**, 115–128.
BOLTON, W. & OAKLEY, K. (1987) A longitudinal study of social support and depression in unemployed men. *Psychological Medicine*, **17**, 453–460.
BOORMAN, T., STANDARDT, S. & SCOTT, J. (1992) Problem based interviewing in general practice. *LINC-UP Bulletin*, **2**, 7–10.
BROWN, G. W. (1989) Depression: a radical social perspective. In *Depression: An Integrative Approach* (eds K. Herbst & E. S. Paykel), pp. 21–44. Oxford: Heinemann Medical Books.
——, BIFULCO, A. & HARRIS, T. O. (1987) Life events, vulnerability and onset of depression – some refinements. *British Journal of Psychiatry*, **150**, 30–42.
—— & HARRIS, T. O. (1978) *Social Origins of Depression: A Study of Psychiatric Disorder in Women*. London: Tavistock.
BURNS, D., SHAW, B. & CROKER, W. (1987) Thinking styles and coping strategies of depressed women: an empirical investigation. *Behaviour Research and Therapy*, **25**, 223–225.
COX, J. L., HOLDEN, J. M. & SAGOVSKY, R. (1987) Detection of postnatal depression – development of the 10 item Edinburgh Postnatal Depression Scale (EPDS). *British Journal of Psychiatry*, **150**, 782–786.
DER, G. & BEBBINGTON, P. (1987) Depression in inner London: a register study. *Social Psychiatry*, **22**, 73–84.
DEW, M. A., DUNN, L. O., BROMET, E. J., *et al* (1988) Factors affecting help-seeking during depression in a community sample. *Journal of Affective Disorders*, **14**, 223–234.
EDWARDS, J. G. (1989) Drug-related depression: clinical and epidemiological reports. In *Depression: an Integrative Approach* (eds K. R. Herbst & E. S. Paykel). Oxford: Heinemann.
VAN DER EYKEN, W. (1982) *Homestart: A Four Year Evaluation*. Leicester: Homestart Consultancy.
FRANK, E., KUPFER, D. J., PEREL, J. M., *et al* (1990) Three year outcomes for maintenance therapies of recurrent depression. *Archives of General Psychiatry*, **47**, 1093–1099.
FREELING, P., RAO, B. M., PAYKEL, E. S., *et al* (1985) Unrecognised depression in general practice. *British Medical Journal*, **290**, 1880–1883.
GASK, L., McGRATH, G., GOLDBERG, D., *et al* (1987) Improving the psychiatric skills of established general practitioners. *Medical Education*, **21**, 362–368.
GOLDBERG, D. & HUXLEY, P. (1980) *Mental Illness in the Community*, pp. 47–122. London: Tavistock.
HARRIS, T. O., BROWN, G. W. & BIFULCO, A. (1986) Loss of parent in childhood and adult psychiatric disorder: the role of lack of adequate parental care. *Psychological Medicine*, **16**, 641–659.
HENDERSON, A. S. (1988) *An Introduction to Social Psychiatry*, pp. 73–156. Oxford: Oxford Medical.
HIRSCHFELD, R. & SHEA, T. (1992) Personality. In *Handbook of Depression* (ed. E. S. Paykel). Edinburgh: Churchill Livingstone.
HOOLEY, J. (1987) The nature and origins of expressed emotion. In *Understanding Major Mental Disorder* (eds K. K. Hahlweg & M. Goldstein), pp. 176–194. New York: Family Process Press.
——, ORLEY, J. & TEASDALE, J. (1986) Levels of expressed emotion and relapse in depressed patients. *British Journal of Psychiatry*, **148**, 642–674.
INGHAM, J., KREITMAN, N., MILLER, P., *et al* (1987) Self-appraisal, anxiety and depression in women – a prospective study. *British Journal of Psychiatry*, **151**, 643–651.
JACOBSON, N. (1984) Marital therapy and the cognitive behavioural treatment of depression. *Behaviour Therapist*, **7**, 143–147.
JENKINS, C. (1976) Psychosocial modifiers of response to stress. In *Stress and Mental Disorders* (eds J. Barret, R. Rose & G. Kerman), pp. 265–278. New York: Raven Press.
JOHNSTONE, A. & GOLDBERG, D. P. (1976) Psychiatric screening in general practice: a controlled trial. *Lancet*, **ii**, 605–608.

JORM, A. F. (1987) *Modifiability of a Personality Trait Which is a Risk Factor for Neurosis*. Psychiatric Association Symposium on Epidemiology and the Prevention of Mental Disorders (Abstracts), September 15–17.
KILCH, L. G., ANDREWS, G. & NEILSON, M. (1988) The long-term outcome of depressive illness. *British Journal of Psychiatry*, **153**, 752–775.
KLERMAN, G. & BARRETT, J. (1973) Clinical and epidemiological aspects of affective disorder. In *Lithium: Its Role in the Psychiatric Research and Treatment* (eds S. Gershon & B. Shopsin), pp. 201–236. New York: Plenum Press.
KRAUSE, N. (1987) Understanding the stress process: linking social support and locus of control beliefs. *Journal of Gerontology*, **42**, 589–593.
LEE, A. S. & MURRAY, R. M. (1988) The long-term outcome of Maudsley depressives. *British Journal of Psychiatry*, **153**, 741–775.
LEHMANN, H. E., FENTON, F. R., DEUTSCH, M., et al (1988) An 11-year follow-up study of 110 depressed patients. *Acta Psychiatrica Scandinavica*, **78**, 57–65.
MCGUFFIN, P., KATZ, R. & BEBBINGTON, P. (1987) Hazard, heredity and depression. A family study. *Journal of Psychiatric Research*, 365–375.
—— & —— (1986) Nature, nurture and affective disorder. In *The Biology of Depression* (ed. J. F. W. Deakin), pp. 26–52. London: Gaskell.
MAGUIRE, P., TAIT, A., BROOKE, M., et al (1980) The effect of counselling on the psychiatric morbidity associated with mastectomy. *British Medical Journal*, **281**, 1454–1456.
——, BROOKE, M., TAIT, A., et al (1983) The effect of counselling on physical disability and social recovery after mastectomy. *Clinical Oncology*, **9**, 319–324.
MELLER, I., FICHTER, M., WEYERER, S., et al (1989) The use of psychiatric facilities by depressives: results of the Upper Bavarian Study. *Acta Psychiatrica Scandinavica*, **79**, 27–31.
MONROE, S. M. (1988) Social factors in depression. *Current Opinion in Psychiatry*, **1**, 165–175.
NEWTON, J. (1988) *Preventing Mental Illness*, pp. 134–196. London: Routledge.
—— & CRAIG, T. (1991) Prevention. In *Community Psychiatry* (eds D. Bennett & H. Freeman), pp. 488–516. Edinburgh: Churchill Livingstone.
PARKER, G., KILOH, L. & HAYWARD, L. (1987) Parental representations of neurotic and endogenous depressives. *Journal of Affective Disorders*, **13**, 75–82.
PARKES, C. M. (1981) Evaluation of a bereavement service. *Journal of Preventative Psychiatry*, **1**, 179–188.
PAYKEL, E. S. (1991) Depression in women. *British Journal of Psychiatry*, **158** (Suppl. 10), 22–29.
——, DIMASCIO, A., KLERMAN, G. L., et al (1976) Maintenance therapy of depression. *Pharmakopsychiatrie Neuro-psychopharmacologie*, **9**, 127–136.
——, MANGEN, S. P., GRIFFITHS, J. H., et al (1982) Community psychiatric nursing for neurotic patients: a controlled trial. *British Journal of Psychiatry*, **140**, 573–581.
—— & COOPER, Z. (1991) Life events and social support. In *Handbook of Affective Disorders*, 2nd Edn. (ed. E. S. Paykel). Edinburgh: Churchill Livingstone.
PEARLIN, L. I. & SCHOOLER, C. (1978) The structure of coping. *Journal of Health and Social Behaviour*, **19**, 2–21.
PERRIS, C., ARRINDALL, W. A., PERRIS, E., et al (1986) Perceived deprived parental rearing and depression. *British Journal of Psychiatry*, **148**, 170–175.
POUND, A., MILLS, M. & COX, T. (1985) A pilot evaluation of Newpin. A home-visiting and befriending scheme in south London. *Newsletter of the Association of Child Psychology and Psychiatry*, October, 2–4.
PRIEN, R. F. (1992) Maintenance treatment. In *Handbook of Affective Disorders*, 2nd Edn. (ed. E. S. Paykel), pp. 419–436. Edinburgh: Churchill Livingstone.
RAPHAEL, B. (1977) Preventative intervention with the recently bereaved. *Archives of General Psychiatry*, **34**, 1450–1454.
ROBINS, L., HELZER, J., WEISSMAN, M., et al (1984) Lifetime prevalence of specific psychiatric disorders in three sites. *Archives of General Psychiatry*, **41**, 949–958.
RORSMAN, B., GRASBECK, A., HAGRELL, O., et al (1990) A prospective study of first incidence depression: the Lundby study 1957–1972. *British Journal of Psychiatry*, **156**, 336–342.
RUTTER, M. (1985) Resilience in the face of adversity: protective factors and resistance to psychiatric disorder. *British Journal of Psychiatry*, **147**, 598–611.
SCOTT, J. (1988) Psychological models of depression. *Current Opinion in Psychiatry*, **1**, 719–724.
—— (1992) Social and community approaches. In *Handbook of Affective Disorders*, 2nd Edn. (ed. E. S. Paykel), pp. 525–534. Edinburgh: Churchill Livingstone.
—— (1993) Chronic depression: can cognitive therapy succeed when other treatments fail? *Behavioural Psychotherapy*, **20**, 25–36.
SHAW, D. M. & KOCH, H. C. (1982) Affective disorders. In *Rehabilitation in Psychiatric Practice*, (ed. R. G. McCreadie), pp. 7–27. London: Pitman.

SMITH, A. & WEISSMAN, M. (1992) Epidemiology. In *Handbook of Affective Disorders*, 2nd Edn. (ed. E. S. Paykel), pp. 111–130. Edinburgh: Churchill Livingstone.

TALBOTT, J. A., CLARK, G. H., SHARFSTEIN, S. S., *et al* (1987) Issues in developing standards governing psychiatric practice in community mental health centres. *Hospital and Community Psychiatry*, **38**, 1198–1202.

TYRER, P., FERGUSON, B. & WADSWORTH, J. (1990) Liaison psychiatry in general practice: the comprehensive collaborative model. *Acta Psychiatrica Scandinavica*, **81**, 359–363.

VAUGHN, C. & LEFF, J. (1976) The influence of family and social factors on the course of psychiatric illness. A comparison of schizophrenic and depressed neurotic patients. *British Journal of Psychiatry*, **129**, 125–137.

WEISSMAN, M. & KLERMAN, G. (1977) Sex differences and the epidemiology of depression. *Archives of General Psychiatry*, **34**, 98–111.

—— & PAYKEL, E. S. (1974) *The Depressed Woman: A Study of Social Relationships*, pp. 154–170. Chicago: University of Chicago Press.

WILLIAMS, J. M. G. (1989) Cognitive treatment for depression. In *Depression: an Integrative Approach* (eds K. R. Herbst & E. S. Paykel). Oxford: Heinemann.

WING, J. K. (1971) Social psychiatry. *British Journal of Hospital Medicine*, **5**, 53–56.

ZUNG, W. W. K., MAGILL, M., MOORE, J., *et al* (1983) Recognition and treatment of depression in a family medicine practice. *Journal of Clinical Psychiatry*, **44**, 3–6.

8 Suicide

KEITH HAWTON

According to official statistics suicide is the cause of approximately 4000 deaths per year in England and Wales. In addition, a large number of 'suicidal' deaths receive coroners' verdicts of 'undetermined cause' or 'accidental' death (Holding & Barraclough, 1978). The true extent of suicide is therefore greatly in excess of official figures. In recent years suicide rates in the UK have undergone significant changes in age and sex patterns. The major change has occurred in males, in whom rates have increased substantially, particularly in the young (Hawton, 1992). Rates of suicide (including deaths from undetermined cause) among men aged 25-44 years in England and Wales rose by a third between 1980 and 1990, the rate in 1990 exceeding that of men aged 65 and over for the first time this century. In males in the age group 15-24 years the rates increased by 85% (Office of Population Censuses and Surveys, 1982, 1991; Charlton *et al*, 1992). Suicide statistics for young men in Scotland and Northern Ireland have changed in parallel with those in England and Wales. Suicide rates in females, however, have markedly declined, especially in the young. Because of the increase in rates in young males, suicide is now one of the leading causes of years of life lost through death.

Rates of attempted suicide (parasuicide or deliberate self-harm) in the UK are among the highest in Europe. Following the massive increase in attempted suicide, especially self-poisoning, during the 1960s and early '70s (Alderson, 1974), there was evidence of a decline in rates in the late 1970s and early '80s (Brewer & Farmer, 1985; Platt *et al*, 1988). However, this decline has probably halted and may even have reversed (Hawton & Fagg, 1992*a*). Although official national figures are unavailable, calculations based on local rates suggest that currently there are at least 100 000 hospital referrals per year in England and Wales because of attempted suicide (Hawton & Fagg, 1992*a*). Many other episodes do not come to medical attention or are not referred to hospital (Kennedy & Kreitman, 1973). Attempted suicide occurs more often in females than males, and principally in young people, two-thirds of cases being under 35 years of age.

Suicide and attempted suicide are closely linked, 1% of hospital-referred attempters dying by suicide within a year of an attempt (a rate 100 times that of the general population) and 40-50% of suicides having a history of attempted suicide.

Prevention

Suicidal behaviour results from many causes, some social and some clinical. Several causes are beyond the scope of clinicians in terms of prevention, which may depend more on large-scale social changes. Nevertheless, it is important that these be brought to the attention of social policy makers. Some factors relate to psychiatric disorders and their prevention in general, topics which have been discussed in other chapters. Here, attention will be paid to the most important factors known to be linked to suicidal behaviour.

Detection and treatment of psychiatric disorders

Studies of suicides have shown that the vast majority of individuals who kill themselves have a psychiatric disorder at the time of death, with depression being the most common specific disorder (47–70%), followed by alcohol dependence (15–27%) and schizophrenia (2–12%) (Robins *et al*, 1959; Dorpat & Ripley, 1960; Barraclough *et al*, 1974). More than one disorder is present in some cases, the combination of depression and alcohol misuse being especially frequent. The pattern may be somewhat different in young suicides, substance misuse and personality problems being particularly common (Marttunen *et al*, 1993).

Psychiatric disorders are less common in attempted suicide patients, with about a third reaching criteria for a formal diagnosis. Depression and alcohol dependence are again especially common, with smaller proportions of patients having anxiety disorders or schizophrenia (Newson-Smith & Hirsch, 1979; Urwin & Gibbons, 1979).

Early detection and adequate treatment of the relevant psychiatric disorders must therefore be an important element in prevention of suicidal behaviour. Earlier studies showed that the majority of people who kill themselves (Barraclough *et al*, 1974) or who make attempts (Hawton & Blackstock, 1976; Bancroft *et al*, 1977) had been in recent contact with doctors, usually the general practitioner, but also a sizeable proportion with psychiatrists. It can therefore be argued that the psychiatric disorders of these individuals would or should have been detected and that perhaps their treatment could have been improved and suicidal behaviour prevented. One must however avoid too readily reaching such a conclusion because, first, it is notoriously difficult to predict who is most at risk of suicidal behaviour (Hawton, 1987), and, second, it must be recognised that some suicides occur in spite of the best efforts of clinicians. Furthermore, it appears that relatively few younger suicides have seen their general practitioners during the weeks before their deaths (Vassilas & Morgan, 1993; Gunnell, 1994).

Depression

The risk of suicide in patients with affective disorder is considerable. Guze & Robins (1970) calculated on the basis of 17 follow-up studies that approximately 15% end their lives by suicide, which is 30 times the general population risk. Barraclough & Pallis (1975) found that patients most at risk were males, older females, those who are single and living alone, and those with a history of attempted suicide. Insomnia, impaired memory and self-neglect were also associated with suicide.

There are specific psychological characteristics which may be amplified in depression and which are also associated with suicide risk. Hopelessness (negative expectations about the future) is the most important, and may be more important than depression itself (Beck *et al*, 1985). It has been postulated by Beck and colleagues that the tendency to become hopeless when depressed varies between individuals and that this tendency is carried over from one depressive episode to another. Thus in assessing any patient with depression it is important to evaluate the patient's attitude to his or her future, as well as enquiring about suicidal ideas and plans. Furthermore, in patients with a clear tendency to become hopeless when depressed and hence to be at especially high risk of suicidal behaviour, particular care should be paid to the prevention and early detection and treatment of future episodes of depression.

Other psychological characteristics that appear to be associated with suicide risk are dichotomous thinking, which is the tendency to categorise events and experiences in either of two extremes (e.g. 'I am good or bad'), rigid thinking and poor problem-solving skills (Weishaar & Beck, 1990). Such characteristics may be amenable to therapeutic interventions, including cognitive behaviour therapy.

In a study of 100 suicides Barraclough *et al* (1974) found that only a minority of the depressives were receiving antidepressant drugs at the time of their death and that in some of those who were, the drugs prescribed were inappropriate in terms of either type or dosage. This emphasises the need for education of doctors, especially general practitioners, about the appropriate use of antidepressants in correct doses. One of the problems here is that some of the antidepressants, especially the older ones, are dangerous in overdose and can cause death (Cassidy & Henry, 1987). While several less dangerous preparations (e.g. serotonergic and tetracyclic antidepressants) are now available many clinicians believe (contrary to results of most research trials) that the older antidepressants remain the most effective. Limiting the amount of medication available to patients at any one time and involvement of relatives and friends in supervision of medication may help reduce the risk of serious overdose.

There is now convincing evidence that prophylactic medication such as lithium carbonate and carbamazepine is effective in reducing episodes of affective disorder, especially in patients with bipolar disorders. Evidence is accumulating that the use of such medication may also have a significant role in the prevention of suicidal behaviour in afflicted individuals (Causemann & Müller-Oerlinghausen, 1988).

Substance misuse

There are extremely strong links between alcohol problems and both suicide and attempted suicide. Therefore prevention of alcohol misuse and early detection and adequate treatment of those who are developing problems must be a major factor in prevention of suicidal behaviour. This also applies to drug misuse, which (together with alcohol misuse) is closely linked to suicidal behaviour in young people (Marttunen *et al*, 1991). The prevention of these disorders is discussed in Chapter 12. Since substance misuse is extremely common in suicide attempters, especially the young, and is a specific risk factor for subsequent suicide (Hawton *et al*, 1993), there is a particular need for there to be close links between general hospital services for suicide attempters and substance misuse services.

Schizophrenia

While schizophrenia makes only a small contribution to the total number of suicides and attempted suicides, the risk of suicidal behaviour in schizophrenia is high with probably at least 10% of patients killing themselves (Miles, 1977). Preventive aspects of schizophrenia are discussed more fully in Chapter 12. There are, however, particular aspects of suicide in schizophrenia which merit attention here.

Those most at risk seem to be relatively young males with a chronic relapsing disorder in which depressive features are common (Roy, 1982). Many such suicides had attained a relatively high level of educational status prior to their illness, were unemployed, tended to retain high, non-delusional expectations of themselves, and yet were largely aware of the effects of their illness and its implications for their future functioning (Drake *et al*, 1984). Suicide in schizophrenia usually occurs during a relatively non-psychotic phase of the illness, but when there are depressive features, especially those of a psychological kind (such as feelings of inadequacy and hopelessness). This picture highlights the need for continuing support of individuals with schizophrenia, especially those who live alone, and attention to their needs in the long-term, not just at times of acute illness. Well-organised community support programmes involving community psychiatric nurses and other professionals able to establish and sustain supportive relationships with such individuals and to organise occupational and social programmes are likely to be very important in suicide prevention in this group. However, such services must have the readily available option of admitting patients for hospital in-patient care at times of crisis such as when a patient becomes acutely psychotic or severely depressed. Adequate hospital facilities are therefore also important in suicide prevention.

The period immediately following discharge from psychiatric in-patient care is a time of very high risk for suicide, both in people suffering from schizophrenia and those with other psychiatric disorders (Goldacre *et al*, 1993). This highlights the need for careful planning of aftercare and early involvement of community support staff, especially community psychiatric nurses.

Physical ill-health

Physical disorders, particularly those of a chronic nature, are common among suicides. This is especially so for elderly males who commit suicide, and in these cases the illness often appears to have contributed to the suicide (Dorpat & Ripley, 1960). Specific conditions that often occur in suicides include peptic ulcer, cardiovascular disease, malignancies and epilepsy (Sainsbury, 1955; Dorpat & Ripley, 1960; Barraclough, 1981; Whitlock, 1986). Physical ill-health is also relatively common in people who attempt suicide (Bancroft *et al*, 1977), with a specific association having been demonstrated in people with epilepsy (Mackay, 1979; Hawton *et al*, 1980). Suicide risk is also, unsurprisingly, greatly increased in people with AIDS or HIV infection (Marzuk *et al*, 1988). Expansion in the AIDS and HIV problem may eventually have a significant effect on suicide rates, especially in the young. Establishment of supportive networks for sufferers may help with their emotional problems and reduce suicide risk.

In view of the high frequency of contact with general practitioners and other clinicians before suicide or suicide attempts, as noted above, the associations of suicidal behaviour with physical disorders highlights the need for doctors to be vigilant for affective disturbance and suicidal thinking in patients with such conditions.

Unemployment and poverty

Both suicide (Platt, 1984) and attempted suicide (Platt & Kreitman, 1984; Hawton & Rose, 1986) are closely associated with unemployment, although the nature of the association is unclear. It could be due to the adverse effects that unemployment can have on mental health (Smith, 1985) or to people with psychiatric disorders and other risk factors for suicidal behaviour being at increased risk of becoming unemployed. The association is clearly complex, with there probably being an indirect causal association between unemployment and suicidal behaviour in a sizeable proportion of cases. In addition to mental health problems, poverty is likely to be another linking factor.

This association between unemployment and suicidal behaviour must be emphasised as one of several good reasons to discourage policy makers from creating economic policies in which increased levels of unemployment are a necessary consequence.

Family problems and marital breakdown

Conflict in families and between partners is common in both suicide attempters (Dorpat *et al*, 1965; Bancroft *et al*, 1977) and people who kill themselves (Bulusu & Alderson, 1984). One reason for the recent increase in young male suicides might be increased family breakdown related to the rapid rise in the divorce rate which occurred among parents of young people in the 1960s and '70s. Increasing divorce rates in the young themselves could also be relevant.

If the incidence of marital and family disharmony and breakdown could be reduced this might have important implications for rates of suicidal behaviour, both now and in the future. Marital and family counselling agencies such as Relate should therefore be supported. Educational measures within schools might also help prepare young people for future relationships, including methods of dealing with conflicts. Where family breakdown is inevitable, support for partners and children, again as provided by agencies such as Relate and conciliation services, might help reduce the resulting trauma.

Control of methods used for suicide

There is good evidence that reducing the availability of specific means of suicide can prevent some suicides and not simply result in replacement of the now unavailable method by another one. The best example in the UK was the 34% reduction in suicide rates between 1963 and 1974 which occurred in parallel with (and almost certainly because of) the gradual change in domestic gas supplies from coal gas to non-toxic North Sea Gas (Kreitman, 1976). Until this time coal gas poisoning had been the most common method of suicide. Reduced prescribing of barbiturates (which are very dangerous in overdose) around this time could also have been a contributory factor.

In the USA, where shooting is the principal method of suicide, the possible effects of restricting gun ownership have been debated (Clarke & Lester, 1989). Research suggests that the effects might not be as great as hoped but that they would be most noticeable in 15–24 year-olds (Sloan et al, 1990). There could however be a compensatory increase in suicide by other means (Rich et al, 1990). Probably the only way of finding out what would result is if gun legislation were introduced on a large scale.

Use of car exhaust has recently become a very common method of suicide, especially in young males (Charlton et al, 1992). While increasing availability of cars may be a relevant factor and is clearly likely to continue, diminishing the toxicity of exhaust by means of highly efficient catalytic converters is likely to prevent some suicides. A simple measure such as changing the shape of exhaust outlets so that airtight attachment of piping is impossible could be another, although this may interfere with the procedure used for testing exhaust emissions.

'Suicide barriers' should be erected on all high bridges and other such sites with a special reputation for suicide. However, it is interesting that, in the USA at least, there has been objection on aesthetic grounds to such steps (Clarke & Lester, 1989).

Some people have argued that the apparent decline in deliberate self-poisoning which occurred in the UK in the early 1980s was due to a reduction in the inappropriate prescribing of psychotropic medication, especially minor tranquillisers, which had become a common response to people presenting in general practice with 'personal problems' (Trethowan, 1975). It has been postulated that prescription medication for such problems, to which a more appropriate response might be support and encouragement of patients with guidance on how they deal with their problems using their own resources, could be a possible factor encouraging people to resort to pills in the face of stress and hence an overdose in the face of overwhelming distress (Hawton & Catalan, 1987). This is difficult to prove, although there is good evidence for parallel increases in deliberate self-poisoning and prescribing of psychotropic medication (Forster & Frost, 1985). In spite of absence of absolute proof, responsible prescribing of psychotropics must be encouraged. Increased availability of more appropriate help for patients with personal problems in the form of counselling in specific problem-solving (Catalan et al, 1984) should facilitate this. Since GPs are under increasing time pressure and are therefore less able than they might have been to give such help themselves, employment of properly trained counsellors in general practice might be a means of providing appropriate help. However, this potentially expensive development so far lacks the support of much needed controlled treatment trials.

Deliberate self-poisoning, especially by the very young, is often highly impulsive (Bancroft et al, 1979; Hawton et al, 1982). Since the substances used for overdoses are frequently those readily available in relatively large quantities in most homes (e.g. analgesics) it has been reasonably argued that reducing the numbers of tablets available over the counter and greater use of blister packs might help prevent self-poisoning, or at least reduce its dangers. This especially applies to paracetamol and paracetamol combinations because self-poisoning with paracetamol has become extremely common in recent years, again especially in the young (Hawton & Fagg, 1992b), and is dangerous, posing significant risk of potentially fatal liver damage. Death from liver damage can occur with an overdose of as few as 25 500 mg tablets of paracetamol, although some patients (e.g. alcoholics with liver damage) may be susceptible to even smaller amounts. At least 100 deaths a year in the UK are due to paracetamol self-poisoning (O'Grady *et al*, 1991). Methionine, which protects against liver damage, can be added to paracetamol. Currently, however, this combination is only available on prescription. Education of the public about the need to keep domestic supplies of medication (including non-prescribed drugs) to a minimum is a further step which should be encouraged.

Media reporting of suicides

There is evidence that media reports of suicides can be associated with further suicides. For example, increases in numbers of suicides have been linked to dramatic newspaper and television programmes about suicides (Gould & Shaffer, 1986). In the south of England, Barraclough *et al* (1977) found a statistical association between local newspaper reports of suicides and further suicides in young males. Possible media effects on attempted suicide have not been studied so much. Platt (1987) found only little evidence for an 'imitation' effect following the overdose of a key female figure in the popular television soap series *Eastenders*. While many of the studies in this field are open to criticism on methodological grounds, the most methodologically sound study provided evidence of a clear effect of media dramatisation of suicide on subsequent suicides, at least in terms of the method used (Schmidtke & Häfner, 1988). Thus following the double broadcast in Germany of a serial in which a 19-year-old man died by suicide on a railway, strong imitation effects were observed, were most marked in young males, lasted longer in this group and corresponded to the audience viewing figures.

The possible influences of the media on suicidal behaviour should be brought to the attention of those responsible for producing the media. One would not want to see the reporting of suicides suppressed (indeed appropriate reporting may be an important element in education of the public about suicide), but straightforward, undramatic factual reporting should be encouraged. The presentation of suicide or attempted suicide in the context of dramas should only be done with expert advice. Any such programme should always be followed by advertisements for help-lines and encouragement for distressed people to seek help through these or other means.

Educational measures

Public

It is important that the public should be as well informed as possible about the facts of mental illness, including suicide. It should, for example, be made clear that some psychiatric conditions carry a relatively high risk of suicide. This might encourage people to provide more support to relatives who are ill. It may also encourage more people to seek help for psychiatric disorder – it is important to note, for example, that while in most of the reported series of suicides psychiatric disorder has been identified in virtually all cases, a sizeable proportion of these had *not* been in recent contact with medical agencies. Lastly, it might make the enormous burden faced by relatives (especially parents) of people who have killed themselves a little easier to bear.

Schools

There are two potential broad school-based strategies towards suicide prevention. The first is specific education and training of young people in general 'life-skills' for coping with stress, conflicts and crises (Sarason & Sarason, 1981). Such programmes have been established in many American schools for some time and are now being introduced in the UK. So far, however, they have been subjected to relatively little evaluation. One study indicated that girls and boys responded differently to the same programme, girls benefiting more (Overholser *et al*, 1990), suggesting that the two sexes may require different types of programme or, preferably, that elements useful for each sex need to be incorporated in the same programme. Focusing this type of programme specifically on suicide prevention, rather than on the development of a broad range of coping skills, does not appear to be effective (Vieland *et al*, 1991).

The second strategy is specific education of teachers concerning the early recognition of children and adolescents with psychiatric disorders and the risk factors for suicidal behaviour. While there are several published examples of such programmes (e.g. Ross, 1987; Ryerson, 1987), so far they appear not to have been evaluated.

Clinicians

There is no doubt that it is important for clinicians in all specialities as well as in general practice to be informed about suicide risk and its assessment and management. The association between physical disorders and suicidal behaviour which was noted above emphasises the need for clinicians to be able to detect affective disorder and signs of hopelessness in patients with physical ill-health. As noted earlier, general practitioners need to be particularly well informed about the nature of depression, and skilled in its detection and treatment. On the Swedish island of Gotland a special postgraduate training programme for GPs about affective disorder not only resulted in increased detection and treatment of patients with this condition, but was followed by a reduction in the local suicide rate, a change which differed from both the long-term trend in Gotland and trends in Sweden as a whole (Rutz *et al*, 1989, 1992). While one must have some reservations about concluding that the education programme was definitely the reason for the decline in the suicide rate, the numbers involved being relatively small, the results are sufficiently impressive to encourage efforts of this kind elsewhere. The Defeat Depression Campaign in this country is a very welcome development in this regard (Paykel & Priest, 1992).

Special services for people at risk

During the 1960s and early '70s there was a great deal of enthusiasm for walk-in crisis centres, particularly in the USA. Assessment of the effects of these centres (admittedly difficult to undertake) has unfortunately not demonstrated much impact on suicide rates (Weiner, 1969; Lester, 1974), with the exception of a promising report of a significant association with reduced suicide rates in young females, the principal users of crisis centres (Miller *et al*, 1984). Establishment and evaluation of carefully designed centres which are attractive to and meet the needs of specific groups of people at risk (especially the young) should be encouraged.

In the UK the Samaritan organisation is the main agency with a specific goal of suicide prevention, its work being based primarily on confidential telephone counselling known as 'befriending'. This organisation undoubtedly attracts suicidal clients (Barraclough & Shea, 1970). However, while an initial study suggested that the Samaritans were effective in preventing suicide (Bagley, 1968), a subsequent and better designed investigation found no evidence of a significant impact of the Samaritans on suicide rates (Jennings et al, 1978). It is possible that such studies are not sensitive enough to detect actual effects. Certainly it would not be appropriate to negate the efforts of the Samaritans on the basis of these results. The Samaritans are likely to be less relevant to the prevention of attempted suicide, however, since Samaritan clients and attempted suicide patients differ considerably (Kreitman & Chowdhury, 1973), the Samaritan clients including a greater proportion of men and more socially isolated individuals. Furthermore, an extensive weekly television series portraying the work of the Samaritans was associated with a very marked increase in the numbers of people seeking help from the Samaritans in Edinburgh but no change in local attempted suicide rates (Holding, 1974).

General hospital services for suicide attempters

Controlled evaluative studies of special services for suicide attempters referred to general hospitals have so far demonstrated some positive benefits for the psychosocial adjustment of women (but not men), yet little or no impact on rates of repetition of attempts (Chowdhury et al, 1973; Gibbons et al, 1978; Gibbons, 1979; Hawton et al, 1981; Hawton et al, 1987; Salkovskis et al, 1990). Design faults, especially inclusion of too broad a range yet insufficient numbers of patients, may be relevant to this disappointing conclusion (Hawton, 1989). The rate of completed suicide among attempters of 1% within one year of an attempt (Hawton & Fagg, 1988), while 100 times that of the general population, is too low for an effect of such services on completed suicide to be detectable in controlled treatment studies. In a naturalistic follow-up study in Finland of people who made attempts of high intent there were fewer subsequent suicides in those who had a psychiatric assessment than in those who were not assessed, although the difference in risk did not attain statistical significance (Suokas & Lönnqvist, 1991). Suicide attempters are a population of patients which surely merits proper general hospital services in which adequate assessment and aftercare are available. Anecdotal evidence unfortunately indicates that good quality services are relatively rare, the services in some hospitals being all but absent. The development of such services and their adequate evaluation should be encouraged.

Limitations of suicide prevention

Suicidal behaviour has been a feature of civilisation throughout history (Alvarez, 1974) and will continue to be so. It is important to acknowledge that mortality by suicide is a major risk in certain psychiatric disorders, just as death is in physical illnesses such as cardiac disease or diabetes. The aim of preventive efforts should be the reduction of this cause of death to the lowest possible level. Total eradication of suicidal behaviour will never be feasible. In education of both clinicians and the public this point should not be omitted, or else a suicidal event is likely to lead to demoralising condemnation of those trying hardest to prevent such an outcome.

The difficulties of identifying those most at risk of suicidal acts should never be underestimated. Even when people at risk are identified, prevention is not easy. A society which rightly demands that there be respect for the principle that its members should be allowed to take responsibility for themselves (except when severely mentally ill) must also accept that such responsibility may include decisions about suicide.

No single means of prevention is by itself likely to have a major lasting impact on the problems of suicide and attempted suicide. The various facets of suicidal behaviour and its prevention which have been discussed should have made it clear that prevention is not the sole responsibility of clinicians. There are much wider responsibilities that society, including economic and social policy planners, should recognise and address.

References

ALDERSON, M. R. (1974) Self-poisoning: what is the future? *Lancet*, **i**, 1040–1043.
ALVAREZ, A. (1974) *The Savage God: A Study of Suicide*. Penguin: London.
BAGLEY, C. R. (1968) The evaluation of a suicide prevention scheme by an ecological method. *Social Science and Medicine*, **2**, 1–14.
BANCROFT, J., SKRIMSHIRE, A., CASSON, J., et al (1977) People who deliberately poison or injure themselves: their problems and their contacts with helping agencies. *Psychological Medicine*, **7**, 289–303.
——, HAWTON, K., SIMKIN, S., et al (1979) The reasons people give for taking overdoses: a further enquiry. *British Journal of Medical Psychology*, **52**, 353–365.
BARRACLOUGH, B. (1981) Suicide and epilepsy. In *Epilepsy and Psychiatry* (eds E. H. Reynolds & M. R. Trimble), pp. 62–76. Edinburgh: Churchill Livingstone.
—— & PALLIS, D. J. (1975) Depression followed by suicide: a comparison of depressed suicides with living depressives. *Psychological Medicine*, **5**, 55–61.
—— & SHEA, M. (1970) Suicide and Samaritan clients. *Lancet*, **ii**, 868–870.
——, BUNCH, J., NELSON, B., et al (1974) A hundred cases of suicide: clinical aspects. *British Journal of Psychiatry*, **125**, 355–373.
——, SHEPPERD, D. M. & JENNINGS, C. (1977) Do newspaper reports of coroners' inquests incite people to commit suicide? *British Journal of Psychiatry*, **150**, 528–532.
BECK, A. T., STEER, R. A., KOVACS, M., et al (1985) Hopelessness and eventual suicide: a 10-year prospective study of patients hospitalised with suicidal ideation. *American Journal of Psychiatry*, **145**, 559–563.
BREWER, C. & FARMER, R. (1985) Self-poisoning in 1984: a prediction that didn't come true. *British Medical Journal*, **290**, 391.
BULUSU, L. & ALDERSON, M. (1984) Suicides 1950–1982. *Population Trends*, **35**, 11–17.
CASSIDY, S. & HENRY, J. (1987) Fatal toxicity of antidepressant drugs in overdose. *British Medical Journal*, **295**, 1021–1024.
CATALAN, J., GATH, D. H., EDMONDS, G., et al (1984) The effects of non-prescribing of anxiolytics in general practice. I: Controlled evaluation of psychiatric and social outcome. *British Journal of Psychiatry*, **144**, 593–602.
CAUSEMANN, B. & MÜLLER-OERLINGHAUSEN, B. (1988) Does lithium prevent suicides and suicide attempts? In *Lithium: Inorganic Pharmacology and Psychiatric Use* (ed N. Y. Birch), pp. 23–24. Oxford: IRL Press.
CHARLTON, J., KELLY, S., DUNNELL, K., et al (1992) Trends in suicide deaths in England and Wales. *Population Trends*, **69**, 10–16.
CHOWDHURY, N., HICKS, R. C. & KREITMAN, N. (1973) Evaluation of an after-care service for parasuicide (attempted suicide) patients. *Social Psychiatry*, **8**, 67–81.

CLARKE, R. V. & LESTER, D. (1989) *Suicide: Closing the Exits*. p. 105. New York: Springer Verlag.
DORPAT, T. L. & RIPLEY, H. S. (1960) A study of suicide in the Seattle area. *Comprehensive Psychiatry*, **1**, 349–359.
——, JACKSON, J. K. & RIPLEY, H. S. (1965) Broken homes and attempted suicide. *Archives of General Psychiatry*, **12**, 213–216.
DRAKE, R. E., GATES, C., COTTON, P. G., et al (1984) Suicide among schizophrenics: who is at risk? *Journal of Nervous and Mental Disease*, **172**, 613–617.
FORSTER, D. P. & FROST, C. E. B. (1985) Medicinal self-poisoning and prescription frequency. *Acta Psychiatrica Scandinavica*, **71**, 657–674.
GIBBONS, J. L. (1979) *The Southampton Suicide Project. Report to the DHSS*. Department of Psychiatry, Southampton.
——, BUTLER, P., URWIN, P., et al (1978) Evaluation of a social work service for self-poisoning patients. *British Journal of Psychiatry*, **133**, 111–118.
GOLDACRE, M., SEAGROTT, V. & HAWTON, K. (1993) Suicide after discharge from psychiatric in-patient care. *Lancet*, **342**, 283–286.
GOULD, S. H. & SHAFFER, D. (1986) The impact of suicide in television movies: evidence of imitation. *New England Journal of Medicine*, **315**, 690–694.
GUNNELL, D. J. (1994) Recent studies of contacts with services prior to suicide – Somerset. In *The Prevention of Suicide* (eds R. Jenkins, S. Griffiths, I. Wylie, et al), pp. 114–120. London: HMSO.
GUZE, S. B. & ROBINS, E. (1970) Suicide among primary affective disorders. *British Journal of Psychiatry*, **117**, 437–438.
HAWTON, K. (1987) Assessment of suicide risk. *British Journal of Psychiatry*, **150**, 145–153.
—— (1989) Controlled studies of psychosocial intervention following attempted suicide. In *Current Research on Suicide and Parasuicide* (eds S. D. Platt & N. Kreitman), pp. 180–195. Edinburgh: Edinburgh University Press.
—— (1992) By their own young hand: suicide is increasing rapidly in young men (Editorial). *British Medical Journal*, **304**, 1000.
—— & BLACKSTOCK, E. (1976) General practice aspects of self-poisoning and self-injury. *Psychological Medicine*, **6**, 571–575.
——, FAGG, J. & MARSACK, P. (1980) Association between epilepsy and attempted suicide. *Journal of Neurology, Neurosurgery and Psychiatry*, **43**, 168–170.
——, BANCROFT, J., CATALAN, J., et al (1981) Domiciliary and out-patient treatment of self-poisoning patients by medical and non-medical staff. *Psychological Medicine*, **11**, 169–177.
——, COLE, D., O'GRADY, J., et al (1982) Motivational aspects of deliberate self-poisoning in adolescents. *British Journal of Psychiatry*, **141**, 286–291.
—— & ROSE, N. (1986) Unemployment and attempted suicide among men in Oxford. *Health Trends*, **18**, 29–32.
—— & CATALAN, J. (1987) *Attempted Suicide: A Practical Guide to its Nature and Management (Second Edition)*, p. 175. Oxford: Oxford University Press.
——, MCKEOWN, S., DAY, A., et al (1987) The evaluation of out-patient counselling compared with general practitioner care following overdoses. *Psychological Medicine*, **17**, 751–761.
—— & FAGG, J. (1988) Suicide and other causes of death following attempted suicide. *British Journal of Psychiatry*, **152**, 359–366.
—— & —— (1992a) Trends in deliberate self-poisoning and self-injury in Oxford, 1976–1990. *British Medical Journal*, **304**, 1409–1411.
—— & —— (1992b) Deliberate self-poisoning and self-injury in adolescents: a study of characteristics and trends in Oxford, 1976–1989. *British Journal of Psychiatry*, **161**, 816–823.
——, PLATT, S., FAGG, J., et al (1993) Suicide following parasuicide in young people. *British Medical Journal*, **306**, 1641.
HOLDING, T. (1974) The BBC 'Befrienders' series and its effects. *British Journal of Psychiatry*, **124**, 470–472.
—— & BARRACLOUGH, B. M. (1978) Undetermined deaths – suicide or accident? *British Journal of Psychiatry*, **133**, 542–549.
JENNINGS, C., BARRACLOUGH, B. M. & MOSS, J. R. (1978) Have the Samaritans lowered the suicide rate? A controlled study. *Psychological Medicine*, **8**, 413–422.
KENNEDY, P. & KREITMAN, N. (1973) An epidemiological survey of parasuicide (attempted suicide) in general practice. *British Journal of Psychiatry*, **123**, 23–34.
KREITMAN, N. (1976) The coal gas story: UK suicide rates 1960–1971. *British Journal of Preventive and Social Medicine*, **30**, 86–93.
—— & CHOWDHURY, N. (1973) Distress behaviour: a study of selected Samaritan clients and parasuicide (attempted suicide) patients. *British Journal of Psychiatry*, **123**, 1–8.

Lester, D. (1974) The effect of suicide prevention centers on suicide rates in the United States. *Health Services Report*, **89**, 37-39.

Mackay, A. (1979) Self-poisoning - a complication of epilepsy. *British Journal of Psychiatry*, **134**, 277-282.

Marttunen, M. J., Aro, M. A., Henriksson, M. M., et al (1991) Mental disorders in adolescent suicide. *Archives of General Psychiatry*, **48**, 834-839.

——, —— & Lönnqvist, J. K. (1993) Adolescence and suicide: a review of psychological autopsy studies. *European Child and Adolescent Psychiatry*, **2**, 10-18.

Marzuk, P., Tierney, H., Tardiff, F., et al (1988) Increased risk of suicide in persons with AIDS. *Journal of the American Medical Association*, **259**, 1333-1337.

Miles, C. P. (1977) Conditions predisposing to suicide: a review. *Journal of Nervous and Mental Disease*, **164**, 231-246.

Miller, H. L., Coombs, D. W., Leeper, J. D., et al (1984) An analysis of the effects of suicide prevention facilities on suicide rates in the United States. *American Journal of Public Health*, **74**, 340-343.

Newson-Smith, J. G. B. & Hirsch, S. R. (1979) Psychiatric symptoms in self-poisoning patients. *Psychological Medicine*, **9**, 493-500.

O'Grady, J. G., Wendon, J., Tan, K. C., et al (1991) Liver transplantation after paracetamol overdose. *British Medical Journal*, **303**, 221-223.

Office of Population Censuses and Surveys (1982) *Mortality Statistics for England and Wales 1980*. London: HMSO (DH2 Series No. 7).

—— (1991) *Mortality Statistics for England and Wales 1990*. London: HMSO (DH2 Series No. 17).

Overholser, J., Evans, S. & Spirito, A. (1990) Sex differences and their relevance to primary prevention of adolescent suicide. *Death Studies*, **14**, 391-402.

Paykel, E. S. & Priest, R. (1992) Recognition and management of depression in general practice: consensus statement. *British Medical Journal*, **305**, 1198-1202.

Platt, S. (1984) Unemployment and suicidal behaviour - a review of the literature. *Social Science and Medicine*, **19**, 93-115.

—— (1987) The aftermath of Angie's overdose: is soap (opera) damaging to your health? *British Medical Journal*, **294**, 954-957.

—— & Kreitman, N. (1984) Trends in parasuicide and unemployment among men in Edinburgh 1968-82. *British Medical Journal*, **289**, 1029-1032.

Platt, S., Hawton, K., Kreitman, N., et al (1988) Recent clinical and epidemiological trends in parasuicide in Edinburgh and Oxford: A tale of two cities. *Psychological Medicine*, **18**, 405-418.

Rich, C. L., Young, J. G., Fowler, R. C., et al (1990) Guns and suicide: possible effects of some specific legislation. *American Journal of Psychiatry*, **147**, 342-346.

Robins, E., Murphy, G. E., Wilkinson, R. H., et al (1959) Some clinical considerations in the prevention of suicide based on a study of 134 successful suicides. *American Journal of Public Health*, **49**, 888-899.

Ross, C. P. (1987) School and suicide: education for life and death. In *Suicide in Adolescence* (eds R. F. W. Diekstra & K. Hawton), pp. 155-172. Dordrecht: Martinus Nijhoff.

Roy, A. (1982) Suicide in chronic schizophrenia. *British Journal of Psychiatry*, **141**, 171-177.

Rutz, W., van Knorring, L. & Walinder, J. (1989) Frequency of suicide on Gotland after systematic postgraduate education of general practitioners. *Acta Psychiatrica Scandinavica*, **80**, 151-154.

——, —— & —— (1992) Long-term effects of an educational programme for general practitioners given by the Swedish Committee for the prevention and treatment of depression. *Acta Psychiatrica Scandinavica*, **85**, 457-464.

Ryerson, D. M. (1987) 'ASAP' - an adolescent suicide awareness programme. In *Suicide in Adolescence* (eds R. F. W. Diekstra & K. Hawton), pp. 173-190. Dordrecht: Martinus Nijhoff.

Sainsbury, P. (1955) *Suicide in London*. Maudsley Monograph No. 1. London: Chapman and Hall.

Salkovskis, P. M., Atha, C. & Storer, D. (1990) Cognitive-behavioural problem solving in the treatment of patients who repeatedly attempt suicide. A controlled trial. *British Journal of Psychiatry*, **157**, 871-876.

Sarason, I. G. & Sarason, B. R. (1981) Teaching cognitive and social skills to high school students. *Journal of Consulting and Clinical Psychology*, **49**, 121-135.

Schmidtke, A. & Häfner, H. (1988) The Werther effect after television films: new evidence for an old hypothesis. *Psychological Medicine*, **18**, 665-676.

Sloan, J. H., Rivara, F. P., Reay, D. T., et al (1990) Firearm regulations and rates of suicide. A comparison of two metropolitan areas. *New England Journal of Medicine*, **322**, 369-373.

Smith, R. (1985) Occupational health. 'I couldn't stand it any more'. Suicide and unemployment. *British Medical Journal*, **291**, 1563-1566.

SUOKAS, J. & LÖNNQVIST, J. (1991) Outcome of attempted suicide and psychiatric consultation: risk factors and suicide mortality during a five-year follow-up. *Acta Psychiatrica Scandinavica*, **84**, 545-549.

TRETHOWAN, W. H. (1975) Pills for personal problems. *British Medical Journal*, **3**, 749-751.

URWIN, P. & GIBBONS, J. L. (1979) Psychiatric diagnosis in self-poisoning patients. *Psychological Medicine*, **9**, 501-507.

VASSILAS, C. & MORGAN, H. G. (1993) General practitioners' contact with victims of suicide. *British Medical Journal*, **307**, 300-301.

VIELAND, V., WHITTLE, B., GARLAND, A., *et al* (1991) The impact of curriculum-based suicide prevention programs for teenagers: an 18-month follow-up. *Journal of the American Academy of Child and Adolescent Psychiatry*, **30**, 811-815.

WEINER, I. W. (1969) The effectiveness of a suicide prevention program. *Mental Hygiene*, **53**, 357-363.

WEISHAAR, M. E. & BECK, A. T. (1990) The suicidal patient: how should the therapist respond? In *Dilemmas and Difficulties in the Management of Psychiatric Patients* (eds K. Hawton & P. Cowen), pp. 65-76. Oxford: Oxford University Press.

WHITLOCK, F. A. (1986) Suicide and physical illness. In *Suicide* (ed A. Roy), pp. 151-170. Baltimore: Williams and Wilkins.

9 Schizophrenia

EVE C. JOHNSTONE and JULIAN P. LEFF

The disorder which came to be known as schizophrenia was separated from the broad mass of functional psychoses by Emil Kraepelin in 1896. Since that time there have been extensive studies of the condition, and despite many inconsistent findings and much remaining uncertainty, some issues have been broadly established. The lifetime risk world-wide is about eight per thousand (Lin & Stanley, 1982). The peak incidence of schizophrenia occurs in early adult life and 75–80% of patients will have their first episode of illness before the age of 45 years (Bland *et al*, 1976). Kraepelin considered that a poor outcome was a validating characteristic of schizophrenia. Not all subsequent authors have agreed with this view and Kraepelin himself acknowledged that some patients did recover, that the degree of impairment in the end state was variable and that the course run to reach that end state varied greatly. He also expressed the idea that since the cause of the disorder was unknown, there could be no rational treatment, and management had to be empirical.

Sadly these generalisations are still widely applicable. Although some factors are known to be contributory, the cause of schizophrenia remains unknown. While treatments have been introduced in the last hundred years which are helpful, these are empirical and there is no treatment which even the most optimistic clinician would recommend as being curative in the generality of cases. The outcome for many remains limited, although the heterogeneity of course and outcome which Kraepelin noted continue to be observed. Determinants of this heterogeneity are not well established.

In general terms, the principal clinical features of the acute episodes are florid, 'positive' psychotic symptoms such as hallucinations, delusions and incoherence of thought. These symptoms usually, but not always, respond reasonably satisfactorily to treatment, but in many cases they are likely to recur, so that the positive symptoms run a relapsing and remitting course, stretching out often over many years. At the same time as this episodic pattern of positive symptomatology is modified by treatment, there is often the development of 'negative' features of loss of verve and animation, inability to respond emotionally or sustain interests, together with paucity of speech and blunting of enthusiasm. These features are relatively stable (Johnstone *et al*, 1987*b*) and relatively unaffected by treatment.

The variable although generally limited outcome of schizophrenia is illustrated by the recent findings of an extensive follow-up study (Johnstone *et al*, 1991). In this investigation 532 patients with schizophrenia were followed up for three to thirteen years after discharge from in-patient care for an index episode. The study showed that in many cases the illness was clearly associated with recurrent or persistent problems, so that patients required a mean of more than five subsequent admissions, usually for relapse. The heterogeneity of most aspects of schizophrenia was very evident from this study, and not all patients fared badly, but unemployment, social difficulties and a restricted lifestyle were common. Many patients had persistent symptoms and a substantial number required much support from relatives. The rates of self-harm, suicide and early death were distressingly high. Various aspects of the behaviour of these patients brought more than 30% of those interviewed into contact with the police. These disappointing findings were obtained even though more than 90% were receiving medical or social support, 45% were under continuous supervision from a consultant psychiatrist, and about 90% were thought to be taking neuroleptic drugs. At the time of last contact in June 1990, less than 10% were receiving in-patient care and less than 1% of either patients or relatives sought the patient's return to in-patient care. Nonetheless, this study does illustrate the severity of the problems associated with this very distressing disorder.

Possibilities for prevention are necessarily limited by our lack of knowledge of the underlying cause or causes of the disorder itself, and indeed of the determinants of the heterogeneity of course. Nonetheless, some facts are known and there are possibilities with regard to primary, secondary and tertiary prevention.

Primary prevention

This depends upon knowledge of the underlying cause; as far as schizophrenia is concerned the cause is as yet unknown but certain factors are thought or known to be contributory.

Genetic factors

It is established that the condition is familial (Zerbin-Rudin, 1972) and adoption studies have shown that the familiality is due to genetic factors and not to shared environment (Heston, 1966; Kety *et al*, 1975). A substantial proportion of schizophrenic patients do not have a family history of the disorder, and the fertility rate of schizophrenic patients is low. This indicates that if genetic factors are a major contributing factor to the generality of schizophrenia, then the mutation rate must be high, or there is a state of balanced polymorphism. For these reasons there seems little scope for prevention under this heading, even if such steps were considered ethical and moral.

Occurrence of schizophrenia-like psychoses

It is well established that certain physical disorders are associated with a psychosis clinically indistinguishable from schizophrenia more often than would be expected by chance (Davison & Bagley, 1969). In one study of 268 patients fulfilling defined criteria for first episodes of schizophrenia, 15 had unsuspected organic illness of definite or possible aetiological significance (Johnstone *et al*, 1987*a*). In this and in a separate study of less specified psychotic illness (Johnstone *et al*, 1988) a number of these organic disorders related to substance misuse, although the majority overall did not. The role of substance misuse in the reported high incidence of psychoses of a schizophrenic nature in Afro-Caribbeans living in the UK is uncertain (Harrison *et al*, 1989). The organic disorders which are unrelated to substance use are varied and the main common thread between them is some tendency to involve the temporal lobes of the brain (Johnstone *et al*, 1987*a*).

It is possible that in this country a very small reduction in the incidence of schizophrenia could be produced by a reduction in temporal lobe disease. This would not be easy to achieve but perhaps successful treatment of middle ear disease in childhood would have some slight effect. It is possible that the effects in developing countries where temporal lobe disease is generally commoner, perhaps as a result of perinatal events, would be rather greater. The extent to which the incidence of schizophrenia would be reduced by control of substance misuse is uncertain, but the majority of schizophrenic patients do not have problems of this nature (Johnstone *et al*, 1991), and even if drug and alcohol use were eliminated, schizophrenia would persist.

Possibility of perinatal trauma

Some studies but not others (Lewis, 1989; Done *et al*, 1991; O'Callaghan *et al*, 1991) have indicated that obstetric or perinatal problems may be associated with the later development of schizophrenia. The very similar incidence of schizophrenia (at least as defined in Schneiderian terms) across a wide range of countries (Sartorius *et al*, 1986) where obstetric and infant mortality vary greatly makes it unlikely that this effect, if present at all, is strong. At present, because the incidence of schizophrenia is so similar in countries where the risks of perinatal problems are so different, it is not possible to suggest what kind of changes in obstetric practice could affect the frequency of the later development of schizophrenia.

Structural brain changes

The presence of structural brain changes, which probably antedate the first evidence of the psychosis and may be developmental, has been demonstrated in populations of schizophrenic patients over the last 15 years by imaging and neuropathological studies (Lewis, 1989; Bruton *et al*, 1990; Johnstone *et al*, 1994).

The fact that these changes have been demonstrated raises the possibility that when their cause has been determined, then possibilities for prevention may become apparent. Until the cause of the changes is known any possibility of preventing schizophrenia through this avenue of investigation remains a future hope rather than a present reality.

Social factors

There is an extensive literature on the possible contribution of parental attitudes and behaviour to the aetiology of schizophrenia. However, there is no scientific evidence which provides strong support for the operation of this factor (Hirsch & Leff, 1975). A number of studies indicate a triggering role for independent life events (Brown & Birley, 1968; Day *et al*, 1987), but since they occur in everyone's life, there can be no specific link with schizophrenia. Furthermore they are, by their nature, almost impossible to avoid, so there is little scope for intervention even if one could identify the person with vulnerability for schizophrenia.

The almost universally high incidence of schizophrenia in immigrant populations is explicable by a variety of factors, including selective migration, stress of migration, stress of living in an alien society, exposure to new environmental pathogens, and an ethnic vulnerability. The last-named is exceedingly unlikely, given the variety of ethnic groups that exhibit raised incidence rates. Research is under way to investigate the various possible aetiological factors, but some at least would open up possibilities of preventive action, e.g. environmental pathogens, societal stress.

Secondary prevention

Drug treatment

The question of whether or not early drug treatment of schizophrenic episodes improves the prognosis is not entirely clear, but it is certainly possible that early treatment in an acute episode of schizophrenia has enduring beneficial effects. In the Northwick Park Study of the treatment of schizophrenic episodes it was found that the most important determinant of relapse within 2 years was duration of illness prior to obtaining neuroleptic treatment ($P<0.0001$) (Crow *et al*, 1986). Indeed, although patients on maintenance neuroleptic treatment were significantly less likely to relapse ($P<0.002$) within 2 years than those on placebo, patients who went onto neuroleptics early and then were on placebo relapsed less than those who commenced treatment late and were maintained on active treatment for 2 years. Possible reasons for these findings are firstly that some feature associated with high risk of relapse tends to delay admission – a slow and insidious onset might lead to later admission and might be independently associated with poor outcome. Similarly, lack of social support (itself perhaps related to insidious onset) could delay hospital admission, but also be related to earlier relapse after discharge. A second, perhaps more arresting explanation is that delay in institution of treatment itself leads to poorer long-term outcome, i.e. that persistence of symptoms untreated by neuroleptic drugs leads to abnormality which cannot be completely reversed by subsequent treatment. The mechanism of such a possibility is unclear but the study of May *et al* (1981) offers some support for the idea of enduring effects of neuroleptic treatments. In this study the trial phase was confined to the period of the patient's first hospital admission, treatment subsequent to discharge being outside the investigators' control. Nevertheless, patients treated with neuroleptic drugs in the trial phase did much better in terms of outcome in the subsequent three years and the group treated initially without drugs, who spent a longer time in hospital in the trial phase, did worse.

These matters require further study, ideally including a trial in which first episode cases are randomly allocated to early and late introduction of neuroleptics, but at present there is certainly a possibility that the early introduction of neuroleptics when schizophrenic symptoms are first evident would reduce the morbidity of this disorder on an enduring basis.

There is no doubt that maintenance neuroleptic treatment is of benefit in reducing the relapse rate of acute schizophrenic episodes (Davis, 1975). Patients are often reluctant to comply with neuroleptics and there may be a price to pay for the reduction in relapse rate (Johnstone et al, 1990). Perhaps for these reasons the possibility of identifying prodromal features of schizophrenia and of aborting relapse by prompt treatment of these have been examined (Herz et al, 1982). Most recent work indicates that this is not as satisfactory as maintenance neuroleptic treatment (Hirsch et al, 1990; Jolley et al, 1990) and has little to offer in preventive terms.

However, for those on maintenance drugs, the prompt recognition of an impending relapse and the rapid implementation of appropriate measures, such as increasing the dose, may reduce the duration of an episode of schizophrenia. For this reason it is probably advantageous to train patients and their relatives to recognise the prodromal signs of a relapse (Birchwood et al, 1989).

Social treatments

Over the past 15 years, several packages of intervention focused on the family of schizophrenic patients have been developed and tested in controlled trials (Goldstein et al, 1978; Falloon et al, 1982; Leff et al, 1982; Hogarty et al, 1986; Tarrier et al, 1988). These studies have shown that for patients living in a stressful family environment, usually defined in terms of high expressed emotion (Vaughn & Leff, 1976) these interventions in combination with maintenance neuroleptic drugs confer an advantage over drugs alone. In the first two years after discharge from hospital, these interventions reduce the relapse rate by about one half, from over 60% to around 33% (e.g. Leff et al, 1990). Despite different names for the interventions, they comprise a common core of components. These include education about schizophrenia, teaching problem-solving skills, improving communication, preventing conflict, reducing contact between patient and relatives, expanding social networks, and lowering expectations (Kuipers et al, 1992). The interventions may be delivered by means of family sessions in the context of a relatives' group. However, the offer of a group on its own leads to poor attendance, and it needs to be used in combination with family sessions (Leff et al, 1989). The problem remains of how to ensure that this form of social treatment is taken up by clinical teams on a country-wide basis, given that it appears to be an effective form of secondary prevention. This problem is currently being tackled by instituting training courses in the necessary skills, which are targeted at community psychiatric nurses, since this cadre of professionals is already visiting patients and their families in their homes.

Tertiary prevention

It is not difficult to argue that the greatest problem of schizophrenia is not the acute psychotic episodes, nor the fact that the relapse of florid episodes may not be preventable, but the slow steady development of a defect characterised by negative symptoms of apathy, loss of will, inability to respond emotionally or to relate to others.

There is no treatment that can reliably be recommended as relieving negative symptoms in the same way that neuroleptics relieve positive symptoms. We really do not know how maintenance neuroleptic treatment designed to reduce the frequency of positive symptoms affects this situation. There is some evidence that there is a price to be paid for the lower relapse rate of higher doses of maintenance neuroleptic treatment in terms of dysphoria and less good social adjustment (Branchey *et al*, 1981; Kane *et al*, 1983; Marder *et al*, 1987). Relapse can only be a negative experience and it has been suggested (Stevens, 1982) that in its course schizophrenia resembles multiple sclerosis, having recurrent attacks with partial remission but increasing deficit. In terms of this idea it would be expected that relapses would in themselves contribute to the development of the defect state. The situation therefore is that on the one hand lower doses of medication are associated with, by some measures, a less severe defect state, and on the other that lower doses of medication are associated with increased levels of relapse which may in themselves lead to a more severe defect state. If these uncertainties could be clarified it is possible that modifications of physical treatment which could limit the handicap of defect symptoms would become evident.

Social treatments

Controversy surrounds the role of social influences in exacerbating or improving negative symptoms in schizophrenia. Original work by Wing & Brown (1970) strongly suggested that negative symptoms waxed and waned with the degree of social stimulation provided by the psychiatric hospital. On the other hand, Johnstone *et al* (1981) found that schizophrenic patients who had spent most of their life in the community were as disabled by negative symptoms as long-term inmates of psychiatric hospitals.

There is no doubt that negative symptoms in some patients improve as the positive symptoms fade, while in others they persist for years. Rehabilitation programmes are built on the premise that negative symptoms can be improved by providing the optimal degree of stimulation and structure. There is evidence that such programmes do benefit positive symptoms (Wing & Freudenberg, 1961), but the evidence for their effect on negative symptoms is less impressive (Wing *et al*, 1972). A major problem in this area of research is the measurement of negative symptoms, which remains unsatisfactory despite the recent proliferation of scales.

An important area of tertiary prevention is the social treatment of persistent psychotic symptoms which are unresponsive to neuroleptic medication. Approaches to increasing the patient's control over delusions and hallucinations by adopting a variety of strategies have been described by a number of clinicians (Boker *et al*, 1989) but the experimental testing of their efficacy is in its infancy. Accounts from patients who have persistent florid symptomatology in the face of adequate neuroleptic medication (Falloon & Talbot, 1981) show that such patients may employ a wide range of strategies to try to cope with the intrusion of their symptoms, and these are successful in some cases. Such strategies include postural changes, specific activities, reduction of sensory inputs, for example by earplugs or listening to loud stimulating music to 'drown out the voices'. The techniques that individual patients employ vary, as does the success associated with them. There is a lack of experimental support for the use of these coping strategies, but individual patients who are not helped by standard methods of treatment may find some of these coping mechanisms helpful. At present there is no reliable means of determining which patients are most likely to be helped or the strategy which has most chance of being useful.

References

BIRCHWOOD, M., SMITH, J. & MACMILLAN, J. F. M. (1989) Predicting relapse in schizophrenia: An early signs monitoring system using patients and relatives as observers. *Psychological Medicine*, **19**, 649–656.

BLAND, R. C., PARKER, J. H. & ORN, H. (1976) Prognosis in schizophrenia: a ten-year follow-up of first admissions. *Archives of General Psychiatry*, **33**, 949–954.

BOKER, W., BRENNER, H. D. & WURGLER, S. (1989) Vulnerability-linked deficiencies, psychopathology and coping behaviour of schizophrenics and their relatives. *British Journal of Psychiatry*, **155** (Suppl. 5), 128–135.

BRANCHEY, M. H., BRANCHEY, L. B. & RICHARDSON, M. A. (1981) Effect of neuroleptic adjustment on clinical condition and tardive dyskinesia in schizophrenic patients. *American Journal of Psychiatry*, **138**, 608–612.

BROWN, G. W. & BIRLEY, J. L. T. (1968) Crises and life changes and the onset of schizophrenia. *Journal of Health and Social Behaviour*, **9**, 203–214.

BRUTON, C. J., CROW, T. J., FRITH, C. D., et al (1990) Schizophrenia and the brain: a prospective clinico-neuropathological study. *Psychological Medicine*, **20**, 285–304.

CROW, T. J., MACMILLAN, J. F., JOHNSON, A. L., et al (1986) The Northwick Park study of first episodes of schizophrenia II. *British Journal of Psychiatry*, **148**, 120–127.

DAVISON K. & BAGLEY, C. R. (1969) Schizophrenia-like psychoses associated with organic disorders of the nervous system: a review of the literature. In *Current Problems in Neuropsychiatry* (ed. R. N. Herrington), pp. 113–184. Ashford, Kent: Headley Brothers.

DAVIS, J. M. (1975) Overview: maintenance therapy in schizophrenia. *American Journal of Psychiatry*, **132**, 1237–1245.

DAY, A., NEILSEN, J. A., KORTEN, A., et al (1987) Stressful life events preceding the acute onset of schizophrenia: a cross-national study from the World Health Organization. *Culture, Medicine and Psychiatry*, **11**, 123–206.

DONE, D. J., JOHNSTONE, E. C., FRITH, C. D., et al (1991) Complications of pregnancy and delivery in relation to psychosis in adult life: data from the British perinatal mortality survey sample. *British Medical Journal*, **302**, 1576–1580.

FALLOON, I. R. H. & TALBOT, R. E. (1981) Persistent auditory hallucinations: coping mechanisms and implications for management. *Psychological Medicine*, **11**, 329–339.

——, BOYD, J. L., MCGILL, C. W., et al (1982) Family management in the prevention of exacerbations of schizophrenia. *Archives of General Psychiatry*, **35**, 169–177.

GOLDSTEIN, M. J., RODNICK, E. H., EVANS, J. R., et al (1978) Drug and family therapy in the aftercare treatment of acute schizophrenia. *Archives of General Psychiatry*, **35**, 169–177.

HARRISON, G., BOLTON, A., NEILSON, D., et al (1989) Severe mental disorder in Afro-Caribbean patients: some social demographic and service factors. *Psychological Medicine*, **19**, 683–696.

HERTZ, M. I., SZYMANSKI, H. V. & SIMON, J. C. (1982) Intermittent medication for stable schizophrenic outpatients: an alternative to maintenance medication. *American Journal of Psychiatry*, **139**, 918–922.

HESTON, L. L. (1966) Psychiatric disorders in foster home reared children of schizophrenic mothers. *British Journal of Psychiatry*, **112**, 819–825.

HIRSCH, S. R. & LEFF, J. P.(1975) *Abnormalities in the Parents of Schizophrenics*. Maudsley Monograph No. 22. Oxford: Oxford University Press.

——, JOLLEY, A. G., MCRINK, A., et al (1990) Trial of brief intermittent neuroleptic prophylaxis for selected schizophrenic out-patients: clinical and social outcome at 2 years. *Schizophrenia Research*, **31**, 40–41.

HOGARTY, G. E., ANDERSON, C. M., REISS, D. J., et al (1986) Family psychoeducation, social skills training, and maintenance chemotherapy in the aftercare treatment of schizophrenia. I. One-year effects of a controlled study on relapse and expressed emotion. *Archives of General Psychiatry*, **43**, 633–642.

JOHNSTONE, E. C., OWENS, D. G. C., GOLD, A., et al (1981) Institutionalisation and the defects of schizophrenia. *British Journal of Psychiatry*, **139**, 195-203.

———, MACMILLAN, J. F. & CROW, T. J. (1987a) The occurrence of organic disease of possible or probable aetiological significance in a population of 268 cases of first episode schizophrenia. *Psychological Medicine*, **17**, 371-379.

———, OWENS, D. G. C., FRITH, C. D., et al (1987b) The relative stability of positive and negative features in chronic schizophrenia. *British Journal of Psychiatry*, **150**, 60-64.

———, COOLING, N. J., FRITH, C. D., et al (1988) Phenomenology of organic & functional psychoses and the overlap between them. *British Journal of Psychiatry*, **153**, 770-776.

———, MACMILLAN, J. F., FRITH, C. D., et al (1990) Further investigation of the predictors of outcome following first schizophrenic episodes. *British Journal of Psychiatry*, **157**, 182-189.

———, FRITH, C. D., LEARY, J., et al (1991) Background, method and general description of the sample in disabilities and circumstances of schizophrenic patients. *British Journal of Psychiatry*, **159** (Suppl. 13), 7-11.

———, BRUTON, C. J., CROW, T. J., et al (1994) Clinical correlates of post-mortem brain changes in schizophrenia: decreased brain weight and length correlated with indices of early impairment. *Journal of Neurology, Neurosurgery & Psychiatry*, **57**, 474-479.

JOLLEY, A. G., HIRSCH, S. R., MORRISON, E., et al (1990) Trial of brief intermittent neuroleptic prophylaxis for selected schizophrenic out-patients: clinical and social outcome at 2 years. *British Medical Journal*, **301**, 837-842.

KANE, J. M., RIFKIN, A. & WOERNER, M. (1983) Low dose neuroleptic treatment of out-patient schizophrenia. *Archives of General Psychiatry*, **40**, 893-896.

KETY, S. S., ROSENTHAL, D., WENDER, P. H., et al (1975) Mental illness in the biological and adoptive families of adopted individuals who have become schizophrenic: a preliminary report based upon psychiatric interview. In *Genetic Research in Schizophrenia* (eds R. R. Fieve, D. Rosenthal & H. Brill), pp. 147-165. Baltimore: Johns Hopkins University Press.

KRAEPELIN, E. (1896) *Psychiatrie*, 5th edn. Leipzig: Barth.

KUIPERS, L., LEFF, J. & LAM, D. (1992) *Family Work for Schizophrenia: A Practical Guide*. London: Gaskell.

LEFF, J., KUIPERS, L., BERKOWITZ, R., et al (1982) A controlled trial of social intervention in the families of schizophrenic patients. *British Journal of Psychiatry*, **141**, 121-134.

———, BERKOWITZ, R., SHAVIT, N., et al (1989) A trial of family therapy v. a relatives' group for schizophrenia. *British Journal of Psychiatry*, **154**, 58-66.

———, ———, ———, et al (1990) A trial of family therapy v. a relatives' group for schizophrenia: two-year follow-up. *British Journal of Psychiatry*, **157**, 571-577.

LEWIS, S. W. (1989) Congenital risk factors for schizophrenia. *Psychological Medicine*, **19**, 5-13.

LIN, T. Y. & STANLEY, C. C. (1962) *The Scope of Epidemiology in Psychiatry*. Geneva: WHO (Public Health Paper).

MARDER, S. R., VAN PATTEN, T. & MINTZ, J. (1987) Low and conventional dose maintenance therapy with flupenthixol decanoate. *Archives of General Psychiatry*, **44**, 518-521.

MAY, P. R. A., TUMA, A. H., DIXON, W. J., et al (1981) Schizophrenia: a follow-up study of the results of five forms of treatment. *Archives of General Psychiatry*, **38**, 776-784.

O'CALLAGHAN, E., SHAM, P., TAKEI, N., et al (1991) Schizophrenia after prenatal exposure to 1957 A_2 influenza epidemic. *Lancet*, **337**, 1248-1250.

SARTORIUS, N., JABLENSKY, A., KATON, A., et al (1986) Early manifestations and first contact incidence of schizophrenia in different cultures. *Psychological Medicine*, **16**, 909-928.

STEVENS, J. R. (1982) Neurology & Neuropathology of Schizophrenia. In *Schizophrenia as a Brain Disease* (eds F. A. Henn & H. A. Nasrallah), pp. 112-147. Oxford: Oxford University Press.

TARRIER, N., BARROWCLOUGH, C., VAUGHN, C., et al (1988) The community management of schizophrenia: a controlled trial of a behavioural intervention with families to reduce relapse. *British Journal of Psychiatry*, **153**, 532-542.

VAUGHN, C. E. & LEFF, J. P. (1976) The measurement of expressed emotion in the families of psychiatric patients. *British Journal of Clinical and Social Psychology*, **15**, 157-165.

WING, J. K. & BROWN, G. W. (1970) *Institutionalism and Schizophrenia*. Cambridge: Cambridge University Press.

——— & FREUDENBERG, R. K. (1961) The response of severely ill chronic schizophrenic patients to social stimulation. *American Journal of Psychiatry*, **118**, 311-322.

WING, L., WING, J. K., GRIFFITHS, D., et al (1972) An epidemiological and experimental evaluation of industrial rehabilitation of chronic psychotic patients in the community. In *Evaluating a Community Psychiatric Service* (eds J. K. Wing & A. M. Hailey), pp. 283-308. Oxford: Oxford University Press.

ZERBIN-RUDIN, E. (1972) Genetic research and the theory of schizophrenia. *International Journal of Mental Health*, **1**, 42-62.

10 Anxiety disorder

PETER TYRER

Anxiety is unlike any other psychological symptom. It is both a necessary drive that is essential for survival as well as a symptom that can cause distress and suffering. This is demonstrated in the Yerkes–Dodson law, named after its initial proponents in 1908 (Figure 10.1). At low levels of anxiety an increase in stress leads to an improvement in performance. As this is normally a desired effect the anxiety is functioning as a drive. However, when maximum performance is being achieved a further increase in anxiety leads to a catastrophic fall in performance and eventually to total disintegration of function. This is the anxiety that should cause concern to mental health professionals and which needs to be both treated and prevented wherever possible.

However, it will be unreasonable to expect to prevent all forms of anxiety, not least because the symptom has such biological value. In particular, anxiety is a frequent accompaniment of all forms of change in life and as such changes are perhaps more common nowadays than they were previously, this is sometimes described as the 'Age of Anxiety'. While for many it may be desirable, and sometimes possible, to escape from what seems to be an increasingly threatening environment, for those that are not able to take such a step a certain level of

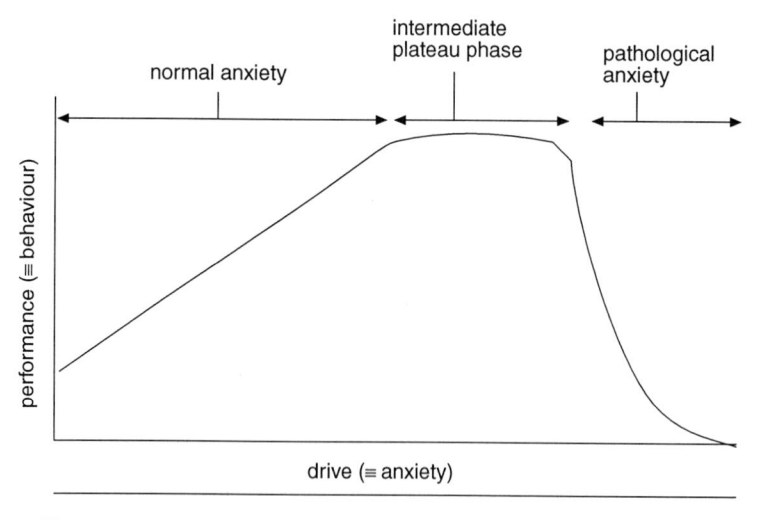

Fig. 10.1. *The relationship between anxiety and performance (the Yerkes–Dodson law)*

anxiety is necessary for effective coping. It is when this coping becomes ineffective that the problem becomes a pathological one.

There are many factors that affect the progression of abnormal to pathological anxiety. Only a minority of people exposed to anxious stimuli will become pathologically anxious and a great deal depends on the specific vulnerability of the person to pathological anxiety. This vulnerability, which is affected by constitutional, probably genetic, factors, personality and early experiences, is difficult to prevent and attempts to create social conditions whereby children grow up in environments which are conducive to good mental health (stimulated by the Mental Hygiene Movement in the United States in the early years of the century) have been largely unsuccessful. However, anxiety differs from its fellow mood, depression, in having many other complicating factors that can be prevented or modified to a greater or lesser extent and can therefore have a major bearing on the incidence of pathological anxiety. One can argue that the potential for preventing anxiety is therefore somewhat greater than that for depression, in which the relationship between the precipitating factors, vulnerability and expression of symptoms is more direct (Paykel, 1978).

In the case of anxiety full primary prevention is impossible; anxiety is necessary to existence and it is the inappropriate persistence and development of normal to pathological anxiety with which mental health professionals are most concerned.

Inter-relationship between anxiety and other neurotic disorders

Anxiety and depression are highly correlated and frequently co-exist in their pathological forms. Successful prevention of anxiety disorders would almost certainly prevent depressive ones to a roughly similar degree, and it is important not to regard any preventive measure as particularly specific.

This perhaps is unexpected, at least to a layman, because anxiety is clearly an emotion associated with danger and threat, whereas depression is more associated with loss. Although there is some evidence that threatening events are more likely to produce anxiety than depression, and loss events more likely to produce depression than anxiety (Finlay-Jones & Brown, 1981), it is not very striking. The more impressive finding (Paykel & Dowlatshahi, 1988) is that mixed types of event are common, and so are mixed symptoms (Tyrer, 1985).

Genetic studies suggest that there is a common origin to anxiety, depressive, panic, phobic and obsessive compulsive disorders (Andrews *et al*, 1990) and the same is true of their progress, response to treatment and outcome (Tyrer, 1985; Tyrer *et al*, 1992). It is quite possible, however, that anxiety is a fundamental driving force in all these disorders and that if we were able to prevent pathological anxiety it could have a salutary effect on all of these. Certainly Freud (1926) thought so in one of his later and most influential papers.

Preventable factors

The influences that commonly are involved in making anxiety pathological in nature are shown in Figure 10.2. It is becoming increasingly realised that there is genetic vulnerability to anxiety. It is generally more marked than depression (Young *et al*, 1971). It has been recognised recently in the identification of the

90 Prevention of specific disorders

```
                    ┌─────────────────────┐
                    │   Normal anxiety    │
                    └─────────────────────┘
                       │              │
                       ▼              ▼
            Factors that are    Factors that are to some
            difficult to prevent  extent preventable
                       │              │
                       ▼              │
                  Genetic             │
                  vulnerability       ▼
                       │         Nature and severity of
                       │         psychosocial stressors
                       ▼              │
                  Specific            ▼
                  vulnerability ──▶ Anticipatory anxiety
                  to anxiety         │
                       │             ▼
                       │        Secondary anxiety
                       ▼
                    ┌─────────────────────┐
                    │ Pathological anxiety│
                    └─────────────────────┘
```

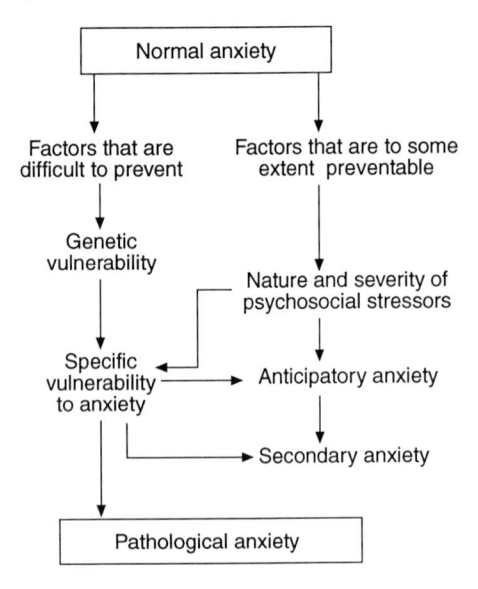

Fig. 10.2. Factors influencing the development of pathological anxiety

anxious personality, which can be sufficiently maladaptive to be regarded as a personality disorder (Mann et al, 1981; World Health Organization, 1992). This position can be accentuated by specific events occurring early in childhood development and Bowlby (1973) emphasised the importance of attachment behaviour in normal development and the significance of separation in creating anxiety. Bowlby postulated that repeated and unresolved separation will make children more likely to have anxiety in later life, but there is no really good evidence that this is the case. If so, one would have expected, for example, much greater prevalence of anxiety disorders in the 1950s and 1960s, particularly in the southeast of England, because of the large number of children who were evacuated, often under highly unpleasant conditions that predispose towards separation anxiety, during the Second World War. However, although such epidemiological data are not available, there is certainly evidence that separation anxiety predisposes to anxious disorders, particularly phobias, in later childhood (Gittelman-Klein & Klein, 1973; Raskin et al, 1982). There may in due course be reasonable data from follow-up of studies such as that in the Isle of Wight (Rutter et al, 1976) that might establish the extent to which anxiety in childhood is associated with anxiety in later life. At present we still rely rather too heavily on the data from Robins (1966) who showed only a relatively small association between child and adult anxiety.

Nature and severity of psychosocial stressors

Anxiety is a product of uncertainty and to some extent those who are vulnerable to anxiety can be protected from pathological anxiety by being placed in relatively constant environments. It is clearly inappropriate for those who are vulnerable to anxiety to indulge in high-risk leisure pursuits such as hang-gliding and climbing cliffs, and to work in occupations such as market trading or high-pressure selling.

Although to a large extent those with a potential for anxiety are sensible enough to avoid activities that could predispose towards anxiety, sometimes they are less aware, and much then depends on skills of personnel officers, friends and advisers, and immediate superiors in detecting signs of anxiety before they become uncontrollable. In particular, the mistake is sometimes made that an anxious or timid person can be made into a strong and brave one by facing up to danger in its various forms. If the underlying personality is genuinely that of a timid and anxious person, this approach is doomed to failure and will only make the problem worse. However, at present it is the absence of employment that is likely to be more anxiety provoking than misplaced employment, and there is little the psychiatric services can do about this.

This does not mean that it is impossible to prevent the impact of some psychosocial stressors. Anxiety is about *perceived* threat, and sometimes the perception is greatly exaggerated. There are many stressors that are experienced at some time in people's lives that can have their impact minimised by preparing the subject for them in advance and thereby preventing pathological anxiety from developing (Table 10.1).

Most of the courses of action suggested in Table 10.1 do not involve the psychiatric services directly. Counselling is increasingly being taken over as one of the responsibilities of clinical psychology services as well as voluntary bodies. Whether this is always wise is far from clear, and there is concern that the diffused nature of counselling covers a wide range of professional competence and incompetence. It is possible that the Royal College of Psychiatrists could take a more active role in defining counselling and setting standards for training.

More responsible dissemination of information about psychiatric problems that can assume epidemic proportions is extremely important. The possibility of the College having its own press office in addition to its public relations committee (or possibly an extension of it) may be a way of dealing with this issue. Alternatively, greater psychiatric input to the Press Council might also help.

Early detection of pathological anxiety

One of the most important parts of secondary prevention is the early detection of disorder so that appropriate action can be taken early in its course. This is not usually considered to be a problem in anxiety disorders, as anxiety as a symptom is normally detected easily and early by patients and doctors. However,

TABLE 10.1
Examples of psychosocial stressors that can have their anxiety-provoking content reduced

Stressor	Anxiety reduction
Hospital admission (childhood)	Opportunities for parental accommodation
Examinations	School and college counselling
Major surgery (particularly cardiac)	Creation of homely rather than clinical ward environment
Diagnosis of serious illness (e.g. cancer, AIDS)	Counselling services needed to explain implications and promote adjustment
Major disaster (earthquake, multiple road accident)	Counselling of above
Public health scare	Responsible reporting by media
Epidemic 'hysteria'	Rapid dissemination of factual information

although symptoms are detected early they are not always treated appropriately, and much of the concern over the apparently excessive prescription of minor tranquillisers such as the benzodiazepines in the 1960s and 1970s was over their inappropriate use in anxiety (Trethowan, 1975).

Now that there are recognised and effective psychological treatments of anxiety that can be given in primary care, early detection could be followed by a more appropriate range of treatments in which non-pharmacological approaches figure prominently, and drug treatment with tranquillisers is put in proper perspective (Lader et al, 1992).

Anticipatory anxiety

It is important to realise that pathological anxiety can be internally generated. When patients have been exposed to external stressful events and become pathologically anxious, the experience is extremely unpleasant and becomes a reason for fear. When placed in the context of intolerable stress all individuals, whether vulnerable or not, will become pathologically anxious in terms of their symptomatology, even though the nature of the stress is such that the symptoms could be regarded as within the range of normal anxiety. If the person subsequently fears the return of that anxiety to a sufficiently great extent the fear will become reality and new symptoms will be created.

This is particularly common in the case of phobic anxiety, in which anxiety symptoms are confined to certain well specified situations. Once the anxiety is linked to a situation the subject learns that whenever that situation is encountered, anxiety will be experienced, simply because it is expected to be. In the minutes, days, or months before the expected exposure to the situation there is ample opportunity for the person to get steadily more anxious because he or she is expecting the worst when the final exposure to the situation takes place.

Anticipatory anxiety can be helped by successful treatment of phobias, particularly by gradual exposure to the feared situation, but, better still, could be prevented by learning methods of controlling anxiety in advance of exposure to the situation. Such methods include physical exercise, relaxation training (with or without traditional aids such as audio tapes), reading accounts of coping with anxiety – best exemplified in Claire Weekes' well known book (1962) – and a balanced lifestyle.

Secondary anxiety

Secondary anxiety is not adequately defined and can have several meanings, and in the context of this subject is largely concerned with secondary prevention. I regard it as 'anxiety about anxiety' in which there is new anxiety generated by the actual symptoms of primary anxiety, which can sometimes turn out to have far-reaching pathological consequences.

One of the reasons that secondary anxiety appears to be relatively common is that, although its psychological manifestations are well recognised, its physical ones are not. A range of symptoms are created by anxiety, mainly due to sympathetic nervous discharge, including tremor, palpitations, feeling faint, sweating, nausea, diarrhoea, stomach churning, dizziness, and muscle tension.

Unless the sufferer realises that all these symptoms can be explained entirely by psychological mechanisms there is a danger that one or more of them can create excessive concern and thereby reinforce existing anxiety. A large number of people who attend medical facilities with cardiac, respiratory, and bowel symptoms, and symptoms of muscle tension such as headache, suggest that there is a strong predilection for anxiety to be mainly confined to the somatic sphere (Tyrer, 1976).

Although it is common for such presentations of anxiety to be regarded as a separate disorder, somatisation disorder or a related somatoform disorder (see Chapter 18) we must not forget that the first manifestation of such somatisation is anxiety. Indeed, studies of patients with marked anxiety symptoms (panic disorder, agoraphobia) have demonstrated clear evidence of somatisation (Fisher & Wilson, 1985; Cameron et al, 1986).

Certainly it is more acceptable to present with organic than with psychological symptoms but I doubt whether this can account for this mode of presentation entirely. There is increasing evidence that those who understand their bodies' physiology the least are most likely to misinterpret their symptoms in this way. Such misinterpretation includes what has now become known as 'catastrophising' (e.g. believing that the onset of palpitations signifies an imminent heart-attack), and somatising (the belief that a bodily symptom is indicative of the physical disease even when it is clearly related to other symptoms of anxiety) (see Chapter 18). This misinterpretation of symptoms is a major cause of continued distress and wasted medical time. Patients repeatedly trek from one medical discipline to another looking for a physical answer to their symptoms, a quest that sometimes becomes as committed as the search for the Holy Grail.

It is hard to escape the conclusion that better education of simple physiology would prevent a great deal of this secondary anxiety and that much suffering in consulting rooms up and down the country could be prevented by better teaching of human biology in our classrooms and physiology by health professionals (Table 10.2). This opinion is supported by one study that showed significant benefit of a single interview concentrating on straightforward physiological explanation to patients with symptoms of somatisation (Smith et al, 1986).

The early stage of development of phobic symptomatology is a form of secondary anxiety. The sequence: anxiety attack→link to situation→fear of situation→phobia can be prevented by a rapid return to the situation where the episode of anxiety occurred. This 'instant' exposure therapy should be widely taught in human biology so that it becomes standard. Interestingly enough, it probably was standard 50 years ago, when facing up to fearful situations in this way was a test of 'moral fibre', but has been lost in this more self-indulgent era.

TABLE 10.2
Prevention of secondary anxiety

Type of anxiety	Main preventive measure
Panic	Better awareness of threat and understanding of sympathetic nervous system
Somatosthenic (somatisation)	Better education of physiology of anxiety (beginning at school), and of general practitioners
Phobias	Education by health visitors, nurses, general practitioners and public health workers of the dangers of responding to anxiety by avoidance

Tertiary prevention

Anxiety tends to be a recurrent rather than a continuously chronic condition and even patients who have apparently persistent symptoms show remarkable fluctuations from day to day and week to week (Tyrer, 1976). The same cannot be said for the secondary behavioural consequences of anxiety, particularly phobias. Phobic patterns of behaviour, once established, are often very difficult to alter, and even successful treatment in a psychiatric setting may be followed by short setbacks or longer term relapse. This is more common with pharmacological than with behavioural treatments (Marks & O'Sullivan, 1989) but can occur with both.

Both agoraphobia and social phobias can progress from a state of mild handicap with only occasional avoidance to a crippled existence in which the sufferer is completely housebound. There is concern from epidemiological data that a large number of patients with agoraphobia (particularly agoraphobia without coexisting symptoms of panic) continue to suffer from their disorders without specialist advice. This has been highlighted recently in elderly patients by Lindesay (1991) who found that despite significant symptomatology and handicap very few patients received any form of specific anti-anxiety or phobic treatment.

As it has now been established that behavioural treatment can be given equally effectively by self-instructional methods as by direct therapist intervention (Ghosh & Marks, 1987) it would help tertiary prevention by leaving details of treatment strategies to be adopted in the event of relapse. These could then be set in motion at the first sign of reemergence of phobic fear and avoidance; this could go a long way towards improving health without any new specialist intervention.

Such strategies could with profit involve the spouses and partners of agoraphobic patients. It has been appreciated for some years that the nature of the close relationships of agoraphobic patients may play a major part in the persistence and development of the phobia (Hafner, 1977; Milton & Hafner, 1979). Partners may therefore create the conditions for relapse by their behaviour and this could be anticipated by preventive strategies being outlined before discharge from psychiatric care.

Prospects for prevention

Prospects for preventing pathological anxiety are reasonably good. Many forms of anxiety, particularly those that are amenable to secondary prevention, have become far less frequent over the years as the population has become more conscious of physiological and bodily function. What used to be called 'anxiety hysteria' (the presentation of anxiety symptoms with complete misunderstanding of their nature and cause) is no longer seen because our knowledge base has improved. In tackling prevention all mental health professionals need to be aware that anxiety usually lies at the base of the maladaptive and inappropriate constructions that together make up the superstructure of neurotic disorder. If we can prevent any of these foundations from being laid down or accreted we can chalk up a significant advance in overcoming psychopathology.

References

ANDREWS, G., STEWART, G., MORRIS-YATES, A., et al (1990) Evidence for a general neurotic syndrome. *British Journal of Psychiatry*, **157**, 6–12.
BOWLBY, J. (1973) *Attachment and Loss, Volume 2. Separation: Anxiety and Anger.* London: Hogarth Press.
CAMERON, O. G., THYER, B. A., NESSE, R. M., et al (1986) Symptom profiles of patients with anxiety disorders. *American Journal of Psychiatry*, **143**, 1132–1137.
FINLAY-JONES, R. & BROWN, G. W. (1981) Types of stressful life events and the onset of anxiety and depressive disorders. *Psychological Medicine*, **11**, 803–815.
FISHER, L. M. & WILSON, G. T. (1985) A study of the psychology of agoraphobia. *Behaviour Research and Therapy*, **23**, 97–107.
FREUD, S. (1926) Inhibitions, symptoms and anxiety. In *Complete Psychological Works, Vol. 20* (trans. J. Strachey, 1959), pp. 75–174. London: Hogarth Press.
GHOSH, A. & MARKS, I. M. (1987) Self-treatment of agoraphobia by exposure. *Behavior Therapy*, **18**, 3–16.
GITTELMAN-KLEIN, R. & KLEIN, D. F. (1973) School phobia: diagnostic considerations in the light of imipramine effects. *Journal of Nervous and Mental Disorders*, **156**, 199–215.
HAFNER, R. J. (1977) The husbands of agoraphobic women and their influence on treatment outcome. *British Journal of Psychiatry*, **131**, 289–294.
LADER, M., BEAUMONT, G., BOND, A., et al (1992). Guidelines for the management of patients with generalised anxiety. *Psychiatric Bulletin*, **16**, 560–565.
LINDESAY, J. (1991) Phobic disorders in the elderly. *British Journal of Psychiatry*, **159**, 531–541.
MANN, A. H., JENKINS, R., CUTTING, J. C., et al (1981) The development and use of a standardized assessment of abnormal personality. *Psychological Medicine*, **11**, 839–847.
MARKS, I. & O'SULLIVAN, G. (1989) Anti-anxiety drug and psychological treatment effects in agoraphobia/panic and obsessive–compulsive disorders. In *Psychopharmacology of Anxiety* (ed. P. Tyrer), pp. 196–242. Oxford: Oxford University Press.
MILTON, F. & HAFNER, J. (1979) Outcome of behaviour therapy for agoraphobia in relation to marital adjustment. *Archives of General Psychiatry*, **36**, 807–811.
PAYKEL, E. S. (1978) Contribution of life events towards causation of psychiatric illness. *Psychological Medicine*, **8**, 245–253.
—— & DOWLATSHAHI, D. (1988) In *Handbook of Life Stress, Cognition and Health* (eds S. Fisher & J. Reason), pp. 241–263. Chichester: Wiley.
RASKIN, M., PEEKE, H. V. S., DICKMAN, W., et al (1982) Panic and generalised anxiety disorder. *Archives of General Psychiatry*, **39**, 687–689.
ROBINS, L. N. (1966) *Deviant Children Grown Up.* Baltimore: Williams & Wilkins.
RUTTER, M., TIZARD, J., YULE, W., et al (1976) Isle of Wight Studies: 1964–1974. *Psychological Medicine*, **6**, 313–332.
SMITH, G. R., MARKHAM, W., MONSON, R. A., et al (1986) Psychiatric consultation in somatization disorder: a randomized controlled study. *New England Journal of Medicine*, **314**, 1407–1413.
TRETHOWAN, W. H. (1975) Pills for personal problems. *British Medical Journal*, **3**, 749–751.
TYRER, P. (1976) *The Role of Bodily Feelings in Anxiety.* Maudsley Monograph No. 23, p. 57. Oxford: Oxford University Press.
—— (1985) Neurosis divisible? *Lancet*, **i**, 685–688.
——, SEIVEWRIGHT, N., FERGUSON, B., et al (1992) The general neurotic syndrome: a coaxial diagnosis of anxiety, depression and personality disorder. *Acta Psychiatrica Scandinavica*, **85**, 201–206.
WEEKES, C. (1962) *Self Help for your Nerves.* London: Angus & Robertson.
WORLD HEALTH ORGANIZATION (1992) *The Tenth Revision of the International Classification of Diseases and Related Health Problems* (ICD-10). Geneva: WHO.
YERKES, R. M. & DODSON, J. D. (1908) The relation of strength of stimulus to rapidity of habit-formation. *Journal of Comparative Neurology and Psychology*, **18**, 459–482.
YOUNG, J. P. R., FENTON, G. W. & LADER, M. H. (1971) Inheritance of neurotic traits: a twin study of the Middlesex Hospital Questionnaire. *British Journal of Psychiatry*, **119**, 393–398.

11 Eating disorders

J. HUBERT LACEY

The reported incidence of the eating disorders has risen dramatically since the early 1960s. The initial response has been to develop treatment programmes and little attention has been given, thus far, to the prevention of these disorders.

It is unclear whether the incidence of eating disorders has actually increased or whether they have been increasingly diagnosed by doctors. Leighton & Millar (1985) reported a threefold increase from 1972 to 1981 in the admission of anorectic patients to psychiatric units in Scotland. The cases of diagnosable anorexia nervosa in Monroe County, New York, more than doubled in the period from 1960 to 1976 (Jones et al, 1980). Pyle et al (1986) found a threefold increase (from 1% to 3.2%) in bulimia from 1980 to 1983 in a college population in the Mid-West. Lacey (1991) reported a similar increase in treatment demand of normal-weight bulimic patients all stemming from a representative 'circumscribed urban catchment area' in southwest London. He reports one new case per year per 1000 women between the ages of 16 and 40.

The American Psychiatric Association (1980) has estimated that approximately one in 250 girls between the age of 12 to 18 have anorexia nervosa. Estimates of the incidence of bulimia range from 1 to 20% depending on the population studied and the strictness with which diagnosis criteria are applied (Halmi et al, 1981; Van Thorre & Vogel, 1985).

Diagnosis, prevalence and incidence are made more difficult by the pathoplasticity of the eating disorders. In the '60s, abstaining anorexia was the most common form of presentation. By the '70s, the bulimic form of anorexia was more common than the abstaining form. During the '80s, normal-weight bulimia became increasingly prevalent until by the end of the decade it was between three and five times more common than anorexia nervosa. Recently the so-called 'multi-impulsive' form of bulimia (where alcohol and drug misuse, repeated stealing, sexual disinhibition, overdosing and other forms of self-damage present fluctuatingly and, often, alternatively with the eating disorder) has become more diagnosed although this form is still representative of only a minority of all normal-weight bulimics.

Risk factors

A number of empirical studies have attempted to isolate various risk factors associated with anorexia nervosa and bulimia, the most salient being demographic characteristics, dieting, family and constitutional predisposition and social–cultural influences.

Demographic characteristics

Both anorexia and bulimia nervosa occur overwhelmingly in women, less than 10% of anorectics being men while normal-weight bulimia in men is extremely rare. Anorectics present between 12 and 20 years, the average being 16 years (Johnson, 1982; Mitchell & Pyle, 1982) while normal-weight bulimia presents up to an age of 25 years (Fairburn & Cooper, 1982; Lacey, 1982) with an average age of onset of the disorder of 18.7 years. Anorexia stems predominantly from the middle or upper social class backgrounds (Garfinkel & Garner, 1982) while bulimia arises equally in all social classes (Lacey, 1991). Only four demographic variables mark out bulimics from the general population from which they stem: sex, age, less likely to be black or Asian, or to be married (Lacey & Dolan, 1988). Both disorders are now being reported in older women; the number of blacks and Asians is increasing whereas 10 years ago, eating disorders among ethnic groups were almost unheard of (Garfinkel & Garner, 1982; Levenkron, 1982).

Personality

There is no universal personality pattern in anorexia nervosa (Yager & Strober, 1985) but anorectics are classically described as introverted, compliant and perfectionistic (Crisp, 1979). Bulimics are described as more extroverted than anorectics and bulimic anorectics are more active interpersonally and sexually than abstaining anorectics. The minority of normal-weight bulimics in the multi-impulsive category has many of the features of the explosive personality of ICD–9 (World Health Organization, 1987) or of the borderline personality (Lacey & Evans, 1986).

Constitutional predisposition

Scott (1986) claimed that the available data suggests a hereditary component but that the precise genetic involvement remains unclear. Strober & Humphrey (1987) hypothesise that there may be an interaction between genetic effects and family environment such that an individual with a genetically-determined predisposition to avoidance behaviour may be differentially sensitive to, and more adversely affected by a family environment that detracts from a sense of self-esteem and self-efficacy. Lacey *et al* (1991) have shown that in a representative catchment area, normal-weight bulimia was significantly more likely to occur in elder or only daughters. The number of reports of anorexia nervosa in twins (Garfinkel & Garner, 1982); a higher-than-normal incidence of affective disorders in the families of anorectics (Gershon *et al*, 1984; Rivinus *et al*, 1984) and bulimics have all indicated a possible genetic component in the development of the eating disorders.

Social and cultural influences

Sub-groups of women who are in professions that require a certain body-weight are more likely to develop eating disorders. The incidence of eating disorders is higher among dancers, models, actresses and athletes than in the general population of women (Garner & Garfinkel, 1980; Joseph et al, 1982; Hamilton et al, 1985). Because at least 90% of eating-disordered patients are women, it is obvious that they are at much greater risk of developing eating disorders than are men. This unequal distribution may prevail because, in our society, thinness in women is associated, not only with greater attractiveness but also with greater 'femininity'. It needs to be noted, however, that while, generally speaking, slimness in women is considered an attractive feature by women, there is no evidence that men, as a whole, hold this opinion.

Dieting

The onset of binge-eating, whether in anorexia nervosa or bulimia, always follows an extended period of severe dieting (Fairburn & Cooper, 1982; Johnson, 1982; Gandour, 1984). In a study of 30 normal-weight bulimic patients (Lacey et al, 1986) found that in 74% of patients, the circumstances immediately preceding the onset of bulimic symptoms involved the inability to maintain a low carbohydrate diet, which led to carbohydrate craving and to binge-eating and purging. Virtually all the main research centres have published research noting that repeated dieting constitutes a risk factor not only for bulimia but also for anorexia nervosa.

Family dynamics

A variety of empirical studies have been aimed at differentiating eating disorder sub-groups from each other on the basis of differences in family interactional patterns. The results of these studies have indicated that there is generally more pathology in the families of normal-weight bulimics and of bulimic anorectics than there is in the families of abstaining anorectics, that is, anorectics without bulimic symptoms (Garner et al, 1983; Kog et al, 1985). Bulimic women report that their parents have poor marital relationships and that their own relationships with their parents are poor. A significant minority of the parents of bulimics have sought help for emotional problems from their general practitioner or have been referred to a psychiatrist. The most common diagnosis for mothers is depression while that for fathers is alcohol misuse. The most frequently described family dynamic is that the bulimic reports, prior to her illness and during adolescence, being used as an 'unofficial therapist' by her mother who is lonely and estranged from her husband.

Descriptions of incest and childhood sexual abuse by the eating-disordered are not new (Abraham & Beumont, 1982; Crisp, 1984) but recently the opinion has gained ground that at a clinical level, these events are commonly reported by such patients. Oppenheimer et al (1985) systematically studied 78 eating-disordered patients of mixed diagnoses. Nearly two-thirds of the women patients described adverse sexual experiences, mostly in childhood, and 36% of the perpetrators were members of the patients' families.

The author (Lacey, 1990) systematically studied 112 consecutive referrals of normal-weight bulimic women from a circumscribed catchment area. He found that only eight patients (7%) reported sexual abuse involving physical contact. Four (3.6%) of these described incest, but only in two cases (1.8%) did the incest occur in childhood. Just over 5% of the sample reported unlawful sexual intercourse in childhood or gross indecency. The prevalences of incest and indecency among normal-weight bulimics is perhaps less than described in other neurotic populations and the notion that there is a relationship between sexual abuse and subsequent disturbed eating must be contentious. Studies do suggest, however, that incest and sexual abuse reported by bulimics is usually in those multi-impulsive patients who also misuse alcohol or drugs as well as food.

Prevention

The necessity for developing some type of prevention programme for eating disorders is beginning to receive more emphasis (Crisp, 1979; Button & Whitehouse, 1981; Chng, 1983; McSherry, 1983; Frey, 1984; Katz, 1985; Smead, 1985; Yager, 1985; Killen *et al*, 1986).

Some researchers have questioned whether a prevention programme for eating disorders is possible. Vandereycken & Meermann (1984) for example, contend that the aetiology of eating disorders is insufficiently determined to develop preventive programmes of substance. Further, it would be difficult, if not impossible, to modify socio-cultural influences such as the emphasis on thinness in women. Katz (1985), on the other hand, considered socio-cultural factors to be the most appropriate target for preventive efforts simply because they are so broadly encompassing. Yager (1985) agreed, stating that because the preoccupation with thinness among women spread so rapidly after the last war, the reversal could occur just as rapidly. Yager argued that it was for the media and fashion industries to depict women at a healthier and more realistic weight, and for the right opinion-leader women to reinforce this value. Such a tactic would threaten vested economic interests as well as the established customs and mores of our society (Albee, 1982). As a result, prevention programmes using such methods would be unlikely to be encouraged or supported, monetarily or otherwise. Smead (1985) emphasised these problems. She contends that the fashion, dietetic and media industries would prove to be powerful antagonists if interventions were directed towards changing various aspects of feminine appearance. She rightly claims that these major industries would not want to have the status quo disrupted. However, she fails to grasp that the media industry has many different 'ideal' female body shapes, each associated with an aspect of femininity, and a shift in emphasis from one to another, may not lead to an overall reduction in trade.

Concern has been expressed that programmes to increase public awareness through education may actually encourage eating disorders (Fairburn & Cooper, 1982; Chiodo & Latimer, 1983; Garner, 1985). Fairburn & Cooper (1982) and Lacey *et al* (1986) have presented evidence that many bulimic patients learn their unhealthy weight-control methods from magazines or television programmes. Withholding knowledge is unlikely to be effective, however, and attempts to do so are almost certain to be self-defeating. Further, the ultimate conclusion of such a view would be that eating disorders cannot be prevented or that the general public is not capable of responding appropriately to such information (Smead, 1985). Similar arguments have been levelled against substance misuse prevention programmes. There might be advantages, therefore, in using some of the principles of these programmes in developing prevention programmes for eating disorders. Certainly, details of anorexia and bulimia nervosa should be firmly part of the medical curriculum.

Based on the risk factors discussed earlier, it is clear that adolescent girls are most at risk for developing anorexia nervosa and young adult women most at risk from bulimia nervosa. It would seem that a prevention programme in schools and colleges would be relevant. Because the proposal for such a programme might be met by resistance from school authorities, careful preparation as well as close co-operation and mutual understanding between school authorities and those proposing the programme would be essential.

Some American authors have outlined extensive programmes aimed at both junior and senior school pupils (Shisslak & Crago, 1987). It appears that the intrusion into the academic timetable would be substantial and it would be suprising if such programmes were welcomed in the UK. Didactic tuition, group meetings, assignments and class discussions are recommended. There is no evidence that such an approach would be effective and concern would undoubtedly be expressed that such intensive 'tuition' might lead to the very illnesses which the programmes are designed to prevent. Undoubtedly, however, education of teachers and school councillors on the prevalence, symptoms and consequences of eating disorders can only help. Physical education instructors and coaches, in particular, need to be alerted to the risk of inadvertently contributing to a student's self-destructive pursuit of thinness. In addition, games and PT instructors might have the best opportunity in identifying pupils who, through the way they treat their bodies, seem to be most at risk of developing an eating or weight disorder. Further, those colleges which deal with dance, drama and modelling students might reasonably be expected to have special presentations on the symptoms and complications of these disorders.

The suggestion that because family relationships can be a factor in the development of an eating disorder, preventive efforts need to be directed towards parents and families, seems fraught with dangers. However, PTA meetings which deal with child health might reasonably include a brief presentation on eating disorders as a part of a general package dealing with behavioural disorders of the young (say, along with those dealing with drug misuse).

Although many studies have shown that the parents of anorectics and bulimics themselves have deviant eating patterns, there have been few prospective studies. Nonetheless at a clinical level, anorectic mothers in particular seem to have problems with their children's dietary management. Although there is no evidence, common sense would indicate that this group should have special attention with long-term management whose primary aim is the prevention of the disorder passing to the next generation. Similarly, the adolescent daughters of alcoholic fathers are another susceptible group.

For the vast majority of the population, however, the main means of counselling and information-sharing would be via the media. Television and radio are both transient and tend to dramatise these disorders for effect. Journalists working on women's magazines seem particularly responsible and are perhaps the best medium by which the profession can outline the symptoms and dangers of these disorders. The danger of dieting at times of emotional stress should be emphasised. As families and the general public begin to learn more about the consequences of anorexia and bulimia, and as girls are encouraged to develop personal values, self-worth and effective expression in the world, there is a greater likelihood that young women will not succumb to such extreme methods of dieting or dietary manipulation.

References

ABRAHAM, S. F. & BEUMONT, P. J. V. (1982) Varieties of psycho-sexual experience in patients with anorexia nervosa. *International Journal of Eating Disorders*, **1**, 10–19.
ALBEE, G. W. (1982) Preventing psychopathology and promoting human potential. *American Psychologist*, **37**, 1043–1050.
AMERICAN PSYCHIATRIC ASSOCIATION (1987) *Diagnostic and Statistical Manual of Mental Disorders* (3rd edn), revised (DSM–III–R). Washington, DC: APA.
BUTTON, E. J. & WHITEHOUSE, A. (1981) Sub-clinical anorexia nervosa. *Psychological Medicine*, **11**, 509–516.
CHIODO, J. & LATIMER, P. R. (1983) Vomiting as a learned weight-control technique in bulimia. *Journal of Behavior Therapy and Experimental Psychiatry*, **14**, 131–135.
CHNG, C. L. (1983) Anorexia nervosa: why do some people starve themselves? *Journal of School Health*, **53**, 22–26.
CRISP, A. H. (1979) Early recognition and prevention of anorexia nervosa. *Developmental Medicine and Child Neurology*, **21**, 393–395.
—— (1984) The psychopathology of anorexia nervosa: getting the 'heat' out of the system. In *Eating and its Disorders* (eds A. J. Stunkard & E. Stellar). New York: Raven Press.
FAIRBURN, C. & COOPER, P. (1982) Self-induced vomiting and bulimia nervosa: an undetected problem. *British Medical Journal*, **284**, 1153–1155.
FREY, D. (1984) The counselor's role in the treatment of anorexia nervosa and bulimia. *Journal of Counselling and Development*, **63**, 248–249.
GANDOUR, M. J. (1984) Bulimia: clinical description, assessment, etiology and treatment. *International Journal of Eating Disorders*, **3**, 3–38.
GARFINKEL, P. E. & GARNER, D. M. (1982) *Anorexia Nervosa: a Multidimensional Perspective*. New York: Brunner/Mazel.
GARNER, D. M. (1985) Iatrogenesis in anorexia nervosa and bulimia nervosa. *International Journal of Eating Disorders*, **4**, 701–726.
—— & GARFINKEL, P. E. (1980) Socio-cultural factors in anorexia nervosa. *Psychological Medicine*, **10**, 647–656.
——, —— & O'SHAUGHNESSY, M. O. (1983) Clinical and psychometric comparison between bulimia in anorexia nervosa and bulimia in normal-weight women. In *Understanding Anorexia Nervosa and Bulimia: Report of the Fourth Ross Conference on Medical Research* (ed. G. J. Bergman), pp. 6–13. Columbus, OH: Ross Laboratories.
GERSHON, E. S., SCHREIBER, J. L., HAMOVIT, J. R., et al (1984) Clinical findings in patients with anorexia nervosa and affective illness in their relatives. *American Journal of Psychiatry*, **141**, 1419–1422.
HALMI, K., FALK, J. & SCHWARTZ, E. (1981) Binge-eating and vomiting: a survey of a college population. *Psychological Medicine*, **11**, 697–706.
HAMILTON, L. H., BROOKS-GUNN, J. & WARREN, M. P.(1985) Socio-cultural influences on eating disorders in professional female ballet dancers. *International Journal of Eating Disorders*, **4**, 465–477.
JOHNSON, C. (1982) Anorexia nervosa and bulimia. In *Promoting Adolescent Health: a Dialog in Research and Practice* (ed. T. Coates), pp. 397–412. Orlando: Academic Press.
JONES, D. J., FOX, M. M., BABIGIAN, H. M., et al (1980) Epidemiology of anorexia nervosa in Monroe Country, New York: 1960–1976. *Psychosomatic Medicine*, **42**, 551–558.
JOSEPH, A., WOOD, I. K. & GOLDBERG, S. C. (1982) Determining populations at risk for developing anorexia nervosa based on selection of college major. *Psychiatry Research*, **7**, 53–58.
KATZ, J. L. (1985) Some reflections on the nature of the eating disorders: on the need for humility. *International Journal of Eating Disorders*, **4**, 617–626.
KENNEDY, S. & GARFINKEL, P. (1985) Anorexia nervosa. In *Psychiatry Update: Annual Review* Vol. 4, (eds R. E. Hales & A. J. Frances), pp. 438–463. Washington, DC: APA.
KILLEN, J. D., TAYLOR, B., TELCH, M. J., et al (1986) Self-induced vomiting and laxative and diuretic use among teenagers. *Journal of the American Medical Association*, **255**, 1447–1449.
KOG, E., VANDEREYCKEN, W. & VERTOMMEN, H. (1985) Towards a verification of the psychosomatic family model: a pilot study of ten families with an anorexia/bulimia nervosa patient. *International Journal of Eating Disorders*, **4**, 525–538.

LACEY, J. H. (1982) The bulimic syndrome at normal body weight: reflections of pathogenesis and clinical features. *International Journal of Eating Disorders*, **2**, 59–66.
—— (1990) Incest, incestuous fantasy and indecency: a clinical catchment area study of normal-weight bulimic women. *British Journal of Psychiatry*, **157**, 399–403.
—— (1991) The treatment demand for bulimia: a catchment area report of referral rates and demography. *Psychiatric Bulletin of the Royal College of Psychiatrists*.
——, COKER, S. & BIRTCHNELL, S. A. (1986) Bulimia: factors associated with its etiology and maintenance. *International Journal of Eating Disorders*, **5**, 475–487.
—— & EVANS, C. D. H. (1986) The impulsivist: a multi-impulsive personality disorder. *British Journal of Addiction*, **81**, 715–723.
—— & DOLAN, B. (1988) Bulimia in British blacks and Asians: a catchment area study. *British Journal of Psychiatry*, **52**, 73–79.
——, GOWERS, S. G. & BHAT, A. (1991) Bulimia nervosa: family size, sibling sex & birth order: a catchment area study. *British Journal of Psychiatry*, **158**, 491–494.
LEIGHTON, K. M. & MILLAR, H. R. (1985) Anorexia nervosa in Glasgow. *Journal of Psychiatric Research*, **19**, 167–170.
LEVENKRON, S. (1982) *Treating and Overcoming Anorexia Nervosa*. New York: Scribner.
MCSHERRY, J. A. (1983) Anorexia nervosa – a preventable illness? *Journal of the Royal Society of Health*, **103**, 207–209.
MITCHELL, J. E. & PYLE, R. L. (1982) The bulimic syndrome in normal weight individuals: a review. *International Journal of Eating Disorders*, **1**, 61–73.
OPPENHEIMER, R., HOWELLS, K., PALMER, R. L., *et al* (1985) Adverse sexual experiences in children with clinical eating disorders. *Journal of Psychiatry Research*, **19**, 357–361.
PYLE, R. L., HALVORSON, P. A., NEUMAN, P. A., *et al* (1986) The increasing prevalence of bulimia in freshman college students. *International Journal of Eating Disorders*, **5**, 631–647.
RIVINUS, T. M., BIEDERMAN, J., HERZOG, D. B., *et al* (1984) Anorexia nervosa and affective disorders: a controlled family history study. *American Journal of Psychiatry*, **141**, 1414–1418.
SCOTT, D. W. (1986) Anorexia nervosa: a review of possible genetic factors. *International Journal of Eating Disorders*, **5**, 1–20.
SHISSLAK, G. & CRAGO, M. (1987) Primary prevention of eating disorders. *Journal of Consulting & Dieting Psychology*, **55**, 660–667.
SMEAD, V. S. (1985) Considerations prior to establishing preventive interventions for eating disorders. *Ontario Psychologist*, **17**, 12–17.
STROBER, M. & HUMPHREY, L. (1987) Familial contributions to the etiology and course of anorexia nervosa and bulimia. *Journal of Consulting and Clinical Psychology*, **55**, 654–659.
VANDEREYCKEN, W. & MEERMANN, R. (1984) Anorexia nervosa: is prevention possible? *International Journal of Psychiatry in Medicine*, **14**, 191–205.
VAN THORRE, M. D. & VOGEL, F. X. (1985) The presence of bulimia in high school females. *Adolescence*, **20**, 45–51.
WORLD HEALTH ORGANIZATION (1987) *The Ninth Revision of the International Classification of Diseases and Related Mental Health Problems* (ICD-9). Geneva: WHO.
YAGER, J. (1985) Afterword. In *Psychiatry Update: Annual Review*, Vol. 4 (eds R. Hales & A. Frances), pp. 516–521. Washington, DC: APA.
—— & STROBER, M. (1985) Family aspects of eating disorders. In *Psychiatry Update: Annual Review*, Vol. 4, (eds R. E. Hales & A. J. Frances), pp. 481–502), Washington, DC: APA.

12 Drug and alcohol-related problems

ANDREW JOHNS and BRUCE RITSON

Given our awareness of the consequences and complications of drug and alcohol misuse, of the difficulties of treatment and of the high mortality rate, it is beyond dispute that prevention is better than cure. Prevention not only benefits the individual but is also crucial for society as a whole. Alcohol misuse is responsible for thousands of accidents on and off the road and a high proportion of injuries and deaths are related to acute intoxication. Drug trafficking is associated with organised crime and threatens social structures and indeed the economies of whole countries. In addition, the increasing spread of HIV is probably the most serious threat to the health of the world and has made the prevention of drug misuse by injection relevant to all countries and cultures.

Although the need for prevention is clear the best course of action is not. As the causes of drug misuse are complex and multi-factorial, it follows that no single intervention is likely to have a dramatic or immediate effect.

All too often, prevention strategies are well-meaning but inappropriate and ill-directed. Startling images of dead or unwell addicts may not square with the more mundane reality of day-to-day drug use. A strategy that attempts to reduce the impact of public drunkenness should be very different to that directed at encouraging safer drinking by young women and in pregnancy. There are also siren-calls for an easy solution. There is on one side a plea for an absolute prohibition on drugs and draconian penalties for misuse while on the other, a demand that state-marketed drugs should be legally available in the high street.

In modern jargon, a comprehensive approach is needed for preventing drug and alcohol-related harm. This demands an appreciation of the diversity of the population at risk, an understanding of causal and risk factors and awareness of the importance of the economic and social environment. Lastly a prevention policy that gives priority to health measures which run roughshod over the prevailing customs and attitudes of a community is unlikely to succeed.

Given that drug and alcohol misuse cannot be eradicated, the traditional distinction between primary, secondary and tertiary prevention is of limited validity. A more useful classification is to consider substance misuse prevention measures under the headings of 'Supply reduction', 'Demand reduction' and 'Harm reduction'.

'Supply' or 'availability' reduction

Strategies to control the availability of drugs of misuse rely on statutory control and law enforcement. In all countries, laws control the production, supply, importation, exportation, sale, prescription and possession of drugs of misuse with the intention of ensuring that there is sufficient to meet any genuine medical need and that none are diverted for illicit use.

Crop-control measures

The main drugs of misuse, i.e. alcohol, tobacco, heroin and cocaine, all have a botanical derivation. It follows that a prevention strategy should incorporate measures to reduce and control the cultivation of these crops in their country of origin. However, the economies of many countries are dependent on these licit or illicit cash crops. Attempts have been made to eradicate cocaine growth in Central and South America and also to introduce crop substitution programmes in countries such as Thailand in order to persuade farmers to grow licit crops instead of the opium poppy.

These interventions have had a limited effect. Opium and cocaine are vastly profitable to deprived rural areas. Many developed and developing regions are highly dependent on the licit income from nicotine, while closer to home, there are considerable Common Market subsidies for the cultivation of vines and tobacco.

Interception and interdiction measures

It has been estimated that despite the efforts of H.M. Customs, only 10–30% of illicitly imported drugs are seized. In 1992, seizures by police and customs amounted to: 550 kg heroin, 2.2 tonnes cocaine, 540 000 doses of LSD, 550 000 doses of ecstasy, 51 tonnes of cannabis and 570 kg of amphetamines. Seizures of Class A drugs rose by 27% over the previous year, largely due to increased ecstasy and LSD seizures (Home Office, 1993). There is concern that the 1992 abolition of internal border controls in Europe will facilitate drugs-trafficking.

The police also expend considerable effort on the interdiction of drugs within this country. The main statutory instrument is the Misuse of Drugs Act (1971) as subsequently amended by the Misuse of Drugs Regulations (1985). The effect of this legislation is to define categories of controlled drugs and to establish restrictions on their licit use, together with sanctions on illicit use. Sections of the Misuse of Drugs Act define a series of offences including unlawful supply, possession with intent to supply, unlicensed import or export of a controlled drug and unlawful production. In 1992 there were 48 900 convictions or cautions for drug offences, over 80% of which related to cannabis (Home Office, 1993).

It has been suggested (Justice, 1991) that as the misuse of heroin and stimulants is of greater concern, that the police should redirect their attention to the supply networks of these drugs. The same report also concluded that it was not in the public interest to remove all sanctions on the use of cannabis.

Controls on prescribed drugs

Many drugs of misuse, such as benzodiazepines, amphetamines, barbiturates, diamorphine and cocaine are available in pharmaceutical preparations. Where such drugs have a legitimate medical purpose, they may be prescribed subject to certain controls which vary according to the perceived misuse potential of the drug and the medical setting. For example, diamorphine can be prescribed by any doctor for the alleviation of severe pain, but a licence is required from the Home Office before it can be prescribed for the treatment of drug dependence.

The medical profession has acted to limit the inappropriate prescribing of psychoactive drugs with the result that the use of barbiturates as hypnotics has ceased. With increasing concern about problems associated with long-term benzodiazepine use, preventive efforts have been aimed at influencing doctors' prescribing habits. Nevertheless, a very high proportion of benzodiazepines continue to be dispensed on repeat prescriptions on a long-term basis (Cooper, 1987). All doctors need to be aware of the need for rational prescribing of psychoactive drugs; this topic should be fully addressed in the undergraduate and postgraduate medical curriculum and doctors also need to be aware of non-prescribing interventions (Ghodse & Khan, 1988). These include the need for public education that there is not 'a pill for every ill' and greater use of relaxation training and other psychological techniques.

Taxation and legislative controls on tobacco and alcohol

Measures which influence price in relation to disposal income have a very clear effect on consumption. The responsiveness of consumption to real price is known as price elasticity and for tobacco smoking the effect can be considerable. An increase of 10% in the real price of cigarettes in the UK and the USA has been associated with a fall in consumption of 5% or more. A European Union initiative has proposed tobacco price increases of 35% in France and 87% in Spain in an attempt to influence consumption (Bosanquet & Trigg, 1991).

Price elasticity also applies to alcohol sales. In 1981 the increase in the excise duty on beer and spirits caused their price to rise faster than the retail price index and average disposable incomes. This rise was associated in the Lothian area with a decline in alcohol consumption of 18% and a reduction in alcohol-related harm of 16%. The reduction in problems was evident among both moderate drinkers and most significantly among heavy and dependent drinkers (Kendell *et al*, 1983).

Because of the powerful influence of fiscal measures of this kind, the Royal College of Psychiatrists (1986) recommended that "government taxation policies should be intentionally employed in the interests of health to ensure that per capita alcohol consumption does not increase beyond present levels and is by stages brought to an agreed lower level". The government appears to have an awareness of this argument: *The Health of the Nation* (Department of Health, 1992*a*) states that health will be one of the factors which the Chancellor will take into account when deciding the level of alcohol duties.

The European Union aims to harmonise tax levels on alcohol between member states. The UK has a higher taxation level than most other members. If the recommendations for harmonisation were adopted in their original form, the price of alcohol in Britain would fall dramatically. It has been estimated that this could give rise to a 12% increase in overall alcohol consumption (Crookes, 1989). It is essential that the public health implications of any such changes in pricing are taken into account.

One final measure which has been discussed by the Royal College of Psychiatrists and recommended by the Faculty of Public Health Medicine, was the exclusion of alcohol from the retail price index. Its presence in the index seems to suggest that alcohol is an essential part of any family budget and discourages rises in alcohol tax which will immediately raise the cost of living index, thereby contributing to an inflationary spiral.

There are many legislative strategies for influencing the availability of tobacco and alcohol. In Britain, it has recently been made an offence to sell single cigarettes to children. Licensing controls have limited the nature and number of outlets and the time and place where alcohol can be bought and drunk. In the past 30 years, progressive liberalisation has greatly increased availability. Recent surveys have not demonstrated much significant impact of consumption arising from recent changes in licensing laws (Duffy & Plant, 1986; Goddard, 1991). This may well be because the availability of alcohol in Britain had already neared saturation point. In the past, controls of availability have been shown to have a significant effect on the level of consumption in a community. The number of outlets of alcohol available can also be controlled and again this may influence consumption. The need to travel long distances to obtain alcohol adds to the cost of the product, but also increases the dangers of drinking and driving.

Age restrictions on consumption are also commonplace. In the USA, when some States reduced the age at which drinking was allowed, there was no demonstrable increase in deaths from drinking and driving (National Highway Traffic Safety Administration Report, 1988).

It seems likely that the consumption of alcohol among teenagers commonly occurs first at home, and then in a clandestine way often in public before the permitted age is reached. It is uncertain whether restricting the availability of alcohol to young people significantly affects their style of drinking at a later age (Bagnall, 1990).

Demand reduction

Despite the best efforts of measures to control supply, alcohol and a wide variety of illicit drugs continue to be widely available in this country. Supply-strategies must therefore go hand-in-hand with attempts to reduce demand.

Educational efforts

The prevention of drug, alcohol and also solvent-related problems is an important task for schools (Johns, 1991). In the USA, programmes have been developed which not only give factual information on drug use, but which also seek to develop self-esteem and interpersonal skills. In Britain, 'substance use and misuse' now feature in the National Curriculum and the effect of this will need to be evaluated.

Alcohol education is often seen as a more comfortable choice than measures to control supply, when considering prevention, but it is not necessarily the more effective strategy. Unfortunately, education has rarely been shown to have a significant impact on attitudes or behaviour. There is evidence that it can influence the knowledge which the public, including young people, possess about alcohol. The Royal College of Psychiatrists has recommended that information about sensible limits of consumption along with information about the danger of specific drinking contexts should be widely disseminated.

Education directed at school children needs to acknowledge that children know about alcohol from the age of 5 onwards, but their attitudes change markedly between 11 and 14 years. Educators have stressed that it is very important for children to acquire confidence in dealing with drinking situations and have the social skills necessary to make sensible choices about their subsequent drinking behaviour.

Education can have different foci being, for instance, specifically concerned with the dangers of drinking and driving, the hazards of drinking during pregnancy or they may be directed at particular occupational groups, for instance as part of an alcohol in employment policy. Some have also used the media as a means of disseminating information about alcohol-related problems and encouraging individuals who are experiencing such problems to seek help. There is also evidence that self-help manuals are both popular and effective (Heather *et al*, 1987). Most health promotion endeavours are now turning away from focusing on 'problems' towards a greater concern with promoting healthy lifestyles. The impact of such campaigns has yet to be tested.

There have also been considerable public health efforts aimed at educating the adult population. It is probable that some of the reduction in cigarette smoking seen over the past two decades, relates to increasing public awareness of the risks in the wake of influential reports by the Royal College of Physicians (1987) and campaigns by the Health Education Council.

Advertising controls

It is hard to assess the impact of advertising on alcohol consumption. Studies have not demonstrated much impact of advertising on overall levels of consumption and some have suggested that the banning of advertisements may paradoxically make alcohol more available and cheaper because of the cost element in advertising. Controls over the targeting of advertising, particularly to young people, seem particularly important, and it is also claimed that the ubiquity of alcohol advertising and the way in which alcohol use is portrayed in the media, may make alcohol seem a desirable and acceptable substance which may encourage misuse. The Advertising Standards Authority has created guidelines to ensure that advertising is not misleading and particularly does not aim at young people. Studies show that teenagers are familiar with the content of drinks' advertising long before they can legitimately drink (Aitken *et al*, 1988).

The possible influence of cigarette advertising on levels of consumption has been a matter of lively debate (Raftery, 1989). However, an authoritative review (Department of Health, 1992*b*) concluded that advertising promotes consumption. There is considerable pressure within the European Union to introduce such a ban, although this has been resisted by the British government.

Community responses

Attempts have been made in other countries to tackle alcohol and drug misuse through 'community development' strategies. This is based on the concept that members of a community can be encouraged to identify more closely with the renovation and development of their area and give priority to developing recreational leisure facilities for young people, with the intention of fostering a climate in which substance misuse is less likely to flourish. As an example, a response to the fear that 'crack' use would spread from nearby New York, civic and community leaders in Boston collaborated with the police, church and schools on an active programme of drug interception and prevention which appears to have been relatively successful (Tippel, 1990). Few such programmes have been attempted or evaluated in this country.

The promotion of alternative leisure pursuits shifts the debate about prevention toward a concern with creating a more healthy environment. Going to the pub is one of the most popular social activities among all age groups in this country. Alternative leisure facilities should be available as should alternative (low priced) low and nonalcoholic beers and wines. At present there is concern that the price differential between alcoholic and low alcohol drinks is not sufficient to provide an incentive to change habits. There are encouraging signs of a greater popularity of low-alcohol beers and a greater range of beverage choices and food available in many licensed premises.

Harm reduction

The last decade has seen a much greater emphasis on the need to prevent or at least reduce the harm associated with alcohol and drug use.

Alcohol problems

There is abundant evidence that when a population increases its per capita consumption, there is an accompanying probability of escalation in many indices of alcohol-related harm. For this reason it is important for individuals to be aware of the level of their alcohol consumption and to have some notion of a 'safe' drinking limit. A man who drinks no more than a spaced 21 units or a woman who similarly consumes 14 units a week is unlikely to experience significant alcohol-related harm (Royal College of Psychiatrists, 1986; Royal College of Physicians, 1987) (a 'unit' of alcohol approximates to half a pint of ordinary strength beer and contains about 10 ml of ethanol). *The Health of the Nation* (Department of Health, 1992*a*) identifies the following targets. The proportion of men drinking more than 21 units a week should reduce from 28% in 1990 to 18% by 2005. The proportion of women drinking more than 14 units a week should reduce from 11% to 7% over the same period.

There are a number of techniques available for identifying individuals who are drinking in a harmful or hazardous way, and evidence of the beneficial effects of simple intervention given at an early stage (Babor *et al*, 1986). Advice about 'sensible' drinking has had a demonstrable effect on subsequent health of problem drinkers in general practice (Wallace *et al*, 1988), among male medical admissions to general hospital (Chick *et al*, 1985) and male and female orthopaedic ward admissions (Elvy *et al*, 1988). This evidence coupled with the current NHS commitment to health promotion should stimulate greater interest in secondary prevention by medical practitioners, but it will require a greater commitment to medical education about alcohol (Glass, 1989) and good specialist support services.

Early detection of alcohol problems has been one goal of Employee Assistance Programmes. In these programmes, supervisors are encouraged to detect and enquire about impaired work performance. Where excessive drinking is found to be an important contributing factor, then the employee has a right to referral for counselling while his or her job is retained. This approach has the advantage of providing motivation for change because the client is rewarded by continued employment for complying with treatment (Hore & Plant, 1981). Health services should be encouraged to take a lead in developing programmes of this kind in the interest of their own staff and as encouragement to other employers.

Preventive strategies which seem to influence target behaviours are often more effective than those of a more global nature. For example, attempting to separate drinking from driving, or drunkenness from attendance at football matches.

The contribution of drinking to road accidents is well known. There is some evidence of a declining level of road traffic accidents in Britain, but there is a surprising reluctance to progress to introducing random breath testing which has proven to be effective in several other countries (Faculty of Public Health Medicine, 1991). Other measures aimed at specific behaviours include local bans on public consumption of alcohol, controls on taking alcohol to sporting events, banning of alcohol on football trains and also measures which show that changes in policing practice may reduce the level of alcohol-related problems (Jeffs & Saunders, 1983).

Tobacco problems

It is not generally appreciated by the smoking public, and frequently denied by the tobacco companies, that nicotine has high dependence potential and smoking cigarettes is a highly addictive habit. This was the firm conclusion reached by the surgeon general of the USA in his 1988 report subtitled 'Nicotine Addiction' which concluded unequivocally that tobacco is addicting, that nicotine is involved in this addiction and that the pharmacological and behavioural processes that determine tobacco addiction are similar to those that determine addiction to drugs such as heroin and cocaine (West & Grunberg, 1991). The same report concluded that tobacco dependence can be treated successfully and that effective interventions include behavioural approaches alone and behavioural approaches combined with pharmacological treatments. In particular, nicotine replacement can reduce tobacco withdrawal symptoms and may enhance the efficacy of behavioural treatment.

Despite the scientific authority behind these statements, it seems that the NHS has never taken seriously the need to reduce harm related to tobacco smoking. Short-lived campaigns have concentrated on reducing smoking in the young. The British government continues to resist attempts to control or eliminate cigarette advertising and tobacco company sponsorship of sporting events. Despite this inertia, *The Health of the Nation* (Department of Health, 1992*a*) identifies the target of reducing smoking prevalence to 20% by the year 2000.

There is a need for every doctor and health care worker to be equipped to give simple and effective advice on tackling nicotine addiction. In essence, this comprises an explanation of the benefits of cessation, with an exploration of behavioural and perhaps prescribing strategies combined with group support if this is available. There is a further need for the application of more intensive and supportive psychological and prescribing techniques to those cigarette smokers who do not respond to straightforward interventions – consideration should be given to establishing smoking clinics in all primary care and hospital settings. There is also a need for further treatment strategies to be innovated and evaluated.

Drug problems

One approach to harm reduction has been to prevent misuse by 'redesigning' the chemical structure or formulation of a drug. Each generation of psychoactive drugs has been accompanied by extravagant claims that it is not addictive. All too often, as use becomes more prevalent, the dependence potential of new drugs becomes apparent. In the USA, pentazocine has been marketed in a combined preparation with the opiate antagonist naltrexone. If the pentazocine is taken orally for analgesia as intended, the naltrexone is inactivated. Should the pentazocine be injected, then the naltrexone would act to reduce the 'high' feeling. In this country, the gel in temazepam capsules has been reformulated to make it more difficult to inject, and oral preparations of methadone cannot be injected without serious health consequences to the user. Similar tactics have been used with solvents, with the introduction of new designs that should lack 'sniffing appeal'.

HIV and risk reduction

It is the spread of AIDS that has forced a re-evaluation of drug prevention policies. The Advisory Council on the Misuse of Drugs states that "HIV is a greater threat to public and individual health than drug misuse" (ACMD, 1988).

The primary goal of work with drug misusers must be to prevent them acquiring or transmitting the virus. While in some cases, this will be achieved through abstinence, for the majority efforts have to focus on risk reduction. At present only a small minority of drug misusers are in touch with treatment services. There is an urgent need for development of community-based services, which demands an expansion of existing provision, together with more active involvement of general practitioners; and for the provision of specialist back-up, to allow management of more difficult problems.

Having established contact with drug misusers, the next step is to help them to avoid acquiring or transmitting HIV. The Department of Health (1992a) has as a target:

> "To reduce the percentage of injecting drug misusers who report sharing injection equipment in the previous four weeks by at least 50% by 1997, and by at least a further 50% by the year 2000 (from 20% in 1990 to no more than 10% by 1997 and no more than 5% by 2000)."

There is a need for all services for drug misusers to give practical and explicit advice on risk reduction including advice on injection technique and sexual practices. Many drug clinics in Britain have established needle exchange schemes in order to provide injecting drug misusers with sterile apparatus and also in an attempt to draw them into treatment. The recent nationwide evaluation of these schemes (Stimson *et al*, 1989) found that such exchanges do reach many of those at risk but find it difficult to sustain contact. Nearly 80% of those attending reduced their level of risk behaviour. However, the schemes failed to attract those drug users engaged in the most risky activities. Increasing attention has also been paid to the role of prescribing in attracting drug misusers to services, as a form of 'bait'.

Low-threshold prescribing schemes can operate as a gateway into services, but there is a need to ensure that this intervention is not only appropriate to the individual patient, but takes into account the possible impact on local patterns of drug users. Lastly, there is a need to develop harm reduction strategies which are appropriate for those in custody. Stimson *et al* (1989) found that among 80 drug users who had not attended needle schemes and who had injected drugs while in prison, 20 had shared injection equipment.

Conclusions

Effective prevention will never be brought about or imposed on a community by actions of health professionals alone. In fact it is essential that the community has a commitment to prevention. There have been some signs of this, usually where a particular type of drug misuse has become so prevalent that local people have made a determined and united response to overcome it. Parallels can be drawn with the increasing social disapproval of smoking which has led to a greater decline in consumption than could ever have been achieved by imposed measures.

The prevention of drug and alcohol-related problems, like the treatment and the conditions themselves, is a long-term process. No single preventive measure is likely to be successful alone, but each makes some contribution to a comprehensive programme.

References

ADVISORY COUNCIL ON THE MISUSE OF DRUGS (1988) *AIDS and Drug Misuse, Part 1*. London: HMSO.
AITKEN, P. P., LEATHER, D. S. & SCOTT, A. C. (1988) Ten to sixteen year-olds' perceptions of advertisements for alcoholic drinks. *Alcohol and Alcoholism*, **23**, 491–500.
BABOR, T., RITSON, B. & HODGSON, R. (1986) Alcohol-related problems in the primary health care setting. *British Journal of Addiction*, **81**, 23–46.
BAGNALL, G. (1990) Alcohol education for 13 year olds – does it work. Results from a controlled evaluation. *British Journal of Addiction*, **85**, 89–96.
BOSANQUET, N. & TRIGG, A. (1991) Smoking and economic incentives in Europe. *British Journal of Addiction*, **86**, 627–630.
CHICK, J., LLOYD, G. & CROMBIE, E. (1985) Counselling problem drinkers in medical wards, a controlled study. *British Medical Journal*, **290**, 965–967.
COOPER, J. (1987) Benzodiazepine prescribing – the aftermath. *Druglink*, **2**, 8–10.
CROOKES, W. (1989) *Alcohol Consumption and Taxation*. Institute for Fiscal Studies No 34 I.F.S. London.
DEPARTMENT OF HEALTH (1992a) *The Health of the Nation: a Strategy for Health in England* (Cm 1986). London: Department of Health.

DEPARTMENT OF HEALTH: ECONOMICS AND OPERATION RESEARCH DIVISION (1992b) *The Effect of Tobacco Advertising on Tobacco Consumption: a Discussion Document Reviewing the Evidence*. London: Department of Health.

DUFFY, J. & PLANT, M. (1986) Scotland's liquor licensing changes, an assessment. *British Medical Journal*, **292**, 33-36.

ELVY, G. A., WELLS, J. E. & BAIRD, K. A. (1988) Attempted referral as intervention for problem drinking in the general hospital. *British Journal of Addiction*, **83**, 83-89.

FACULTY OF PUBLIC HEALTH MEDICINE (1991) *Alcohol and the Public Health*. London: Macmillan.

GHODSE, H. & KHAN, I. (Eds) (1988) *Psychoactive Drugs: Improving Prescribing Practices*. Geneva: World Health Organization.

GLASS, I. (1989) Undergraduate training in substance abuse in UK. *British Journal of Addiction*, **84**, 197-202.

GODDARD, E. (1991) *Drinking in England and Wales in the Late 1980s*. London: HMSO.

HEATHER, N., MACPHERSON, F., ALLSOP, S., et al (1987) Effectiveness of a controlled drinking self-help manual one year follow-up. *British Journal of Clinical Psychology*, **25**, 279-287.

HOME OFFICE (1993) *Home Office Statistical Bulletin: Statistics of Drug Seizures and Offenders dealt with, United Kingdom*. Issue 30/93. London: Home Office.

HORE, B. D. & PLANT, M. A. (Eds) (1981) *Alcohol Problems in Employment*. London: Croom Helm.

JEFFS, B. N. & SAUNDERS, W. M. (1983) Minimising alcohol-related offences by enforcement of the existing licensing legislation. *British Journal of Addiction*, **78**, 67-77.

JOHNS, A. (1991) Volatile solvent abuse and 963 deaths. *British Journal of Addiction*, **86**, 1053-1056.

JUSTICE (1991) *Drugs and the Law*. London: Justice.

KENDELL, R. E., DE ROUMANIE, M. & RITSON, E. B. (1983) The effect of economic changes on Scottish drinking habits 1978-82. *British Journal of Addiction*, 365-379.

NATIONAL HIGHWAY TRAFFIC SAFETY ADMINISTRATION (1988) *Alcohol Involvement in Fatal Accidents*. Report HS807268. NHSTA, Washington.

RAFERTY, J. (1989) Advertising and smoking - a smouldering debate? *British Journal of Addiction*, **84**, 1241-1246.

ROYAL COLLEGE OF PHYSICIANS (1987) *A Great and Growing Evil. The Medical Consequences of Alcohol Abuse*. London: Tavistock.

ROYAL COLLEGE OF PSYCHIATRISTS (1986) *Alcohol our Favourite Drug*. London: Tavistock.

STIMSON, G. V., DOLAN, K., DONOGHUE, M. C., et al (1989) Syringe exchange schemes: a report and some commentaries. *British Journal of Addiction*, **84**, 1283-1290.

TIPPEL, S. (1990) *Cocaine use: The U.S. Experience and the Implications for Drug Services in Britain*. London: Community Drug Project.

WALLACE, P., CUTLER, S. & HAINES, A. (1988) Randomised controlled trial of general practitioner intervention in patients with excess alcohol consumption. *British Medical Journal*, **297**, 663-668.

WEST, R. & GRUNSBERG, N. E. (1991) Implications of tobacco use as an addiction. *British Journal of Addiction*, **86**, 485-488.

III. Prevention in psychiatric specialities

13 Child psychiatry

ISSY KOLVIN

The classic approach to prevention of psychiatric problems in childhood was based upon the work of Caplan (1964), who described three different levels of prevention – primary, secondary and tertiary. In theory, prevention is an attractive and powerful concept and in relation to it, phrases such as 'cure is costly – prevention is priceless' were coined.

Primary prevention

The appealing concept of preventing emotional and developmental problems in young children has galvanised a range of programmes with varying degrees of success. Those of a primary preventive nature are discussed with a focus on a target group or population at risk in early childhood. In this context McGuire & Earls (1991) pose some key questions.

(a) Which psychiatric problems can be prevented? They suggest that particular attention should be given to antisocial behaviour and delinquency which can be predicted in the school years.

(b) What strategies have a measurable and meaningful effect? One useful distinction is between intervention with the child (direct) or intervention with parents (indirect). Risk factors are those that when present, increase the likelihood of the child developing a psychiatric disorder (Garmezy, 1983) or induce in the child developmental delays (Werner & Smith, 1982); perinatal anomalies (Neligan *et al*, 1976); difficult temperamental styles (Thomas & Chess, 1977) and chronic illness (Cadman *et al*, 1986).

Risk factors in the family include being in care of social agencies (Rutter, 1989); family dysfunction including alcoholism (Quinton *et al*, 1984); parental psychiatric illness (Rutter & Quinton, 1984); social disadvantage and poverty (Kolvin *et al*, 1990) and criminality (West & Farrington, 1982). Again protective factors that modify the child's response to some environmental hazard have to be taken into account (Rutter, 1979, 1985). Some of these risk factors are sex specific, but it is even more important to note that for the problem to emerge, there needs to be an interaction between pre-disposing factors (risk factors) and co-existing family or relational stresses (triggering events) (McGuire & Earls, 1991). For instance, family deprivation, but especially multiple deprivation in the first five years of life, is a powerful predictor of delinquency and criminality (Kolvin *et al*, 1988).

(c) What extent of intervention is necessary to produce significant change? An earlier notion was that brief interventions could influence outcome in the medium or even longer term. Thus the relevance of the older model of 'medical inoculation' needs to be examined in relation to the more modern 'nutritional' model (Scarr & Weinberg, 1986), which implies that a longer duration of therapy is necessary to sustain improvement (McGuire & Earls, 1991). Allied to this is the concept of 'dosage', that is the extent of input to sustain change.

(d) Do such factors as timing or duration of the intervention influence effectiveness? There is the other widely accepted psychoanalytic view that earlier is better. Finally, McGuire & Earls (1991) offer evidence of the importance of neurobiological maturation as another possible mediating factor.

From their review McGuire & Earls offer a number of conclusions. First, a range of programmes has proved more successful in changing child than parental behaviour. For instance, in relation to families at risk, when teenage mothers were exposed to educational intervention, their children had higher mental and motor developmental quotients at 2 years than were found in controls but there were no differences at 5–8 years (Stone et al, 1988). This and other studies suggest that an inoculation model is not effective when multiple risk factors are present. However, some studies do not fully support the above conclusion (Johnson & Walker, 1987). Studies of the effects of social support and advice to single parents of low socio-economic status, especially when such support is of adequate duration and intensity (Provence & Naylor, 1983), can be effective in changing behaviour of parents and their male but not female children.

Second, as indicated above, boys in at risk environments may respond more dramatically to preventive intervention than girls.

Third, that intervention programmes can change intelligence, but it is noteworthy that they can change behaviour more radically than intelligence. For instance, the study by Campbell et al (1986) in Carolina of at risk families, as represented by young mothers (17 or under), low socio-economic status and low income and psychosocial problems with their children, allocated to day-care programmes for 15 months, found that intellectual development was moderately alterable (Ramey et al, 1984). Further studies on this population suggest that greater attention needs to be devoted to ways of maintaining beneficial effects once achieved – and that early prevention may be more effective than later prevention (McGuire & Earls, 1991). Furthermore, in this study increasing intervention led to increasing improvement compared with controls.

Fourth, it is unlikely that brief methods of enhancing infant responsiveness will substantially improve the academic achievements of socially disadvantaged children and thus society will have to envisage continuing intervention over at least the junior school years.

Fifth, there are serious questions about the utility of parental counselling which has been criticised as containing the potential of undermining parental confidence (Clements, 1985) or even as being unhelpful (Cadman et al, 1987). McGuire & Earls (1991) tentatively suggest that more attention should be given as to how to elicit more effective parenting through parent training; although there is no systematic evidence of effectiveness of counselling, there is some evidence of the utility of specific parental training.

Sixth, only a few programmes have addressed themselves to parent type intervention. One of these, NEWPIN (Cox et al, 1991) seeks to alleviate maternal depression by supporting families with young children and this aims to prevent child abuse. There is preliminary evidence of helpful involvement in the programme and further data will be available in due course. Finally Nicol (1993) has looked at different types of intervention in a population of toddlers whose mothers were screened for maternal depression and explored different types of help to parents. Mothers' groups proved popular; family therapy was less favoured.

Seventh, no review can be undertaken without comments on the Head Start programmes (Darlington *et al*, 1980) which were comprehensive stimulatory and compensatory programmes for pre-school disadvantaged children. It is well known that initial IQ gains rapidly washed out, but subsequent long-term follow-up suggests a more promising general social and emotional (rather than specific cognitive and academic) outcome, in terms of better peer socialisation, lesser frequency and severity of offending, and better employment records.

Secondary prevention

Early secondary prevention is where children are considered to be 'at risk' before symptoms or problems become evident, but not prominent, and these are not necessarily associated with impairment in the social, family, educational or personal sense. Late secondary is where the symptoms/problems are demonstrably evident and are associated with impairment where the service delivery is intended to prevent continuation or progression. Over the last decade there have been some reservations about the utility of secondary preventive approaches, particularly the over-optimism regarding achievements.

With regard to those influential ideas that emerged between the 1960s and 1980s there was particular interest in early secondary preventive activities. Programmes were initiated that aimed at identifying children who were considered to be at grave risk of developing abnormally; service delivery was intended to prevent dysfunction from becoming severe or overt (Kolvin *et al*, 1981/6).

The concept of 'at risk'

The notion of early secondary prevention also includes the concept of 'at risk'. In order to establish an early secondary prevention programme it is desirable to have a method of identifying children 'at risk' so that the highest proportion of those who actually need help (high sensitivity) are included but at the same time those falsely identified as 'at risk' (i.e. high specificity) are excluded (Upshur, 1990). Over the last decade it has been appreciated that risk has multiple components. For instance, Tjossem (1976) advances a tripartite classification of risk, which can be modified to be appropriate for child psychiatry: the categories are behavioural/educational, social-environmental, and biological, and are not mutually exclusive.

However, the identification of children at risk is more easily described than achieved. It is often found that many children who are actually in need of help are not identified by the screening methods utilised, while an even larger number of those who do not need help may be included. Furthermore, a concept of risk that relies on behavioural and educational criteria alone is too narrow and will tend to omit important and stressful socio-demographic and family factors and independent or inter-related biological factors. The children may be at risk in many senses, with little official intervention. Further there is good evidence that social (Neligan *et al*, 1976) and mother–infant interaction (Beckwith, 1984) are more powerful predictors of outcome in low birth weight children than the low birth weight *per se*. Thus, over the last three decades, the concept of risk has grown more complex and the inclusion of broader social and also biological factors in at risk indices indicates the difficulty in identifying which children may benefit from appropriate prevention (Upshur, 1990). Hence Upshur argues that simple screening methods will not be sufficiently sensitive or specific to detect both children and families in need of services. However, attempts to achieve comprehensive cover of all classes of risk factors and which reject single factor models, have yet to prove that they are pragmatic and effective. Single class risk prevention in child psychiatry has already demonstrated its utility (Kolvin *et al*, 1981/6; Kolvin *et al*, 1990).

Specific primary and early secondary prevention programmes

Commonly prevention programmes have focused on inner-city social disadvantage. It has been argued that in such circumstances, early prevention is likely to be more cost-effective than attempting intervention when the effects of deprivation have become deeply ingrained. However, there are four main qualifications to this argument: first, this is true only if the methods of prevention prove to be inexpensive and brief; second, the screening programme must be equally expeditious and inexpensive; third, that the preventive programme does not have any adverse consequences; fourth, the preventive endeavours must be evaluated adequately before attempting to obtain political commitment in such programmes; finally, there are questions concerning the targeting of resources – should they be aimed at the behaviour and scholastic achievements of the children at risk, at their families, or at their social environment.

Preventive programmes have to go beyond an examination of the effects of intervention by exploring the ways in which adverse effects of deprivation are mitigated or mediated. What are the processes and mechanisms that influence changes in behaviour of children? The factors to be explored should cover both the prevention programme itself and a range of other influences, such as the characteristics of the social and family environment and also influences that technically fall into the primary preventive category – namely the schools, their characteristics, the impact of the quality of organisation of academic programmes (Rutter *et al*, 1979) and finally the social characteristics of the school (Moos, 1978; Kolvin *et al*, 1981/6). These issues are best exemplified in relation to some specific prevention programmes.

Recent work indicates that in disadvantaged infant school children, changes in behaviour over time are profoundly influenced by the nature of the children's environment (Kolvin *et al*, 1990). The severity and chronicity of deprivational factors correlated significantly with improvement in behaviour, especially in relation to changes in conduct disorder and hyperactivity. Such findings suggest that in this area, the politician's attitudes and policies about social issues are likely to be as important or even more important than any secondary prevention programmes. Thus, the introduction of innovative social and economic measures as a primary preventive tool should complement any secondary preventive measures by the psychologist or sociologist (Kolvin et al, 1990). This recent research provides some clues about other operative processes and mechanisms. For instance, it was found that more important than the influence of deprivation itself was the personality of mothers and the quality of their resilience in the face of family and environmental adversity – that is, how well did she cope with her life circumstances. Other crucial maternal influences were the quality of her involvement with and stimulation of her children and the thought she gave to her child-rearing practices.

Thus, both social, environmental and family factors are powerful influences on changes of behaviour of children in deprived families, and these influences seem to be mediated through the quality of care and stimulation provided by the main care giver. Hence thought needs to be given as to how social case-workers can help families improve their parenting and problem-solving skills, how politicians can contribute to the modification of the social environment and how educationists can devise ways of optimising school environments as a contribution to mitigating the effects of social and family deprivation on the mental health of chidren.

Late secondary prevention or intervention

Previously, clinicians who have conducted psychotherapy with children and adolescents have done so without the evidence that their activities were validated by sound research. Yet clinicians continued to practice psychotherapy, guided presumably by their own experiences within the context of therapy. But over the last decade it has proved possible to provide evidence at the research level also for the clinician's assumptions (Kolvin et al, 1981/6, 1988). Kolvin and colleagues have argued that positive evidence does exist (based on work conducted in Newcastle) – and additionally, that pessimistic conclusions have in the past been based on inadequate and misleading data. To place this argument on a sound footing, it is essential to address some fundamental issues concerning what constitutes good research evidence.

Criteria for good outcome research

There is considerable variability in methodological criteria across psychotherapy research studies. In an important review, Epstein & Vlok (1981) presented a list of accepted criteria so as to provide a framework for their own evaluation. The main criteria included:

(a) Rigorous and clearly thought out assumptions, questions and procedures
(b) Adequate size of research sample
(c) Random assignment to experimental and control group
(d) Clear description of patient sample to allow generalisation
(e) Post-treatment evaluation and long-term follow-up
(f) Multiple and valid measurement, and sources of assessment

The nature of the control group

With regard to the above, the nature of the control group is important. One of the basic assumptions in psychotherapy research is that the control group will allow systematic investigation of the degree of spontaneous change in untreated patients. Given the possibility that even one diagnostic interview may be of therapeutic benefit in conveying support and reassurance (Meltzoff & Kornreich, 1970) with supposedly 'untreated' controls, in community-based research it is clearly difficult to maintain a rigorous separation between subjects who are 'treated' and those who are not. However, bias may be minimised with no-contact control groups, in which subjects have no knowledge of their inclusion. However, the notion that patients who do not receive formal psychotherapy such as no treatment or waiting list controls, remain without help from other sources has not been substantiated. Many people in search of psychological help do not choose mental health professionals but obtain help from other sources (Gurin et al, 1960). A more accurate representation of psychotherapy evaluation research is that, frequently, formal therapy is being compared with other forms of help of an unknown kind. Finally, treatment dropouts do not constitute adequate controls because selective factors such as motivation may determine continuation and a variety of negative factors may precipitate termination, as may positive factors such as seeing themselves as sufficiently well to no longer need help.

The early reviews that appeared to lead to a discrediting of psychotherapy with adult patients (Eysenck, 1952) were soon paralleled by reviews of child psychotherapy (Levitt, 1957, 1963). In a series of reviews starting 25 years ago, Levitt cites an outcome in child guidance cases at the end of treatment of one-third improved, one-third partly improved, and one-third not improved with similar rates for both treated and untreated cases. Somewhat better rates of improvement were observed at follow-up than at termination of treatment (three-quarters of cases as against two-thirds). Despite serious questions being raised about Levitt's evidence and conclusions, his contention of one-third 'improved', one-third 'partly improved' and one-third 'not improved' became the hallmark against which other therapies were judged. Thus, in the 1970s, the argument which psychotherapy researchers had to confront was that there was essentially no difference in outcome between treated and untreated groups – some 66% of both tended to show improvement. It was suggested that the base rate for spontaneous recovery was so impressive that psychotherapy was not worthwhile as children would improve irrespective; thus, a reliable baseline for spontaneous recovery is crucial.

The Newcastle research makes a useful contribution towards resolution of this complex area (Kolvin et al, 1981/6, 1988; Kolvin, 1990) (see also the next section). In these studies two control groups of disturbed children were identified, for which base rates could be calculated: these consisted of a random sample of 'maladjusted' controls in ordinary schools, aged 11–12 years and a random sample of 'at risk' controls aged 7–8 years, again in ordinary schools. The outcome pattern for the younger group proved similar to that shown by the older group; the large numbers increase the robustness of the results. The combination of control groups yields a sizeable sample of 144 untreated controls (Kolvin et al, 1990). The rate of good outcome after three years proved to be only 41%. These results probably constitute an optimistic estimate of spontaneous improvement. For example, there may have been possible therapeutic contamination of the controls within schools, through the numerous contacts with the controls or their families by research workers.

In addition, certain controls may have obtained help elsewhere. However, against the background of results of the early reviews on spontaneous remission, these are unexpected findings but are consistent with more recent reports. For instance Tramontana's 10-year survey of outcome data with psychiatrically disturbed adolescents (Tramontana, 1980) reveals only four studies with adequate control groups and reasonably sound methodology, with sample size sufficiently large to encourage confidence in results, and which also had follow-up data. When the outcomes of these four studies are combined (Kolvin, 1990), there is a 63% rate of good outcome for the treated cases and 42% for the controls. His analysis leads Tramontana to suggest that the change process in spontaneous remission is not random, but rather there are complex, but systematic, factors operating to produce changes in the absence of formal psychotherapy. He argues that describing it as spontaneous remission merely reflects our ignorance about such factors.

A study by Miller *et al* (1972) was comparable in methodology to the Newcastle treatment-comparison study. Two treatments, namely psychotherapy and systematic desensitisation were evaluated with phobic children. Multiple measures were employed, and assessments were also available at follow-up. While both treatments did better than controls, they did not differ from each other. Most importantly, from the point of view of the present discussion, only 34% of untreated cases had a successful outcome.

The findings examined in this section point consistently to the need for a downward revision of the traditional two-thirds estimate of spontaneous improvement of untreated cases. This represents an important shift in the standpoint of comparison for treatment studies. But what of treatment itself? Can it be shown to be effective?

Is therapy effective?

An example of research programmes that have addressed themselves to this question are the Newcastle studies (Kolvin *et al*, 1981/6, 1988), which go some way towards providing a positive answer. Data are available on several different treatment regimes from two separate studies.

The community-based study which involves school-based intervention, was undertaken with 547 children identified by screen procedures, and about whom individual information was gathered from parents, teachers and individual and group assessments (Kolvin *et al*, 1981/6). Two sets of therapy studies were undertaken – one with junior and one with senior school children. The children were randomly allocated by school class to the various treatment regimes, including a non-treatment regime. Major follow-ups were undertaken 18 and 36 months after the baseline assessments. The treatment regimes, with their principal characteristics, were as follows:

(a) Behaviour modification in secondary schools
(b) Group therapy was applied in both primary and secondary schools and conducted by social workers with small groups, with an emphasis on non-directive principles derived from Axline (1947) and Rogers (1952).
(c) Parent counselling – teacher consultation was applied in primary and secondary schools. Interventions consisted of consultation by social

workers with teachers of identified children, casework with the parents, and attempts to link the home and school.
(d) Nurture work – this was applied in primary schools and consisted of a compensatory and enrichment programme. Teacher-aides were the principal mediators of the procedures.

The study of *seriously disturbed children* was undertaken on a number of groups (Wrate et al, 1985), but the data of concern here are those pertaining to children who attended hospital for treatment either on an out- or in-patient basis, and the screened control group attending ordinary schools who showed comparable psychiatric disturbance both in the quantity of symptoms and the severity of the disorders.

Examining the results some 30–36 months after the start of treatment programmes, the following pattern emerged. Combining the untreated control groups derived from the school studies (Kolvin et al, 1981/6), the base rate for controls of good plus moderate outcome was 41%; the pattern for parent counselling – teacher consultation does not differ significantly from the controls; this base rate was exceeded by some 25% in the case of the nurture work, by 32% in the case of behaviour modification, and by about 35% in the case of group therapy (Kolvin et al, 1988). When combining the data on controls from the clinical and community studies, the base rate is higher, but the broad pattern remains with a similar wide difference between the rates for controls and that obtained with hospital-based clinical referrals (Kolvin et al, 1988).

It is important to try to locate such beneficial changes on the dimension of time. It is commonly believed that patients respond gradually to psychotherapeutic help, with the maximum response being achieved by the end of treatment. Thereafter, patients may reach a plateau, or, with the cessation of therapeutic support, the effects of treatment may begin to dissipate. Examining outcome across assessment points, it was intriguing to find that treatment effects continued to increase for some 18 months after the end of treatment. The failure of the controls to 'catch up' by the end of our follow-up period also suggests that positive processes had been set in motion by therapy.

One of the most attractive ideas to emerge from recent psychotherapy research is whether different types of disorders respond to different kinds of treatment. These concepts of specificity, which are so important in adult disorders, do not appear to be supported by the Newcastle work. There was no consistent evidence of specificity, namely a better response of conduct or neurotic disorders to different treatment or management programmes. Where treatment was effective, it proved to be more so for neurotic and less so for conduct disorders, but there was no particular treatment which was more effective for one or the other.

Comment

The authors of the Newcastle studies conclude that treatment can be effective and that some forms are more effective than others. Thus, nurture work, group therapy and behaviour modification showed significantly better outcome than controls. Parent counselling – teacher consultation proved ineffective, and children in this regime did not do better than untreated controls.

A major theme of the Newcastle studies has been the crucial status of information on untreated controls in evaluating therapy outcome. The results of the Newcastle studies and other reviews in relation to therapy with adolescents (Tramontana, 1980) suggest that therapy researchers have for too long been misled by inflated spontaneous remission rates, against which the impact of their own helping efforts seemed almost inevitably trivial. Levitt's pessimistic estimates seem strangely at odds with clinical experience and findings from longitudinal research that a significant proportion of difficulties in childhood and adolescence do persist. For instance, in the Isle of Wight follow-up study (Graham & Rutter, 1973) of children with psychiatric disorder at 10 years, three-quarters of those with conduct disorders and nearly half (46%) of those with emotional disorders still had handicapping psychiatric disorders in adolescence. There is much other evidence that disorders involving aggressive and anti-social behaviour are likely to persist to a greater extent than emotional disorders (Robins, 1979).

Another theme that the Newcastle studies has helped to highlight is the importance of follow-up assessments once treatment has ended. The findings suggest that therapy may set in motion processes that have effects long after termination and these may go undetected if provision is not made for long-term follow-up. This has been a particular weakness of behaviour modification research where the often unwarranted assumption has been made that withdrawal of reinforcement procedures will lead to the loss of treatment gains, in the absence of programming for reinforcement (MacMillan, 1983). The positive follow-up results reported here are not new: they are consistent with those of Wright *et al* (1976).

As well as considering the notion of the trajectory of change, it is also important to consider other ways in which time is a relevant factor in therapy. Duration of treatment is an important element. For many reasons it is essential to identify forms of therapy that give rise to good outcome in the briefest possible time and hence are the most economic (Strupp, 1978). The Newcastle studies endorse the utility of some shorter term treatments and this is consistent with the findings of others (Luborsky & Spence, 1978; Strupp, 1978) who have indicated that the majority of patients respond positively with brief intervention. An allied question is the importance of frequency of sessions of psychotherapy: type, rather than intensity of treatment, seems to be the critical factor in intervention.

The issue also arises about the central involvement of parents in treatment. They may be given treatment in their own right or be seen as a vehicle through which therapy is applied. However, there is good evidence that involving the child directly in therapy is important (Kolvin *et al*, 1981/6).

Thus, there is now substantial evidence that community-based prevention and intervention approaches help both children who are psychiatrically disturbed and those at risk for disturbance. It is anticipated that in the future research workers will be addressing themselves to ascertaining what other forms of intervention might be helpful and also studying the processes of therapy in endeavours to improve the ability to predict outcome.

Major authoritative reviews also suggest that the available evidence indicates a superiority of psychotherapy over controls (Tramontana, 1980). Such advances must not blind the researcher to monitor as well any deleterious effects of intervention, such as have been described in the Cambridge–Somerville study of delinquency (McCord, 1978).

The targets in late secondary prevention

Who do we target – the index subjects – the children at risk, or those who are symptomatic or the parents or the family? Or do we focus early on behavioural and not on cognitive abilities? Also, how do we screen to identify 'at risk' children with high probability or vulnerability for dysfunction and furthermore what is the cost of the screening? What measures of outcome should be employed? Some reviews and recent research have indicated that a small number of measures at limited points in time may lead to crucial changes being missed (Epstein & Vlok, 1981; Bell et al, 1989). The above suggests that multiple outcome measures should be used. Further, the benefits of intervention are not always in the expected area. Additionally, the outcome should be studied at multiple points in time as 'sleeper effects' (delayed effects) of treatment may occur (Bell et al, 1989).

The future in child and adolescent psychotherapy research

First and foremost it is not possible to ignore the appeal that research must address itself to the critical question of which set of procedures are effective when applied to what kinds of children, with what kinds of problems, as practised by what sorts of therapist (Barrett et al, 1978). Also, an understanding is necessary of the more fundamental processes that are being explored by psychodynamic therapy (Barnett et al, 1991) as has been addressed in adult psychotherapy research. Further, there is a need to explore the therapeutic alliance in relation to outcome. Fourth, a range of measures need to be developed to facilitate the exploration of deeper psychic structures in order to obtain some idea of meaningful change and not merely symptom reduction (Malan, 1975).

Finally, curtailment of follow-up at the end of treatment may lead to a failure to detect so called 'sleeper effects' (Bell et al, 1989); long-term follow-up is essential.

Prevention of suicide in teenagers

A final question concerns suicide which by 1980 ranked second as a cause of death among males aged 15 to 24 in the USA (Shaffer et al, 1988). Are effective means of primary or secondary prevention available? Recently Taylor et al (1992) have reviewed the literature. A major primary prevention thrust in the USA has been the development of general school-based programmes, aimed at heightening awareness of the problems, with the hope that school staff and peers will be able to have access to those teenagers at risk. These approaches are complemented by programmes to improve the teenager's coping abilities. However, as Shaffer et al (1988) point out, predicting which teenagers in the general population may commit suicide is likely to be a costly and inefficient exercise, as it consists of the prediction of rare events from common ones (Eisenberg, 1990).

Nevertheless, such arguments have less force when focusing on populations at high risk, such as those teenagers who have previously been the subject of deliberate self-harm. In these circumstances, in theory at least, secondary prevention/intervention programmes, analogous with those which have been utilised in relation to maladjusted children in ordinary schools (Kolvin et al, 1981/6), are likely to prove less expensive and more efficacious. Unfortunately, the available evidence suggests that these crises services have limited impact, for three main reasons (Shaffer et al, 1988): there is a low utilisation rate in the suicide-prone population; often there are serious questions about the quality of the advice that is offered; and even where crisis advice is offered, there is evidence from the USA (Shaffer et al, 1988) and the UK (Wrate & Kolvin, 1978) that further attendance and the response to advice and offers of help tends to be poor.

Prevention in childhood

The public health model

The original concepts of primary and early secondary prevention have been borrowed from public health approaches to child health problems. In public health the changes in the pattern of serious chronic disorders have emphasised the need for primary prevention through identification of causal processes, as well as the need for early secondary prevention to identify problems as early as possible and to ensure that disability is minimised. However, in the UK, child health has improved enormously since the Second World War, with many infectious diseases and other conditions having been controlled or prevented. Thus previously damaging or life threatening conditions, such as rheumatic fever, have largely disappeared from Western European countries (Taylor, 1990).

Such concepts of prevention do not necessarily carry over well into the mental health field. Eisenberg (1984) has summarised the situation well by pointing out that there are a diversity of problems which necessitate different prevention models. For instance, in preventing pellagra the solution was a macro-economic-social model and the essential ingredients are improved living standards and improved diets.

A general public health model may be necessary, aimed at disease control, of say, water or foodborne infection. In other cases the public health model may be aimed at specific disease control (for instance, in venereal diseases). Of crucial importance is the public health *vaccination model* against polio, pertussis, measles and rubella – this is a quick fix prevention endeavour.

In relation to the above prevention strategies, cost–benefit analyses have to be considered – that balance the cost of the current programme with future savings in medical care in individuals at risk for morbidity. Yet, it is to be remembered that the so called cost benefits may prove illusory – for instance, in the United States deinstitutionalisation was heralded as cost saving but it has been found that often the exercise consists of shifting costs between sectors rather than providing actual savings.

The rationale for disease prevention in childhood is sound as even physical disorders may have major psychological or psychiatric implications. For instance brain damage may not only give rise to handicap and psychopathology but may also increase the individuals vulnerability to other adverse life experiences (Rutter, 1985).

It is also well known that socioeconomic disadvantage and maternal smoking jointly are linked to low birth weight, and the attendant inadequacy of intra-uterine nutrition was linked to higher rates of neonatal mortality and psychiatric morbidity. In one major study socioeconomic disadvantage by far outweighed the contribution of perinatal biological factors in the determination of cognitive and behavioural dysfunction (Neligan *et al*, 1976). However, the fuller availability of good obstetric and neonatal care has been shown to reduce the effects of these adverse experiences (Hawdon *et al*, 1990). Unfortunately endeavours to discourage smoking in the general population have only been moderately successful but there is the suggestion that they are more likely to be successful when they specifically target pregnant women (Eisenberg, 1984).

An allied issue is excess alcohol intake in pregnancy which can give rise to the foetal alcohol syndrome, consisting of growth retardation, central nervous system, cardiac and craniofacial anomalies (Streissguth *et al*, 1983). Eisenberg points out that while public health information programmes dramatically reduced alcohol use in pregnancy, it had only marginal effects on heavy drinkers in the first trimester of pregnancy (Streissguth *et al*, 1983). Congenital rubella with its high risk for mental handicap and autism can be reduced by target vaccination for post-pubertal girls. A variety of neonatal screening programmes are now available such as for phenylketonuria which allow the early institution of treatment programmes. Finally appropriate safety checks and measures can reduce motor vehicular accidents or at least the severity of attendant injuries, accidental overdosage and even a decrease in lead blood levels and their consequent effects on intelligence, learning and behaviour.

It is not surprising that the vaccination model has become the paradigm for prevention (Eisenberg, 1984) and it is likely that this model heavily influenced Gerald Caplan's elaboration of his concept of prevention. However, there remain a number of qualifications but most important – do 'quick fixes' work in reducing psychiatric morbidity? First, does any prevention confer long-term immunity to later stress? Following Erikson, some theorists have argued that successful negotiation of one psychological developmental stage may make successful passage of the next more likely, but this cannot be ensured (Eisenberg, 1977*a*, *b*). Furthermore, good child-rearing practices at one stage of child development may be essential, but are not necessary conditions for subsequent healthy development, nor is there evidence of enduring effects. For instance, the 'Head Start' programmes launched in the USA in the 1960s initially gave rise to considerable optimism. The intention was to interrupt cycles of disadvantage, and the biggest initial gains were in formal education achievements and cognitive abilities, but in neither of these target areas were persistent gains demonstrated. Subsequently the programmes gave rise to considerable pessimism because of the lack of persistence of the effect. However, more recent findings from long-term studies have provided evidence of latent benefits many years after enrolment. These were mainly of the child being more capable of utilising school provisions (Darlington *et al*, 1980). This gives rise to the question of mechanisms by which such time limited interventions begin to have an effect so many years later. Eisenberg (1984) speculates whether it is a consequence of parental involvement, giving them a greater sense of authority, combined with more modern attitudes and motivation of parents. Thus a crucial question is whether one should wait for preliminary evidence of efficacy before launching a prevention programme. But economy is often the hidden agenda behind such prevarications. Further, he points out that "children are exquisitely sensitive to time and they cannot be put into suspended animation while we divert resources into other areas" (Eisenberg, 1984).

Some conclusions

Prevention can be a victim of its own success (Eisenberg, 1984). This is particularly true of many of the public health measures. But as a consequence there may be an attendant increase in the developmental new chronic disorders at the other end of the age spectrum. But what about prevention of psychiatric and psychological morbidity in childhood? Preventive intervention has been shown to be justified for the majority of subjects. Administrators will want wider justification in terms of economic savings but the public and parents may well see justification in terms of improvement in quality of life for the children and their families.

Most of the prevention endeavours have been aimed at intelligence and yet there is good evidence that interventive prevention can influence behaviour more readily than intelligence (McGuire & Earls, 1991).

Further, in respect of behaviour, some argue that early pre-school-based intervention is better than late (Ramey *et al*, 1984) but systematic research has demonstrated that school-based intervention can have significant effects (Kolvin *et al*, 1981/6). The latter research also indicates that direct interventions (directly with the child) may have powerful influences.

However, the schools themselves cannot be ignored as previous work has indicated the significant contribution of the school culture and style of teaching in relation to gains in achievement and also behaviour (Rutter *et al*, 1979). This suggests that ways need to be sought of optimising the school environment as a contribution to mitigating the effects of family deprivation (Kolvin *et al*, 1990).

Finally, there is good evidence to show that the individual differences in maternal personality and care of children, despite equivalent levels of family deprivation, have powerful influences on how children subsequently function. Thus as important as deprivation is a mother's resilience in the face of adversity. These factors must be seen as crucial protective factors in the face of family adversity (Kolvin *et al*, 1990). However social factors were fundamentally potent and hence the politician's attitude towards economic and social policy may be more important in introducing innovative measures as primary preventive tools than any secondary preventive measures by the psychologist or sociologist.

References

AXLINE, V. M. (1947) *Play Therapy*. Boston: Houghton Mifflin.
BARNETT, R. J., DOCHERTY, J. P. & FROMMELT, S. M. (1991) A review of child psychotherapy research since 1963. *Journal of the American Academy of Child and Adolescent Psychiatry*, **30**, 1–14.
BARRETT, L. C., HAMPE, I. E. & MILLER, L. C. (1978) Research on child psychotherapy. In *Handbook of Psychotherapy and Behavior Change* (2nd Edn.) (eds S. L. Garfield & A. E. Bergin), pp. 411–436. New York: Wiley.
BECKWITH, L. (1984) Parent interaction with their preterm infants and later mental development. *Early Child Development and Care*, **16**, 27–40.
BELL, V., LYNE, S. & KOLVIN, I. (1989) Play group therapy: processes and patterns and delayed effects. In *Needs and Prospects of Child and Adolescent Psychiatry* (eds M. H. Schmidt & H. Remschmidt). pp. 149–164. Stuttgart: Hogrefe & Huber.

CADMAN, D., CHAMBERS, L. W., WALTER, S. D., et al (1987) Evaluation of public health pre-school child development screening: the process and outcomes of a community program. *American Journal of Public Health*, **77**, 45–51.
––––, BOYLE, M., OFFORD, D. R., et al (1986) Chronic illness and functional limitation in Ontario. Findings of the Ontario child health study. *Canadian Medical Association Journal*, **135**, 761–767.
CAMPBELL, F. A., BREITMAYER, B. & RAMEY, C. T. (1986) Disadvantaged single teenage mothers and their children: consequences of free educational day care. *Family Relations*, **35**, 63–68.
CAPLAN, G. (1964) *Principles of Preventive Psychiatry*. London: Tavistock.
CLEMENTS, J. (1985) Update – training parents of mentally handicapped children. *Newsletter of the Association of Child Psychology and Psychiatry*, **7**, 2–9.
COX, A. D., POUND, A., MILLS, M., et al (1991) Evaluation of a home visiting and befriending scheme for young mothers: NEWPIN. *Journal of the Royal Society of Medicine*, **84**, 217–220.
DARLINGTON, R. B., ROYCE, J. M., SNIPPER, A. S., et al (1980) Pre-school programs and later school competence of children from low-income families. *Science*, **208**, 202–208.
EISENBERG, L. (1977a) Psychiatry and society: a psychobiological overview. *New England Journal of Medicine*, **297**, 1230.
–––– (1977b) Development as a unifying concept in psychiatry. *British Journal of Psychiatry*, **131**, 225.
–––– (1984) Prevention, rhetoric and reality. *Journal of the Royal Society of Medicine*, **77**, 268–280.
–––– (1990) Public policy: risk factor or remedy? In *Risk Factors and the Prevention of Child Psychiatric Disorders* (eds D. Shaffer, I. Phillips & N. Enzer), p. 138. Washington, DC: ADAMHA.
EPSTEIN, N. D. & VLOK, L. A. (1981) Research on the results of psychotherapy: a summary of evidence. *American Journal of Psychiatry*, 1027–1035.
EYSENCK, H. J. (1952) The effects of psychotherapy. An evaluation. *Journal of Consulting Psychology*, **16**, 319–324.
GARMEZY, N. (1983) Stressors of childhood. In *Stress, Coping and Development in Children* (eds N. Garmezy & M. Rutter), pp. 43–84. New York: McGraw-Hill.
GRAHAM, P. & RUTTER, M. (1973) Psychiatric disorder in the young adolescent: a follow-up study. *Proceedings of the Royal Society of Medicine*, **66**, 1226–1229.
GURIN, G., VEROFF, J. & FELD, S. (1960) *Americans View Their Mental Health: A Nationwide Survey*. New York: Basic Books.
HAWDON, J. M., HEY, E., KOLVIN, I., et al (1990) Born too small – is outcome still affected? *Developmental Medicine and Child Neurology*, **32**, 943–953.
JOHNSON, D. L. & WALKER, T. (1987) The primary prevention of behavior problems in Mexican-American children. *American Journal of Community Psychology*, **15**, 375–385.
KOLVIN, I. (1990) Newcastle community based prevention and intervention studies. In *Early Detection of Psychiatric Disorders in Children* (ed. H. Van Engeland), pp. 67–84. Amsterdam: Swets & Zeitlinger.
––––, GARSIDE, R. E., NICOL, A. R., et al (1981/6) *Help Starts Here: The Maladjusted Child in the Ordinary School*. London: Tavistock.
––––, MACMILLAN, A., NICOL, A. R., et al (1988) Psychotherapy is effective. *Journal of the Royal Society of Medicine*, **81**, 261–266.
––––, MILLER, F., FLEETING, M., et al (1988) Social and parenting factors affecting criminal offence rates. Findings from the Newcastle Thousand Family study (1947–1980). *British Journal of Psychiatry*, **152**, 80–90.
––––, CHARLES, R., NICHOLSON, R., et al (1990) Factors in prevention in inner city deprivation. In *The Public Health Impact of Mental Disorder* (eds D. Goldberg & D. Tantam), pp. 115–123. Stuttgart: Hogrefe & Huber.
LEVITT, E. (1957) The results of psychotherapy with children: an evaluation. *Journal of Consulting Psychology*, **21**, 189–196.
–––– (1963) Psychotherapy with children: a further evaluation. *Behaviour Research and Therapy*, **60**, 326–329.
LUBORSKY, L. & SPENCE, D. P. (1978) Quantitative research and psychoanalytic therapy. In *Handbook of Psychotherapy and Behavior Change* (2nd Edn.) (eds S. L. Garfield & A. E. Bergin), pp. 331–368. New York: Wiley.
MACMILLAN, A. (1983) The effectiveness of behaviour modification procedures in secondary schools with limited teacher training and consultation time. University of Newcastle upon Tyne: PLO/Thesis.
MALAN, D. H. (1975) (Reprint) *A Study of Brief Psychotherapy*. London: Tavistock Plenum.
MCCORD, J. (1978) A thirty year follow-up of treatment effects. *American Psychologist*, **33**, 284.
MCGUIRE, J. & EARLS, F. (1991) Prevention of psychiatric disorder in early childhood. *Journal of Child Psychology and Psychiatry*, **32**, 129–154.
MELTZOFF, J. & KORNREICH, M. (1970) *Research in Psychology*. New York: Atherton Press.

MILLER, L. C., BARRETT, C. I., HAMPE, E., *et al* (1972) Comparison of reciprocal inhibition, psychotherapy and waiting list controls for phobic children. *Journal of Abnormal Psychology*, **79**, 269-279.
Moos, R. H. (1978) A typology of junior high and high school classrooms. *American Educational Research Journal*, **15**, 53-66.
NELIGAN, G. A., KOLVIN, I., SCOTT, D., *et al* (1976) *Born too Soon or Born too Small*. London: Spastics International Medical.
NICOL, R., STRETCH, D. & FUNDUDIS, T. (1993) *Preschool Children in Troubled Families: Approaches to Intervention and Support*. Chichester: Wiley.
PROVENCE, S. & NAYLOR, A. (1983) *Working with Disadvantaged Parents and Children: Scientific Issues and Practice*. New Haven, CT: Yale University Press.
RAMEY, C. T., YEATES, K. O. & SHORT, E. J. (1984) The plasticity of intellectual development: insights from preventive intervention. *Child Development*, **55**, 1913-1925.
ROBINS, L. N. (1972) Follow-up studies of behaviour disorders in children. In *Psychopathological Disorders of Childhood* (eds H. C. Quay & J. S. Werry). New York: Wiley.
ROGERS, C. R. (1952) *Client-Centred Therapy*. Boston: Houghton Mifflin.
RUTTER, M. (1979) Protective factors in children's responses to stress and disadvantage. In *Primary Prevention of Psychopathology, Vol. 3, Social Competence in Children* (eds M. W. Kent & J. E. Rolf), pp. 49-74. Hanover, NH: University Press of New England.
—— (1982) Prevention of children's psychosocial disorders: myth and substance. *Pediatrics*, **70**, 883-894.
—— (1985) Resilience in the face of adversity. Protective factors and resistance to psychiatric disorder. *British Journal of Psychiatry*, **147**, 598-611.
—— (1989) Psychiatric Disorder in Parents as Risk Factors for Children. Prevention Monograph US Department of Health and Human Services.
——, MAUGHAN, B., MORTIMORE, P., *et al* (1979) *Fifteen Thousand Hours: Secondary Schools and Their Effects on Children*. London: Open Books; Cambridge, Mass: Harvard University Press.
—— & QUINTON, D. (1984) Parental psychiatric disorder: effects on children. *Psychological Medicine*, **14**, 853-880.
SCARR, S. & WEINBERG, R. A. (1986) The early childhood enterprise, care and education of the young. *American Psychologist*, **41**, 1140-1146.
SHAFFER, D., GARLAND, A., GOULD, M., *et al* (1988) Preventing teenage suicide: a critical review. *American Journal of Child and Adolescent Psychiatry*, **27**, 675-687.
STONE, W. L., BENDELL, R. D. & FIELD, T. M. (1988) The impact of socioeconomic status on teenage mothers and children who received early intervention. *Journal of Applied Developmental Psychology*, **9**, 391-408.
STREISSGUTH, A. P., DARBY, B. L., BARR, H. M., *et al* (1983) Comparison of drinking and smoking patterns during pregnancy over a six-year interval. *American Journal of Obstetrics and Gynecology*, **145**, 716-724.
STRUPP, H. H. (1978) Psychotherapy research and practice: an overview. In *Handbook of Psychotherapy and Behavior Change* (2nd Edn.) (eds S. L. Garfield & A. E. Bergin), pp. 3-22. New York: Wiley.
TAYLOR, B. (1990) *Prevention in Childhood*. Working party paper, pp. 143-165. Royal College of Psychiatrists.
TAYLER, P. J., BURTON, K. & KOLVIN, I. (1992) Suicidal behaviour in children and adolescents. In *Recent Advances in Clinical Psychiatry* No. 7 (ed. K. Granville-Grossman). Edinburgh: Churchill Livingstone.
THOMAS, A. & CHESS, S. (1977) *Temperament and Development*. New York: Brunner/Mazel.
TJOSSEM, T. (1976) Early intervention: issues and approaches. In *Intervention Strategies for High Risk Infants and Young Children* (ed. T. Tjossem), pp. 3-33. Baltimore: University Park Press.
TRAMONTANA, M. G. (1980) Critical review of research on psychotherapy outcome with adolescents 1967-1977. *Psychological Bulletin*, **2**, 429-450.
UPSHUR, C. C. (1990) Early prevention as preventive intervention. In *Handbook of Early Childhood Intervention* (eds S. J. Meisels & J. P. Shonkoff), pp. 633-650. Cambridge: Cambridge University Press.
WERNER, E. E. & SMITH, R. S. (1982) *Vulnerable, but Invincible: A Longitudinal Study of Resilient Children and Youth*. New York: McGraw-Hill.
WEST, D. & FARRINGTON, D. (1982) *Delinquency: Its Roots. Careers and Prospects*. London: Heinemann Educational.
WRATE, R. M. & KOLVIN, I. (1978) A child psychiatry consultation service to paediatricians. *Developmental Medicine and Child Neurology*, **20** (Suppl), 347-356.
——, ——, GARSIDE, R. F., *et al* (1985) Helping seriously disturbed children. In *Longitudinal Studies in Child Psychology and Psychiatry* (ed. A. R. Nicol), pp. 265-318. Chichester: Wiley.
WRIGHT, D. M., MOELIS, I. & POLLAK, L. J. (1976) The outcome of individual psychotherapy increments at follow-up. *Journal of Child Psychology and Psychiatry*, **17**, 275-285.

14 Mental handicap

KENNETH DAY

The term mental handicap covers a wide range of individuals and conditions and the broad classification into severe and mild mental handicap has relevance both in terms of clinical features and causation.

Severe mental handicap is a pathological condition resulting from abnormal development of or damage to the brain. The overall prevalence rate is around 3 per 1000 with age-specific rates ranging from 2.5 per 1000 in the 0–4 years age group to 1 per 1000 in the over 65s (Fryers, 1984). A large number of causative biomedical factors are known and can be precisely pinpointed in about 50% of cases (Hagberg & Hagberg, 1984). Recent advances in human genetics and medical science have substantially increased the potential for primary and secondary prevention with the promise of even greater breakthroughs in the next decade. Prevalence rates, however, remain relatively constant, reductions in the birth incidence of specific conditions like Down's syndrome being balanced by increased survival of severely damaged infants and a general increase in the life expectancy of mentally handicapped people (*Lancet*, 1990).

The prevalence of mild mental handicap is intrinsically linked to social and economic conditions and rates vary in different communities at different times (Clarke & Clarke, 1984; Richardson, 1990). Less than half of the one million or more people estimated to be mildly intellectually handicapped (IQ 70 or less) in the UK are currently receiving special services, but the proportion is steadily increasing as opportunities for unskilled work progressively decline and everyday life becomes increasingly complex. Biomedical factors, similar to those causing severe mental handicap, can be identified in about a third of cases (Hagberg & Hagberg, 1985) but the majority are due to the normal biological distribution of intelligence within the population (Clarke, 1985). Adverse socio-cultural factors including poor maternal and child care, faulty child-rearing practices and a generally underprivileged home environment play a significant contributory role in most cases (Birch *et al*, 1970; Richardson, 1987). Prevention and amelioration are more dependent upon socio-political factors than medical advances. The influence of prolonged social learning and delayed maturation on eventual social adjustment has been highlighted by Clarke & Clarke (1984).

The maintenance of prevalence rates over time emphasises the importance of tertiary prevention. The World Health Organization's definitions of 'impairment' as the fault in an organ or body system, 'disability' as the consequent loss of function and 'handicap' as the resulting social disadvantage, provides a useful conceptual framework (World Health Organization, 1980). The scope for prevention of secondary disabilities and amelioration of social handicap has increased enormously in recent years with the shift from institutional care to an 'ordinary life' model of care in the community (*Better Services for the Mentally Handicapped*, 1971; *National Health Service and Community Care Act*, 1990). Advances in education, care and management together with improvements and developments in service provision have enabled increasing numbers of mentally handicapped people to lead more independent and fulfilled lives. Other important developments include improved diagnosis and treatment of psychiatric and behaviour disorders, autism and epilepsy; advances in technical aids to independence, and the development of specialised services for groups with special needs like the psychiatrically disordered, the multiply handicapped and the elderly.

Primary prevention

Primary preventive measures include positive family planning, genetic counselling, protection of the foetus from teratogenic agents, improved maternal health and improvements in perinatal and child care.

Genetic counselling

Genetic disorders are responsible for more than half of all miscarriages, a quarter of perinatal deaths and three-quarters of severe handicapping conditions (Burn, 1988). Chromosome abnormalities account for nearly 40% of cases of severe mental handicap (Down's syndrome 36%, other aneuploidies 2–3%), Fragile X syndrome for 6% and other single gene disorders (although individually rare) for 5–7% (Lavoxa *et al*, 1977; Hagberg & Hagberg, 1985).

The remarkable advances in molecular biology and molecular genetics over the last decade, particularly the development of recombinant DNA technology and chromosome banding, has revolutionised the practise of clinical genetics (Weatherall, 1991). Over 1500 autosomal genes and 300 X-linked genes have been identified or located (Wahlstrom, 1990) many of which are clinically useful in the detection of carriers and prenatal diagnosis. In the field of mental handicap these include tuberose sclerosis, phenylketonuria, peripheral neurofibromatosis, Hurler's syndrome, Lesch–Nyhan syndrome, and Tay–Sachs disease. The genetic basis of syndromes of previously unknown aetiology like Prader–Willi and Angelmann's syndrome have been identified and the possibility of somatic gene therapy for certain conditions draws ever closer (Weatherall, 1991).

A major advance has been the discovery of the Fragile X syndrome now known to be responsible for about 6% of severely and 10% of mildly mentally handicapped males and 50% of all sex linked causes of intellectual handicap (Sutherland, 1979; Blomquist *et al*, 1982, 1983). Eighty per cent of affected males and a third of the female carriers are mentally handicapped (Webb *et al*, 1986; Thake *et al*, 1987; Simon *et al*, 1990). The potential for prevention through population screening, carrier detection and prenatal diagnosis has recently been considerably boosted by the identification of the Fragile X gene and its mode of transmission (Connor, 1991). Programmes to raise public and professional awareness are required (Keenan *et al*, 1992; Turner *et al*, 1992) as the majority of affected people are, at the moment, undiagnosed (Rogers & Simensen, 1987).

Prevention of Down's syndrome by genetic counselling is limited to the 2.4% of cases due to a translocation abnormality inherited from one or other parent: 21q/21q translocations carrying a 100% risk of recurrence and DG translocations a 16% risk if the mother is the carrier and a 5% risk if the father is the carrier. Trisomy 21, which occurs spontaneously, has a recurrence risk of less than 1%.

Genetic counselling for the many known genetic and chromosomal causes of mental handicap is only possible at present after the birth of one affected child within the family. Carrier identification and risk prediction have been substantially improved by advances in molecular genetics, the development of computer-based family pedigrees and long-term monitoring of high risk families. Preconceptual screening is currently limited to certain conditions in high risk groups like Tay–Sachs disease in Ashkenazi Jews (Kaback, 1985), but the development of cheap and easy to administer techniques including blood spots and amplifying DNA using polymerase chain reactions from mouth washes may ultimately permit routine preconception screening for carriers of common genetic disorders (Burn, 1988).

Environmental causes

A wide variety of environmental factors acting before, during and after birth are known to cause mental handicap and many are potentially preventable (Hunter *et al*, 1980; Berg, 1985). Berg (1985) has drawn attention to the need to distinguish between causes and associations, and to the more subtle influences of environmental hazards on mental development, and warns against making over-simplistic links – the causal relationship between malnutrition in infancy and intellectual impairment is a good example (Richardson, 1984). A fundamental relationship between socio-economic and family factors and biomedical risk factors like low birth weight, has also been repeatedly demonstrated (Aylward *et al*, 1989*a*, *b*; Robertson *et al*, 1990).

The dangers of foetal damage due to ionising radiation and teratogenic drugs are well documented and have been largely eradicated as a consequence of improved professional and public awareness, increased stringency in the use of diagnostic X-ray in early pregnancy, the preliminary testing of drugs for human use and the protection of industrial workers (Berg, 1985). Exposure to nuclear irradiation carries a high risk of mental retardation in first trimester foetuses and of radiation induced genetic damage (Yamazaki *et al*, 1954; Yamazaki, 1966) and the consequences of nuclear catastrophies like Chernobyl have yet to be fully assessed (Holowinsky, 1993).

Positive family planning, better obstetric care, hospital deliveries and maternal and foetal monitoring have substantially decreased the incidence of birth trauma and perinatal morbidity and mortality. Intensive care of very low birth weight babies has reduced the incidence of pathological sequelae, but cerebral palsy, intellectual impairment and mental handicap still occur in 12–20% (Illsley & Mitchell, 1984; McCormick, 1985). Cases of mental handicap due to the bacterial infections have been virtually eradicated, although constant vigilance is necessary in light of the recent reports of rising numbers of cases of syphilis and drug-resistant tuberculosis (Watson, 1993). Salt iodisation programmes have successfully eliminated endemic cretinism (Eastman & Phillips, 1988): an increase in the iodine content of salt has recently become necessary because of the overall reduction in salt consumption in the general population for health reasons (Konig et al, 1985).

Vaccination of girls aged 10–14 years has achieved only limited success in reducing the incidence of the congenital Rubella syndrome – an important preventable cause of both physical and mental handicap (Smithells et al, 1985). The recently introduced combined measles, mumps and rubella vaccine (MMR) given to all infants of both sexes between the ages of 1 and 2 years, together with pertussis immunisation, should ultimately provide the total herd immunity necessary to completely eradicate Rubella syndrome and mumps, measles and pertussis encephalitis (Department of Health, 1992a). A number of other infections currently pose greater threats to the foetus. Cytomegalovirus infection, which occurs in 0.5 to 2.5% of infants (Hanshaw, 1983), causes mental handicap in at least 10% of those infected (Peckham et al, 1983): preventive vaccination is a future possibility (Lancet, 1983). Neurological abnormalities including mental handicap and sensory deficits are common in congenital toxoplasmosis, which has an incidence of 1 per 20 000 live births; termination is usually recommended for proven foetal infection in the first and second trimester but a recent study concluded that antiparasitic treatment can prevent severe congenital toxoplasmosis and that termination is only necessary in the event of intrauterine death or sonographic evidence of hydrocephalus (Berribi et al, 1994). Maternal listeriosis, an uncommon disease which can seriously harm the foetus, can be prevented by avoiding high risk foods during pregnancy (Department of Health, 1992b).

Congenital HIV infection is a growing problem and has been found to occur in 2 to 2.5 per 1000 live births in the USA (Walker & Messenger, 1992). Maternal drug abuse, low birth weight and prematurity are common complications and the incidence of developmental delay, frank mental handicap, progressive encephalopathy and other neurological disabilities is high (Ultmann et al, 1985; Epstein et al, 1986; Belman et al, 1988; Cogo et al, 1990).

An association between neural tube defects, the cause of 5% of cases of severe mental handicap (Lavoxa et al, 1977), and folate deficiency during pregnancy was established more than a decade ago (Laurence et al, 1980) and the specific preventive role of daily preconceptual folic acid supplements in women who have already had one affected child has recently been unequivocally demonstrated (MRC Vitamin Study Group, 1991). A folate rich diet together with folic acid supplements is now recommended for all women prior to planned conception and during the first 12 weeks of pregnancy (Department of Health, 1992c), but the extent to which this will prevent first occurrences is uncertain: a large scale study is currently underway in China.

Man's long established tradition of using drugs socially can pose problems for the foetus. Smoking during pregnancy is one cause of low birth weight babies (Berg, 1985). Prevention will depend upon the success of anti-smoking campaigns in changing the attitudes and habits of the younger generation and of mothers-to-be. The foetal alcohol syndrome (a combination of developmental delay, growth retardation, neurological abnormalities and characteristic facial dysmorphology) is caused by moderate to heavy alcohol consumption (1–8 units daily) during the first trimester and has a worldwide incidence of 1–2 per 1000 live births (Waterson & Murray-Lyon, 1990; Spohr et al, 1993). An alcoholic mother has a 20–50% risk of giving birth to a child with the foetal alcohol syndrome (Hagberg & Hagberg, 1985). Education programmes to increase public awareness of the risk are important but more specific prevention presents enormous challenges because of the difficulties in identifying and influencing the target group. Screening tests have been developed (World Health Organization, 1993) and some success has been reported in the use of special maternal health teams to trace and support women at high risk in reducing alcohol intake (Larsson, 1983). The extent to which illicit drug taking during pregnancy, an increasing problem in the western world, can cause foetal abnormality is uncertain but LSD, marijuana and cocaine have all been implicated in the causation of chromosome abnormalities and impaired foetal growth (Balson, 1972; Tylden, 1973; Zuckerman et al, 1989). Lifestyle, malnutrition and an increased incidence of low birth weight and preterm babies are important additional factors increasing the risk of foetal abnormality and mental handicap in alcohol misusers and drug takers (Lifschitz et al, 1985; Zuckerman et al, 1989).

Head injury in babies, infants and children is a significant cause of permanent neurological impairment and mental handicap (Smith & Hanson, 1974; Buchanan & Oliver, 1977; Akuffo & Sylvester, 1983). The use of bicycle helmets and seat belts and improvements in car design coupled with health education programmes have to some extent successfully reduced the incidence of accidental head injury, but the prevention of non-accidental head injury remains a major social challenge. Cases of mental handicap due to mercury and lead poisoning, neonatal meningoencephalitis, neonatal hypoglycaemia and venous sinus thrombosis due to inadequate fluid intake in acute gastroenteritis still occur, particularly in disadvantaged families and social groups (Black et al, 1982).

Early intervention

The adverse influence of early deprivation in infancy upon subsequent cognitive performance is well established (Clarke, 1983). Heroic attempts have been made in the USA over the past 30 years to protect children at risk of mild developmental and educational retardation, by providing intensive high quality pre-school intervention programmes from birth through infancy in families selected as being of high risk on the basis of low maternal intelligence (Clarke & Clarke, 1985). The intensively supported children in these programmes achieved superior IQ scores and educational performance at school entry compared to control groups, but these differences were not sustained at follow up (Garber & Hebber, 1977, 1982; Clarke & Clarke, 1985). Nevertheless, the enthusiasm for early intervention continues. Ramey and colleagues have recently reported lasting benefits in intellectual performance and school achievement despite a degree of 'washout' at 12 year follow up in one project (Ramey & Haskins, 1981; Ramey & Ramey, 1992), the most powerful effects being found in those children whose mothers were functioning in the mild to borderline mental handicap range (Martin et al, 1990; Ramey & Ramey, 1992).

Secondary prevention

Secondary prevention is now possible for an increasing number of conditions through (i) prenatal diagnosis and selective termination of affected pregnancies and (ii) neonatal, and in some cases prenatal identification, of affected babies and active treatment.

Prenatal diagnosis

Advances in molecular genetics, together with refinements in the techniques of amniocentesis, ultrasonic imaging and foetoscopy have substantially improved the safety and accuracy of prenatal diagnosis in the second trimester of pregnancy and chorionic villus sampling is increasingly enabling the diagnosis of genetic disease during the first trimester (*Lancet*, 1991). The number of conditions which can be detected prenatally is steadily expanding and diagnosis is now possible earlier and earlier in pregnancy, enabling earlier and safer termination and reducing social and psychological stress (Ward, 1984). Pre-implantation analysis of '*in vitro*' or '*in vivo*' fertilised ova, to ensure that only normal pregnancies are initiated, is now a reality for couples with a high risk of producing a baby with serious genetic disease, and gene replacement therapy for certain conditions is an imminent possibility (Weatherall, 1991).

Amniocentesis and prenatal diagnosis is routinely offered to all women 35 years of age and over (in whom the risk of Down's syndrome is 1 in 400 or more) and to those with a family history of Down's syndrome. One hundred per cent uptake with termination would achieve a 30% reduction in the incidence of Down's births (Mikkelsen *et al*, 1990), but in practice less than half of the women at risk take up the offer (Wald *et al*, 1988). A safe and effective primary screening test for Down's syndrome which can be offered to all pregnant women has just become available. This utilises the recently discovered association between an increased risk of Down's syndrome and abnormally low alpha fetoprotein (AFP) and unconjugated oestriol levels and higher than normal human chorionic gonadotrophin levels in maternal serum. The pioneers of this test have calculated that 60% of affected pregnancies will be identified with no increase in the amniocentesis rate and recommend that maternal serum screening should be routine for all pregnant women (Wald *et al*, 1988, 1992). In a three year demonstration project involving over 1200 women, uptake for screening was 74%, the detection rate 48% and the false positive rate 4.1%; 75% of screen positive women accepted amniocentesis and there was a 90% acceptance of termination in the eleven found to have an affected pregnancy (Wald *et al*, 1992).

Raised maternal serum alpha fetoprotein (AFP) levels have been found to be a reliable indicator of neural tube defects. Up to 85% of cases can be detected using a combination of maternal serum AFP, AFP levels in amniotic fluid and diagnostic ultrasound (Ferguson Smith, 1988) and incidence halved by good antenatal screening programmes (Atkins & Hey, 1991). Prenatal screening for the Fragile X syndrome presents more difficulties, requiring a blood sample from the foetal umbilical cord, as the syndrome cannot yet be readily identified in DNA or chromosome preparations from chorion villus sampling or fibroblast culture from amniotic fluid (*Lancet*, 1986a).

A large number of inherited metabolic diseases including phenylketonuria, galactosaemia, Lesch–Nyhan syndrome, maple syrup urine disease, Hunter's syndrome, Hurler's syndrome and Tay–Sachs disease can now be identified prenatally. Diagnosis is currently limited to the subsequent pregnancies of the parents and siblings of an affected person. Brain damage (kernicterus) due to rhesus haemolytic disease has been virtually eliminated through routine maternal screening, the administration of anti-D gamma globulin, early exchange transfusion and the immunisation of rhesus negative mothers after the birth of the first child. Bilirubin encephalopathy due to immature liver functioning, however, continues to be a risk in low birth weight babies.

Neonatal screening

The routine screening of all neonates using the simple heel prick test developed originally for phenylketonuria (Guthrie & Susi, 1963), permits the early detection and immediate treatment of sporadic congenital hypothyroidism, hyperbilirubinaemia and a growing number of inborn errors of metabolism.

Phenylketonuria (PKU) affects 0.05 to 0.2 per 1000 live births and can be effectively treated with a phenylalanine free diet (Smith *et al*, 1990*a*). Evidence is mounting in favour of lifelong treatment, even in those where a significant degree of mental handicap has already occurred, replacing the previous practice of terminating the diet in the teens (Koch *et al*, 1987; Naughten, 1989; Thompson *et al*, 1990) and recent work suggests that knowing the specific genotype enables a more accurate estimate to be made of the patient's future dietary needs (Okano *et al*, 1991). Women with PKU require a phenylalanine-free or low diet during pregnancy and preferably preconceptually to reduce the risk of foetal brain damage due to maternal hyperphenylalanaemia (Koch *et al*, 1990; Smith *et al*, 1990*b*). Other detectable metabolic disorders with the potential for special dietary treatment are galactosaemia, homocystinuria, maple syrup disease, tyrosaemia and histidinuria. So far the results are far less satisfactory than in PKU, although some success has been reported in galactosaemia and in the treatment of lysosomal storage diseases by bone marrow transplantation (Stern, 1985).

Tertiary prevention

For mentally handicapped people and their families, prevention and amelioration of secondary disabilities and social handicaps is the main priority.

Radical changes in the philosophy of care in the developed countries over the past 30 years have substantially enhanced the possibilities for mentally handicapped people of all ability levels to lead more normal and fulfilled lives. The emphasis today is on the individual and enabling him or her to live as 'ordinary' a life as possible – a philosophy reflected in the massive shift from segregated institutional care to integrated care in the community. Much has been achieved. In the UK, the number of mentally handicapped people in long-term hospital care has been halved since 1971 through active resettlement programmes and there has been a corresponding growth in the range and extent of support networks, educational services, training placements and day and residential services in the community

(Office of Health Economics, 1986). Cessation of all long stay hospital care by the year 2000 is the goal (*National Health Service and Community Care Act*, 1990).

While many mentally handicapped people have undoubtedly benefited from these changes, implementation has not been without problems and there is continuing concern about the adequacy of resourcing of community services, the paucity of systematic evaluation and of their appropriateness for certain groups (Day, 1986, 1988). There is also a growing appreciation of the need to provide specialised services for mentally handicapped people with special needs like the multiply handicapped, the mentally ill, the behaviourally disturbed, offenders, and the ageing and elderly (Royal College of Psychiatrists, 1986; Department of Health and Social Security, 1984, 1989).

At an individual level, many studies have demonstrated the value of early intervention, individual programme planning, the keyworker system and small group living in an ordinary environment. Advances in medical treatment, the use of electronic aids to assist independence and the development of alternative methods of communication have all substantially increased the potential for the amelioration of secondary disabilities like motor and sensory impairments, epilepsy and systemic disease which frequently co-exist and often constitute a greater disability to the individual than the underlying mental handicap (Department of Health and Social Security, 1972; Report of the Jay Committee, 1979; Beange & Bauman, 1991). Health promotion is a growing concept in the care of the disabled (Pope, 1992) and regular monitoring of health status is now recognised as an essential part of management – particularly in the elderly and severely mentally handicapped (Day, 1987; Beange & Bauman, 1991). Sadly, however, mentally handicapped people are still sometimes discriminated against in the competition for health services.

Psychiatric disorder

Mentally handicapped people are more prone to psychiatric disorders than the general population and prevalence rates are particularly high in the severely mentally handicapped (Rutter *et al*, 1976; Corbett, 1979; Gostason, 1985; Lund, 1985; Gillberg *et al*, 1986; Reiss, 1990). Predisposing factors include organic brain damage, epilepsy, sensory impairments, communication difficulties and a range of psychosocial factors. Diagnosis and treatment requires special skill and experience because of atypical presentation and communication difficulties and the unique nature of many of the problems presented (Royal College of Psychiatrists, 1986; Reiss, 1990; Day, 1993).

The scope for prevention is considerable. Mentally handicapped people are as, if not more, vulnerable to life events and personal and environmental stress as the general population (Gilson & Levitas, 1987) and may respond with behavioural disturbance (Ghaziuddin, 1988), psychotic breakdown (Varley, 1984) and reactive depression and anxiety (Day, 1985). The death of the last caring relative is a particularly potent life event for middle aged and elderly mentally handicapped people and a frequent cause of depression (Day, 1985; James, 1986; McLoughlin, 1986). More sensitive preparation for residential care when ageing parents can no longer cope (Carter, 1984; Seltzer & Seltzer, 1985) and the early provision of bereavement counselling would substantially reduce morbidity (Hollins & Sireling, 1991).

The implementation of care in the community has been paralleled by a growth in the incidence of neurotic disorder (Day, 1985; Lund, 1985) and drug and alcohol problems (Krishef & Dinitto, 1981; Edgerton, 1986). Great care is needed in assessing the level of support required by an individual in the community. Poorly conceived community care schemes can bring more stresses than benefits and a high frequency of victimisation, financial and health worries and socialisation has been revealed in some studies (Flynn, 1988). Ineffective social interaction and social isolation have been shown to be important psychosocial correlates of depression in the mentally handicapped (Reiss & Benson, 1985).

Behaviour disorders account for some 50% of psychiatric morbidity and are particularly common in the severely handicapped. They may be manifestations of mental illness, physical discomfort or social distress and frustration, the behavioural phenotype of a genetic syndrome like Prader–Willi or Rett's or a learned behavioural response. Impaired comprehension and communication skills, severe sensory deficits, organic brain damage and faulty management are frequently underlying or contributory factors. The potential for prevention is considerable, through early intervention and advice on management to parents and carers, the correction or amelioration of communication and sensory impairments, and the early and accurate diagnosis and prompt treatment of underlying mental illness. All mentally handicapped people presenting with severe behaviour problems should have a thorough psychiatric and medical assessment.

Behaviour disorder in the mildly mentally handicapped frequently takes the form of antisocial acts involving conflict with the law. As in the general population, it is frequently associated with a range of adverse psychosocial factors (Richardson et al, 1985; Koller et al, 1987; Day, 1990). Prevention depends upon breaking the 'cycle of deprivation' and amelioration requires intensive intervention (Day, 1988, 1990). Antisocial sexual behaviour tends to be over-represented and appears in the main to be a consequence of normal sexual impulses in the absence of opportunities for normal outlets compounded by sexual naïvety and poor adaptive skills (Day, 1994). More enlightened approaches to the sexuality of mentally handicapped people and the routine provision of sex education programmes in schools and adult facilities (Craft, 1987) should reduce the incidence of this problem in the future.

The past 20 years has seen an increasing recognition of the extent of psychiatric disorder in mentally handicapped people, considerable improvements in diagnostic and treatment techniques and an increase in the number of trained psychiatrists and specialised psychiatric services (Day, 1988, 1993; Day & Jancar, 1991). Nevertheless, treatable psychiatric conditions continue to go undiagnosed – the elderly and severely mentally handicapped are particularly at risk (Day, 1985; Patel et al, 1993) and there is an urgent need to educate parents and carers, train first line professionals in the basic elements of the psychiatry of mental handicap, and expand specialist services.

Family adjustment

Amelioration of family psychopathology is another important aspect of tertiary prevention. The diagnosis of mental handicap is a major family crisis which can affect the mental health of parents and siblings and radically alter family life

(Gath, 1978; Bagenholm & Gillberg, 1991). Adolescence, a move into residential care and other lifespan events present additional stresses. Studies by Wilkin (1979) and Dupont (1980, 1986) graphically illustrate the burden on families of coping with a severely mentally handicapped child, the level of care required being the major determinant of the amount of stress experienced by the family irrespective of other factors. This burden has been considerably eased over the past 20 years by the provision of parent counselling and support networks, the development of home-based teaching programmes, an emphasis on parental involvement in training, improvements in educational services and the growth of respite care and financial help (Carr, 1984, 1985).

The majority of families make a positive adjustment (Carr, 1985; Hollins, 1989; Russell, 1990; Fraser & Rao, 1991; Ramey, 1991), responding with 'resilience and unique adaptive functioning' (Dyson, 1991). Family social climate and relationships are key factors influencing adjustment (Flynt & Wood, 1989; Frey *et al*, 1989; Seltzer *et al*, 1991). Where family adjustment problems do occur they can have a profound effect on the life and development of both the handicapped child and the family. Faulty adjustment is a common antecedent of behaviour problems (Koller *et al*, 1987; Gath, 1990). The potential for preventive intervention has yet to be fully exploited and much more attention needs to be paid in clinical practice and research to the identification and provision of help to families at risk. Psychiatrists have an important role in this process in the education and training of staff and through direct therapeutic work with families as well as in research. There is scope for closer collaboration between psychiatrists and general practitioners, obstetricians and health visitors who are in the best position to identify families at risk. Currently psychiatric assistance is rarely sought until the problems have become well entrenched.

Developing countries

Patterns of prevalence and aetiology of mental handicap in developing countries vary considerably according to social, cultural, religious and economic factors (Belmont, 1981; Fryers, 1984). Severely damaged infants rarely survive and mildly mentally handicapped people are scarcely visible where schooling is poor or non-existent, illiteracy high and a prevailing rural economy provides plenty of opportunities for unskilled work. Endemic cretinism, the major infections, malnutrition and patterns of consanguineous marriage in isolated communities – all now largely eradicated in the developed countries – are the principal causes of mental handicap. Maternal HIV infection is rapidly becoming a significant cause, particularly in Central and East Africa where up to 10% of women of childbearing age are sero-positive and a third of the surviving babies are severely mentally retarded (N'Galey *et al*, 1988; Ntaba *et al*, 1988). Clarke & Clarke (1981) have drawn attention to the phenomenon of 'reversible retardation' consequent upon gross physical and social deprivation during conditions of war, famine and epidemic disease, and to the importance of identifying and treating such children who may remain overlooked in orphanages and institutions.

Reductions in family size, general improvements in living standards, improvements in maternal and child nutrition, basic public health measures, the control of communicable diseases and the establishment of equitable primary health care infrastructures are the major preventive measures. The extent to which these can be achieved depends essentially upon the general economic and social development and political stability of the country concerned. The scope for specific prevention programmes is limited. The cost–benefits in developed countries of maternal and neonatal screening programmes for congenital abnormalities rarely, if ever, apply in the developing countries. The success of vaccination programmes depends crucially upon the quality of primary health care services. Endemic cretinism, the single largest cause of severe mental retardation in the world with millions at risk in Asia, South America and Africa (World Health Organization, 1985, 1993), can be prevented simply and cheaply, but food and water iodisation programmes are not always easy to introduce or maintain (*Lancet*, 1986b; Hetzel, 1989; World Health Organization, 1993). The most efficient strategy for reducing the incidence of Down's and other genetic syndromes is the reduction of pregnancies in older mothers through family planning programmes (World Health Organization, 1993) but long established cultural traditions limit their success.

In most developing countries service provision is poorly developed or non-existent, there is no tradition of institutional care and mentally handicapped people live with their families (Sartorius, 1984). The United Nations, in collaboration with the World Health Organization and the United Nations Educational, Scientific and Cultural Organization (UNESCO), has initiated numerous projects world-wide. These include the development of simple screening tests for use by first line workers (World Health Organization, 1992); special education projects (Mittler & Serpell, 1985); Community Based Rehabilitation (CBR) which aims to provide support and training for mentally handicapped people and their families using trained locally based community workers (O'Toole, 1987); manuals for the guidance of families and helpers, and educational and mobility aids (Mittler & Serpell, 1985; Fryers, 1989; Helander *et al*, 1990). The World Health Organization publication *Mental Retardation: Facing the Challenge* (1985) gives advice on all aspects of prevention, rehabilitation and service provision with a special emphasis on developing countries. A more recent publication gives specific advice to professionals, mid-level workers and the general public on the prevention of iodine deficiency, Down's syndrome, the foetal alcohol syndrome and phenylketonuria (World Health Organization, 1993).

Issues in prevention

Scientific and technological advances, together with improvements in medical diagnosis and treatment are increasingly improving the opportunities for primary, secondary and tertiary prevention.

The extent to which the many measures now available can be successfully implemented depends crucially upon the effective dissemination and application of existing knowledge and the development of appropriate service and organisational infrastructures (Mittler, 1984). It requires clear national health care policies, the nationwide availability of key services including genetic counselling clinics and pregnancy risk information, good obstetric and neonatal care, general public health measures and health education programmes.

General societal changes can exert an important influence upon the prevalence and incidence of mental handicap. For example, the reduction in late pregnancies due to more effective contraception has had a far greater impact in reducing the birth frequency of Down's syndrome than antenatal screening programmes (Wynn-Griffiths, 1973) and has also reduced the incidence of other genetic disorders and causative factors associated with this high risk age group. On the other hand, there has been an increase in illegitimate and teenage pregnancies and in the use of tobacco, alcohol and illicit drugs by women of reproductive age – all associated with a higher risk of low birth weight babies, poor utilisation of prenatal care and child abuse (Baumeister & Kupstas, 1990).

Biological risk factors rarely operate independently and socioeconomic, family and other factors have a significant influence in both their expression and the subsequent developmental outcome (Baumeister & Kupstas, 1990). Social disadvantage is associated with lower levels of uptake of immunisation programmes, fewer hospital deliveries and an increased incidence of low birth weight babies (McFarlane & Mugford, 1984) and reductions in the incidence of the discrete biomedical disorders has exposed a 'new morbidity' of poor child care, deprivation, abuse and injury (Baumeister & Kupstas, 1990). This requires an ecological approach to prevention which takes account of the complex interaction between biomedical and socioeconomic factors and of the interaction between the mentally handicapped individual and his environment (Richardson, 1987; Coulter, 1992). Prevention policies need to address the development of specific strategies which break the 'cycle of deprivation' and prevent the cumulative effects of disadvantage and deprivation being passed from generation to generation (Birch *et al*, 1970; Brown & Madge, 1982) and the more general issue of improvements in the socioeconomic status and health of the population, particularly women of reproductive age (Wynn & Wynn, 1979).

In most countries prevention strategies for mental handicap are enmeshed in general public health programmes. The World Health Organization (1985) recommends the setting of specific national targets for the prevention of severe mental handicap. Alberman (quoted in Office of Health Economics, 1986) has suggested that a 20% reduction in the births of severely mentally handicapped children would be a realistic goal over a 5–10 year period in the UK. Crocker (1992) has provided a comprehensive and detailed list of outcome indicators for the evaluation of prevention programmes. In the UK a major contribution to tertiary prevention is the recently published *Protocol for Investment in Health Gain* (Welsh Office NHS Directorate, 1992) which sets specific targets in relation to the physical and mental health of mentally handicapped people and the amelioration of secondary handicap due to physical disabilities. Jenkins *et al* (1994) have compiled a list of health service requirements and outcome indicators for the elderly mentally handicapped.

Certain preventive measures, particularly genetic screening and selective termination, gene therapy and the immediate management of severely damaged babies raise major ethical and moral issues for parents, professionals and society in general (Singer, 1983; Weatherall, 1991; Department of Health, 1992*d*; Versluys, 1993) and create conflicting values in the competition for and allocation of health care resources (Adams, 1984; Gill *et al*, 1987; Wald *et al*, 1992; Chapple *et al*, 1987).

References

ADAMS, M. (1984) Socioethical issues in the management of developmental disability. In *Perspectives and Progress in Mental Retardation* (Vol. I) (ed. J. M. Berg), pp. 3–10. Baltimore: University Park Press.

AKUFFO, E. O. & SYLVESTER, P. E. (1983) Head injury and mental handicap. *Journal of the Royal Society of Medicine*, **545**, 9–76.

ATKINS, A. F. J. & HEY, E. N. (1991) The northern regional foetal abnormality survey. In *Antenatal Diagnosis of Foetal Abnormalities* (eds J. O. Drife & D. Donnai), pp. 13–30. London: Springer-Verlag.

AYLWARD, G. P., VERHULST, S. J. & BELL, S. (1989a) Correlation of asphyxia and other risk factors with outcome: a contemporary view. *Developmental Medicine and Child Neurology*, **31**, 329–340.

——, PFEIFFER, S. I., WRIGHT, A., et al (1989b) Outcome studies of low birth weight infants published in the last decade: a meta-analysis. *Journal of Paediatrics*, **115**, 515–520.

BAGENHOLM, A. & GILLBERG, C. (1991) Psychosocial effects on siblings of children with autism and mental retardation: a population based study. *Journal of Mental Deficiency Research*, **35**, 291–301.

BALSON, P. J. (1972) Damage to chromosomes by drugs. *Adverse Drug Reaction Bulletin*, **37**. Newcastle upon Tyne: Newcastle Regional Hospital Board.

BAUMEISTER, A. A. & KUPSTAS, F. (1990) The new morbidity: implications for prevention and amelioration. In *Combatting Mental Handicap: A Multidisciplinary Approach* (eds P. L. C. Evans & A. D. B. Clarke), pp. 46–72. Bister, Oxon: AB Academic.

BEANGE, H. & BAUMAN, A. (1991) Health care for the developmentally disabled. Is it necessary. In *Key Issues in Mental Retardation Research* (ed. W. I. Fraser), pp. 154–162. London: Routledge.

BELMAN, A. L., DIAMOND, G., DIXON, D., et al (1988) Paediatric acquired immuno deficiency syndrome. *American Journal of Diseases of Children*, **142**, 29–35.

BELMONT, L. (1981) Severe mental retardation across the world: epidemiological studies. *International Journal of Mental Health*, **10**, 85–99.

BERG, J. M. (1985) Physical determinants of environmental origin. In *Mental Deficiency: The Changing Outlook* (4th Edn) (eds A. M. Clarke, A. D. B. Clarke & J. M. Berg), pp. 99–134. London: Methuen.

BERRIBI, A., KOBUCH, W. E., BESSIERES, M. H., et al (1994) Termination of pregnancy for maternal toxoplasmosis. *Lancet*, **334**, 36–39.

BETTER SERVICES FOR THE MENTALLY HANDICAPPED (1971) Cmnd 4683. London: HMSO.

BIRCH, H. G., RICHARDSON, S. A., BAIRD, D., et al (1970) *Mental Subnormality in the Community: a Clinical and Epidemiological Study*. Baltimore: Williams & Wilkins.

BLACK, D., MORRIS, J., SMITH, C., et al (1982) *Inequalities in Health: The Black Report*. New York: Penguin.

BLOMQUIST, H. K., GUSTAVSON, K. H., NORDANSON, I., et al (1982) Fragile site X chromosomes and X linked mental retardation in severely mentally retarded boys in a northern Swedish county: a prevalence study. *Clinical Genetics*, **24**, 393–398.

——, ——, et al (1983) Fragile X syndrome in mildly mentally retarded children in a northern Swedish county: a prevalence study. *Clinical Genetics*, **25**, 147–152.

BROWN, M. & MADGE, N. (1982) *Despite the Welfare State*. London: Heinemann Educational.

BUCHANAN, A. H. & OLIVER, J. E. (1977) Abuse and neglect as a cause of mental retardation: a study of 140 children admitted to subnormality hospitals in Wiltshire. *British Journal of Psychiatry*, **131**, 458–467.

BURN, J. (1988) Clinical genetics: a review. *Journal of the Royal College of Physicians*, **22**, 212–225.

CARR, J. (1984) Family processes and parental involvement. In *Scientific Studies in Mental Retardation* (eds J. Dobbing, A. D. B. Clarke, J. Corbett, et al), pp. 443–456. London: The Royal Society of Medicine & Macmillan.

—— (1985) The effect on the family of a severely mentally handicapped child. In *Mental Deficiency: The Changing Outlook* (4th Edn) (eds A. M. Clarke, A. D. B. Clarke & J. M. Berg), pp. 512–548. London: Methuen.

CARTER, G. (1984) Why are the mentally handicapped admitted to hospital? *British Journal of Psychiatry*, **145**, 283–288.

CHAPPLE, J. C., DALE, R. & EVANS, B. G. (1987) The new genetics: will it pay its way? *Lancet*, i, 1189–1192.

CLARKE, A. M. (1985) Polygenic and environmental interactions. In *Mental Deficiency: The Changing Outlook* (4th Edn) (eds A. M. Clarke, A. D. B. Clarke & J. M. Berg), pp. 267–290. London: Methuen.

—— & CLARKE, A. D. B. (1981) Problems of applying behavioural measures in assessing the incidence and prevalence of mental retardation in developing countries. *International Journal of Mental Health*, **10**, 76–84.

―― & ―― (1984) Social influences in the aetiology and prevention of mild retardation. In *Scientific Studies in Mental Retardation* (eds J. Dobbing, A. D. B. Clarke, J. Corbett, *et al*), pp. 25–42. London: The Royal Society of Medicine & Macmillan.

―― & ―― (1985) Lifespan development and psychosocial intervention. In *Mental Deficiency: The Changing Outlook* (4th Edn) (eds A. M. Clarke, A. D. B. Clarke & J. M. Berg), pp. 440–464. London: Methuen.

COGO, P., LAVERDA, A. M., ADES, A. E., *et al* (1990) Neurological signs in young children with human immune deficiency virus infection. The European collaborative study. *Paediatric Infections Disease Journal*, **9**, 402–406.

COMMITTEE OF ENQUIRY INTO MENTAL HANDICAP NURSING CARE (THE JAY COMMITTEE) REPORT (1979) Volumes I & II (1979) Cmnd 7468-1. London: HMSO.

CONNOR, J. M. (1991) Cloning of the gene for the Fragile X syndrome: implications for the clinical geneticist. *Journal of Medical Genetics*, **28**, 811–813.

CORBETT, J. A. (1979) Psychiatric morbidity and mental retardation. In *Psychiatric Illness and Mental Handicap* (eds P. Snaith & F. E. Jones), pp. 11–25. London: Gaskell.

COULTER, D. L. (1992) An ecology of prevention for the future. *Mental Retardation*, **30**, 363–369.

CRAFT, A. (1987) *Mental Handicap and Sexuality: Issues and Perspectives*. Tunbridge Wells: Costello Press.

CROCKER, A. C. (1992) Data collection of the evaluation of mental retardation prevention strategies: the fateful 43. *Mental Retardation*, **30**, 303–317.

DAY, K. (1985) Psychiatric disorder in the middle aged and elderly mentally handicapped. *British Journal of Psychiatry*, **147**, 660–667.

―― (1986) Developing services for the mentally handicapped: some practical considerations. In *The Provision of Mental Health Services in Britain: The Way Ahead* (eds G. Wilkinson & H. Freeman), pp. 111–120. London: Gaskell.

―― (1987) The elderly mentally handicapped in hospital: a clinical study. *Journal of Mental Deficiency Research*, **31**, 131–146.

―― (1988) Mental handicap and community care. *British Journal of Hospital Medicine*, **40**, 249.

―― (1990) Mental retardation: clinical aspects and management. In *Principles of Forensic Psychiatry* (eds R. Bluglass & P. Bowden), pp. 399–418. Edinburgh: Churchill Livingstone.

―― (1993) Mental health services for people with mental retardation: a framework for the future. *Journal of Intellectual Disability Research*, **37** (Suppl. 1), 7–16.

―― (1994) Male mentally handicapped sex offenders: a clinical study. *British Journal of Psychiatry*, **165**, 630–639.

―― & JANCAR, J. (1991) Mental handicap and the Royal Medico-Psychological Association: a historical association 1841–1991. In *150 years of British Psychiatry 1841–1991* (eds G. E. Berrios & H. Freeman), pp. 268–278. London: Gaskell.

DEPARTMENT OF HEALTH (1989) Needs and responses: services for adults with mental handicap who are mentally ill, who have behaviour problems or who offend. Stanmore: Department of Health leaflets Unit.

―― (1992*a*) *Immunisation Against Infectious Disease*. Department of Health, Welsh Office, Scottish Home and Health Department, DHSS Northern Ireland. London: HMSO.

―― (1992*b*) *The Diagnosis and Treatment of Suspected Listeriosis in Pregnancy: Report of a Working Group*. Standing Medical Advisory Committee. Heywood, Lancashire: Health Publications Unit.

―― (1992*c*) *Folic Acid and the Prevention of Neural Tube Defects: Report from an Expert Advisory Group*. Department of Health, Scottish Office Home and Health Department, Welsh Office and Department of Health and Social Services Northern Ireland. Heywood, Lancashire: Health Publications Unit.

―― (1992*d*) *Report of the Committee on the Ethics of Gene Therapy*. London: HMSO.

DEPARTMENT OF HEALTH & SOCIAL SECURITY (1972) *Census of Mentally Handicapped Patients in Hospital in England and Wales at the end of 1970*. London: HMSO.

―― (1984) Helping mentally handicapped people with special problems: report of a DHSS study team. London: DHSS.

DUPONT, A. (1980) A study concerning the time related and other burdens when severely handicapped children are reared at home. *Acta Psychiatrica Scandinavica*, **62** (Suppl. 285), 249–257.

―― (1986) Socio-psychiatric aspects of the young severely mentally handicapped children on families. *British Journal of Psychiatry*, **148**, 227–234.

DYSON, L. I. (1991) Families with young children with handicaps: parental stress and family functioning. *American Journal of Mental Retardation*, **95**, 623–629.

EASTMAN, C. J. & PHILLIPS, D. I. W. (1988) Endemic goitre and iodine deficiency disorder – aetiology, epidemiology and treatment. *Clinical Endocrinology and Metabolism*, **2**, 719–735.

EDGERTON, R. B. (1986) Alcohol and drug use by mentally retarded adults. *American Journal of Mental Deficiency*, **90**, 602–609.

EPSTEIN, L. G., SHARER, L. R., OLESKE, J. M., et al (1986) Neurologic manifestations of human immunodeficiency virus infection in children. *Paediatrics*, **78**, 678–687.

FERGUSON-SMITH, M. A. (1987) Neural tube defects and Down's syndrome: a success and a failure. In *Screening for Foetal and Genetic Abnormality*, pp. 44–46. London: Kings Fund Forum.

FLYNN, M. C. (1988) *Independent Living for Adults with a Mental Handicap: a Place of My Own*. London: Cassell.

FLYNT, S. & WOOD, T. (1989) Stress and coping of mothers of children with moderate mental retardation. *American Journal of Mental Retardation*, **94**, 278–283.

FRASER, W. I. & RAO, J. M. (1991) Recent studies of mentally handicapped young peoples behaviour. *Journal of Child Psychology and Psychiatry*, **32**, 79–108.

FREY, K., GREENBERG, M. & FEWELL, R. (1989) Stress and coping among parents of handicapped children: a multidimensional approach. *American Journal of Mental Retardation*, **94**, 240–249.

FRYERS, T. (1984) *The Epidemiology of Severe Intellectual Impairment: the Dynamics of Prevalence*. London: Academic Press.

—— (1989) *List of Resources for Training Community Rehabilitation Workers*. Geneva: WHO.

GARBER, H. & HEBER, R. (1977) The Milwaukee project: indications of the effectiveness of early intervention in preventing mental retardation. In *Research to Practice in Mental Retardation* (Vol. 1) (ed. P. Mittler), pp. 119–128. Baltimore: University Park Press.

—— & —— (1982) Modification of predicted cognitive development in high risk children through early intervention. In *How and How Much Can Intelligence Be Increased* (eds D. K. Detterman & R. Sternberg), pp. 131–137. Norwood, NJ: Ablex.

GATH, A. (1978) *Down's Syndrome and the Family: the Early Years*. London: Academic Press.

—— (1990) Down's syndrome children and their families. *American Journal of Medical Genetics* (Suppl.), **7**, 314–316.

GHAZIUDDIN, M. (1988) Behaviour disorder in the mentally handicapped – the role of life events. *British Journal of Psychiatry*, **152**, 683–686.

GILL, M., MURDAY, V. & SLACK, J. (1987) An economic appraisal of screening for Down's syndrome in pregnancy using maternal age and serum alpha fetoprotein concentration. *Social Science and Medicine*, **24**, 725–731.

GILLBERG, C., PEARSON, E., GRUFMAN, E., et al (1986) Psychiatric disorders in mildly and severely mentally retarded urban children and adolescents: epidemiological aspects. *British Journal of Psychiatry*, **149**, 68–74.

GILSON, S. F. & LEVITAS, A. S. (1987) Psychosocial crises in the lives of mentallly retarded people. *Psychiatric Aspects of Mental Retardation Reviews*, **6**, 22–31.

GOSTASON, R. (1985) Psychiatric illness among the mentally retarded: a Swedish population study. *Acta Psychiatrica Scandinavica* (Suppl.), **318**, 1–117.

GUTHRIE, R. & SUSI, A. A. (1963) A simple phenylalanine method for detecting phenylketonuria in a large population of newborn infants. *Paediatrics*, **32**, 338–343.

HAGBERG, B. & HAGBERG, G. (1984) Aspects of prevention of pre-, peri- and post-natal brain pathology in severe and mild mental retardation. In *Scientific Studies in Mental Retardation* (eds J. Dobbing, A. D. B. Clarke, J. A. Corbett, et al), pp. 43–56. London: Royal Society of Medicine & Macmillan.

—— & —— (1985) Neuropaediatric aspects of prevalence, aetiology, prevention and diagnosis. In *Mental Deficiency: The Changing Outlook* (4th Edn) (eds A. M. Clarke, A. D. B. Clarke & J. M. Berg), pp. 326–355. London: Methuen.

HANSHAW, J. B. (1983) Cytomegalovirus. In *Infections & Diseases of the Foetus and NewBorn Infant* (eds J. S. Remington & J. O. Klein), pp. 104–142. Philadelphia: W. B. Saunders.

HELANDER, E., NELSON, S., MENDIS, P., et al (1990) *Training in the Community for People with Disabilities*. Geneva: WHO.

HENTZEL, B. S. (1989) *The Story of Iodine Deficiency*. Oxford: Oxford University Press.

HOLLINS, S. (1989) The family and the mentally handicapped person. *Current Opinion in Psychiatry*, **2**, 623–628.

—— & SIRELING, L. (1991) *Working Through Loss with People Who Have Learning Disabilities*. Windsor, Berkshire: Nfer-Nelson.

HOLOWINSKY, I. Z. (1993) Chernobyl nuclear catastrophe and the high risk potential for mental retardation. *Mental Retardation*, **31**, 35–40.

HUNTER, A. G. W., EVANS, J. A., THOMPSON, D. R., et al (1980) A study of institutionalised mentally retarded patients in Manitoba: 1. Classification and preventability. *Developmental Medicine and Child Neurology*, **22**, 145–162.

ILLSLEY, R. & MITCHELL, R. J. (1984) *Low Birth Weight*. Chichester: Wiley.

JAMES, D. H. (1986) Psychiatric and behaviour disorders amongst older severely mentally handicapped inpatients. *Journal of Mental Deficiency Research*, **30**, 341–345.

JENKINS, R., BROOKSBANK, D. & MILLER, E. (1994) Ageing in mental deficiency: the development of health care outcome indicators. *Journal of Intellectual Disability Research*, **38**, 257–264.

KABACK, M. M. (1985) Annual update of TSD carrier detection and prenatal diagosis experience. International Tay-Sachs Disease Testing Quality Control and Data Collection Centre. (Quoted in Crocker, 1992).

KEENAN, J., KASTNER, T., NATHANSON, R., et al (1992) A statewide public and professional education programme on Fragile X syndrome. *Mental Retardation*, **30**, 355–361.

KOCH, R., AZEN, C. G., HURST, N., et al (1987) The effects of diet discontinuation in children with phenylketonuria, US collaborative study. *European Journal of Paediatrics*, **146** (Suppl. 1), 12–16.

——, HANLEY, W., LEVY, H., et al (1990) A preliminary report of the corroborative study of maternal phenylketonuria in the United States and Canada. *Journal of Inherited Metabolic Diseases*, **13**, 641–650.

KOLLER, H., RICHARDSON, S. A. & KATZ, M. (1987) Antecedents of behaviour disturbance in mildly mentally retarded young adults. *Uppsala Journal of Medical Science*, (Suppl.) **44**, 105–110.

KONIG, M. P., MORDASINI, C., KOHLER, H., et al (1985) Diagnostic value of the measurement of iodine in urine and blood. In *Thyroid Disorders Associated with Iodine Deficiency and Excess* (eds R. Hall & J. Kobberling). *Serono Symposium Series*, **22**, 137–143. New York: Raven Press.

KRISHEF, C. H. & DINITTO, D. M. (1981) Alcohol abuse among mentally retarded individuals. *Mental Retardation*, **19**, 151–156.

LANCET (1983) Editorial. Congenital cytomegalovirus infection. *Lancet*, **i**, 801–802.

—— (1986a) Editorial. Preventive screening for Fragile X syndrome. *Lancet*, **ii**, 1191–1192.

—— (1986b) Editorial. Prevention and control of iodine deficiency disorders. *Lancet*, **ii**, 433–434.

—— (1990) Editorial. Declining mortality from Down's syndrome – no cause for complacency. *Lancet*, **335**, 888–889.

—— (1991) Editorial. Chorion villus sampling: valuable addition or dangerous alternative? *Lancet*, **337**, 1513–1515.

LAURENCE, K. M., JAMES, N., MILLER, M., et al (1980) Increased risk of recurrence of pregnancies complicated by foetal neural tube defects in mothers receiving poor diets and possible benefits of dietary counselling. *British Medical Journal*, **281**, 1592–1594.

LAVOXA, R., RIDLER, M. A. C. & BOWEN-BRAVERY, M. (1977) An aetiological survey of the severely retarded Hertfordshire children who were born between January 1st 1965 and January 31st 1967. *American Journal of Medical Genetics*, **1**, 75–86.

LARSSON, G. (1983) Prevention of foetal alcohol effects – an antenatal programme for early detection for pregnancies at risk. *Acta Obstetrica et Gynecologica Scandinavica*, **62**, 171–178.

LIFSCHITZ, M. A., WILSON, G. S., SMITH, E. O., et al (1985) Factors affecting head growth and intellectual function in children of addicts. *Paediatrics*, **101**, 269–274.

LUND, J. (1985) The prevalence of psychiatric morbidity in mentally retarded adults. *Acta Psychiatrica Scandinavica*, **72**, 563–570.

MACFARLANE, A. & MUGFORD, M. (1984) *Birth Counts: Statistics of Pregnancy and Childbirth*. London: HMSO.

MARTIN, S. L., RAMEY, C. T. & RAMEY, S. L. (1990) The prevention of intellectual impairment in children of impoverished families: the findings of a randomised trial of educational day care. *American Journal of Public Health*, **80**, 844–847.

MCCORMICK, M. C. (1985) The contribution of low birth weight to infant mortality and childhood morbidity. *New England Journal of Medicine*, **312**, 89–90.

MCLOUGHLIN, I. J. (1986) Bereavement in the mentally handicapped. *British Journal of Hospital Medicine*, **36**, 256–260.

MIKKELSEN, M., POULSEN, H. & NIELSEN, K. G. (1990) Incidence, survival and mortality in Down's syndrome in Denmark. *American Journal of Medical Genetics*, (Suppl. 7), 75–78.

MITTLER, P. (1984) Evaluation of services and staff training. In *Scientific Studies in Mental Retardation* (eds J. Dobbing, A. D. B. Clarke, J. A. Corbett, et al), pp. 547–567. London: Royal Society of Medicine & Macmillan.

—— & SERPELL, R. (1985) Services: an international perspective. In *Mental Deficiency: The Changing Outlook* (eds A. M. Clarke, A. D. B. Clarke & J. M. Berg), pp. 715–787. London: Methuen.

MRC VITAMIN STUDY GROUP (1991) Prevention of neural tube defects: results of the Medical Research Council Vitamin Study Group. *Lancet*, **338**, ii, 131–137.

NATIONAL HEALTH SERVICE AND COMMUNITY CARE ACT (1990) London: HMSO.

NAUGHTEN, E. R. (1989) Continuation versus discontinuation of diet in phenylketonuria. *European Journal of Clinical Nutrition*, **43**, 7-12.

N'GALY, B., RYDER, R. W., FRANCIS, H., *et al* (1988) HIV prevalence in Zaire 1984-1988. (Abstract) 4th International Conference on AIDS. Stockholm.

NTABA, H. M. LIOMBA, G. N., SCHMIDT, H. J., *et al* (1988) HIV prevalence in hospital patients and pregnant women in Mulawe. (Abstract) 4th International Conference on AIDS. Stockholm.

OFFICE OF HEALTH ECONOMICS (1986) Mental handicap: partnership in the community. *Studies of Current Health Problems*, No. 83. Office of Health Economics, London.

OKANO, Y., EISENSMITH, R. C., GÜTTER, F., *et al* (1991) Molecular basis of phenotypic heterogenicity in phenylketonuria. *New England Journal of Medicine*, **324**, 1232-1238.

O'TOOLE, B. (1987) Community based rehabilitation (CBR): problems and possibilities. *European Journal of Special Needs Education*, **2**, 177-190.

PATEL, P., GOLDBERG, D. & MOSS, S. (1993) Psychiatric morbidity in older people with moderate and severe learning disability II: the prevalence study. *British Journal of Psychiatry*, **163**, 481-491.

PECKHAM, C. S., COLEMAN, J. C., HURLEY, R., *et al* (1983) Cytomegalovirus infection in pregnancy: preliminary findings from a prospective study. *Lancet*, **i**, 1352-1355.

POPE, A. M. (1992) Preventing secondary conditions. *Mental Retardation*, **30**, 347-354.

RAMEY, C. T. & HASKINS, R. (1981) The modification of intelligence through early experience. *Intelligence*, **5**, 5-17.

―――― & RAMEY, S. L. (1992) Effective early intervention. *Mental Retardation*, **30**, 337-346.

RAMEY, S. L. (1991) The family. *Current Opinion in Psychiatry*, **4**, 678-682.

REISS, S. (1990) The prevalence of dual diagnosis in community based day programmes in the Chicago metropolitan area. *American Journal of Mental Retardation*, **94**, 578-585.

―――― & BENSON, B. A. (1985) Psychosocial correlates of depression in mentally retarded adults. 1. Minimal support and stigmatisation. *American Journal of Mental Deficiency*, **89**, 331-337.

RICHARDSON, S. A. (1984) The consequences of malnutrition for intellectual development. In *Scientific Studies in Mental Retardation* (eds J. Dobbing, A. D. B. Clarke & J. Corbett, *et al*), pp. 233-250. London: Macmillan.

―――― (1987) The ecology of mental handicap. *Journal of the Royal Society of Medicine*, **80**, 203-206.

―――― (1990) For whom is amelioration and secondary prevention intended in mild mental handicap? In *Combatting Mental Handicap* (eds P. L. C. Evans & A. D. B. Clarke), pp. 135-144. Bister, Oxon: AB Academic.

――――, KOLLER, H. & KATZ, M. (1985) Relationship of upbringing to later behaviour disturbance of mildly mentally retarded young people. *American Journal of Mental Deficiency*, **90**, 1-8.

ROBERTSON, C. M. T., ETCHES, P. C. & KYLE, J. M. (1990) Eight years school performance and growth of pre-term, small for gestational age infants: a comparative study with subjects matched for birth weight and gestation age. *Journal of Paediatrics*, **116**, 19-26.

ROGERS, R. C. & SIMENSEN, R. J. (1987) Fragile X syndrome: the common aetiology of mental retardation. *American Journal of Mental Deficiency*, **91**, 445-449.

ROYAL COLLEGE OF PSYCHIATRISTS (1986) Psychiatric services for mentally handicapped adults and young people. *Psychiatric Bulletin*, **10**, 321-322.

RUSSELL, J. A. O. (1990) Families of children with severe disabilities. *Current Opinion in Psychiatry*, **3**, 634-638.

RUTTER, M., TIZARD, J., YULE, W., *et al* (1976) Isle of Wight Studies 1964-1974. *Psychological Medicine*, **7**, 313-332.

SARTORIUS, N. (1984) Mental retardation – a world view. In *Scientific Studies in Mental Retardation* (eds J. Dobbing, A. D. B. Clarke, J. Corbett, *et al*), pp. 573-580. London: Royal Society of Medicine & Macmillan.

SELTZER, M. M. & SELTZER, S. B. (1985) The elderly mentally retarded: a group in need of service. In *Gerontological Social Work Practice in the Community* (eds G. Getzei & J. Mellor), pp. 99-119. New York: Haworth Press.

SELTZER, G. B., BEQUIN, A., SELTZER, M. M., *et al* (1991) Adults with mental retardation and their ageing mothers: impacts of siblings. *Family Reactions*, **40**, 1-8.

SIMON, V. A., ABRAMS, M. T., FREUND, L. S., *et al* (1990) The Fragile X phenotype: cognitive, behavioural and neurobiological profiles. *Current Opinion in Psychiatry*, **3**, 581-586.

SINGER, P. (1983) Sanctity of life or equality of life. *Paediatrics*, **72**, 128-129.

SMITH, I., BEASLEY, M. G. & ADES, A. E. (1990a) Intelligence and quality of dietary treatments in phenylketonuria. *Archives of Diseases of Children*, **65**, 472-478.

――――, GLOSSOP, J. & BEASLEY, M. (1990b) Fetal damage due to maternal phenylketonuria: effects of dietary treatments and maternal phenylalanine concentrations around the time of conception. *Journal of Inherited Metabolic Disease*, **13**, 651-657.

SMITH, S. M. & HANSON, R. (1974) 134 battered children: a medical and psychological study. *British Medical Journal*, **3**, 660-670.
SMITHELLS, R. W., SHEPHARD, S., HOLZE, L., *et al* (1985) National Congenital Rubella Surveillance Programme. 1.7.71-30.6.84. *British Medical Journal*, **291**, 40-41.
SPOHR, H. L., WILLMS, J. & STEINHAUSEN, H. C. (1993) Prenatal alcohol exposure and long term developmental consequences. *Lancet*, **341**, 907-910.
STERN, J. (1985) Biochemical aspects. In *Mental Deficiency: The Changing Outlook* (4th Edn) (eds A. M. Clarke, A. D. B. Clarke & J. M. Berg), pp. 135-212. London: Methuen.
SUTHERLAND, G. R. (1979) Heritable fragile sites on human chromosomes. *American Journal of Human Genetics*, **31**, 125-148.
THAKE, A., TODD, J. & WEBB, T. (1987) Children with Fragile X chromosomes in schools for the mildly mentally retarded. *Developmental Medicine and Child Neurology*, **29**, 711-719.
THOMPSON, A. J., SMITH, I., BRENTON, D., *et al* (1990) Neurological deterioration in young adults with phenylketonuria. *Lancet*, **336**, 602-605.
TURNER, G., ROBINSON, H., LAING, S., *et al* (1992) Population screening for Fragile X. *Lancet*, **339**, 1210-1213.
TYLDEN, E. (1973) The effects of maternal drug abuse on the foetus and infant. *Adverse Drug Reaction Bulletin*, **38**. Newcastle upon Tyne: Newcastle Regional Hospital Board.
ULTMANN, M. H., BELMAN, A. L., RUFF, H. A., *et al* (1985) Developmental abnormalities in infants and children with acquired immune deficiency syndrome (AIDS) and AIDS related complex. *Developmental Medicine and Child Neurology*, **27**, 563-571.
VARLEY, C. K. (1984) Schizophreniform psychoses in mentally retarded adolescent girls following sexual assault. *American Journal of Psychiatry*, **141**, 593-595.
VERSLUYS, C. (1993) Ethics of neonatal care. *Lancet*, **341**, 794-795.
WAHLSTROM, J. (1990) Gene map of mental retardation. *Journal of Mental Deficiency Research*, **34**, 11-27.
WALD, N. J., CUCKLE, H. S., DENSEM, J. W., *et al* (1988) Maternal serum screening for Down's syndrome in early pregnancy. *British Medical Journal*, **297**, 883-887.
——, KENNARD, A., DEMSEN, J. W., *et al* (1992) Antenatal maternal serum screening for Down's syndrome: results of a demonstration project. *British Medical Journal*, **305**, 391-394.
WALKER, D. K. & MESSENGER, K. P. (1992) Quoted In: CROCKER, A. C. Data collection of the evaluation of mental retardation prevention strategies: the fateful 43. *Mental Retardation*, **30**, 305-317.
WARD, R. H. T. (1984) First trimester chorionic villus sampling. In *Prenatal Diagnosis* (eds C. H. Rodeck & K. H. Nicolaides), pp. 99-103. London: Royal College of Obstetricians and Gynaecologists.
WATERSON, E. J. & MURRAY-LYON, I. M. (1990) Preventing alcohol related birth damage: a review. *Social Science and Medicine*, **30**, 349-364.
WATSON, J. (1993) Tuberculosis in Britain today. *British Medical Journal*, **306**, 221-222.
WEATHERALL, D. J. (1991) *The New Genetics and Clinical Practice* (3rd Edn) Oxford: Oxford University Press.
WEBB, T. B., BUNDEY, S. & THAKE, A. (1986) The frequency of the Fragile X chromosome amongst schoolchildren in Coventry. *Journal of Medical Genetics*, **23**, 396-399.
WELSH OFFICE NHS DIRECTORATE (1992) *Mental Handicap (Learning Disabilities) Protocol for Investment in Health Gain*. Cardiff: Welsh Health Planning Forum, Welsh Office.
WILKIN, D. (1979) *Caring for the Mentally Handicapped Child*. London: Croom Helm.
WORLD HEALTH ORGANIZATION (1980) *International Classification of Impairments, Disabilities and Handicaps*. Geneva: WHO.
—— (1985) *Mental Retardation: Meeting the Challenge*. WHO Offset Publications, No. 86. Geneva: WHO.
—— (1992) *Assessment of People with Mental Retardation*. Geneva: WHO.
—— (1993) Guidelines for the primary prevention of mental, neurological and psychosocial disorders. *2. Mental Retardation*. Geneva: WHO.
WYNN, A. & WYNN, M. (1979) *Prevention of Handicap and the Health of Women*. London: Routledge & Keegan Paul.
WYNN-GRIFFITHS, G. (1973) The prevention of Down's syndrome (Mongolism). *Health Trends*, **5**, 59-60.
YAMAZAKI, J. N. (1966) A review of the literature on the radiation dosage required to cause manifest CNS disturbances from *in utero* and postnatal exposure. *Paediatrics* (Suppl.), **37**, 877-897.
——, WRIGHT, S. W. & WRIGHT, P. M. (1954) Outcome of pregnancy in women exposed to the atomic bomb in Nagasaki. *American Journal of Diseases of Children*, **87**, 448-465.
ZUCKERMAN, B., FRANK, D. A., HINGSON, R., *et al* (1989) Effects of maternal marijuana and cocaine use on fetal growth. *New England Journal of Medicine*, **320**, 762-768.

15 Old age psychiatry

DAVID J. JOLLEY

The elderly represent an important group within the population. The number of old people within the UK has increased progressively from 1900, when there were 1.7 millon people over the age of 65, to the present where there are over 8.8 million in this age group. This increase is projected to continue – by the middle of the 21st century there will be in excess of 12 million old people in the UK. The proportion of the population within this age bracket has increased from 4.7% to 15.8% and will rise to over 20%. Within the elderly population the proportion aged over 75 and over 85 have increased disproportionately and will continue to do so (Family Policy Studies, 1991).

The prevalence of disabling psychiatric disorder is relatively high in late life. Some people develop new psychiatric disorders within old age while others have survived into late life with established chronic or relapsing psychiatric disorder (Eastwood & Corbin, 1985). About one-third of all admissions to psychiatric care involve people over the age of 65, as do one-third of referrals to community orientated psychiatric services. Almost two-thirds of resident patients in psychiatric care are currently over the age of 65 (Benbow & Jolley, 1992). Most psychiatric morbidity within old age is managed in non-psychiatric arenas. The elderly with mental disorders are making heavy demands upon informal carers (Levin *et al*, 1989), domiciliary support services (Foster *et al*, 1976), as well as residential care and other hospital services (Kay *et al*, 1970). Thus success in the prevention of psychiatric disorder among the elderly will have substantial benefits not only for individuals but also for the dynamics and economics of welfare and health care delivery for the nation.

Disorders arising in the senium

Depression and other neurotic disorders

Depressive mood is the commonest psychiatric disorder of late life, affecting of the order of 15% of the 65 year age group. Severe biological depressives are less common constituting 1–2% (Eastwood & Corbin, 1985). Anxiety states *per se* or phobias have received less attention but may be more important than has been realised hitherto (Lindesay, 1991). The misery, anxiety, loss of confidence, loss of weight, loss of sleep, loss of tolerance and resilience to other stresses associated with affective disorder mean that health and abilities may not be regained after apparent recovery from physical illness. There is increased dependence upon others for personal and psychological support, for housekeeping, fetching and carrying. There is a requirement for prolonged treatment, rehabilitation and long-term institutional care.

Unresolved depression is associated with reduced life expectancy, death usually occurring from natural causes, less frequently from suicide (Barraclough *et al*, 1974; Murphy *et al*, 1988).

Aetiology

The onset and maintenance of depressed mood is associated with change, particularly change which represents loss to the individual (Murphy, 1982). Retirement, move of home, bereavement, and, most markedly, physical ill health are associated with depression.

Strategies for prevention

Primary: Prevention of physical ill health and programmes to prepare people for the inevitable changes associated with late life such as retirement, and losses by bereavement, should, in theory, reduce the incidence of depressive mood and other affective changes. Action research is lacking.

Secondary prevention: The early detection of people suffering from mood disorders could be enhanced by screening or surveillance of people suffering from ill health, recently bereaved, recently moved home etc. Action research is limited.

Tertiary prevention: There is good evidence that individuals can be helped to recover from depression and other affective disorders once they have been identified. Treatments include psychological and physical treatment methods (Post, 1982). Maintenance of good mood requires ongoing surveillance and treatment and this is associated with decreased morbidity and probably a decreased mortality (Baldwin & Jolley, 1986).

Dementia

Dementia is a syndrome characterised by an acquired impairment of memory and other cognitive functions, change of personality, and a progressive erosion of personal and social skills. In the later stages patients become severely debilitated and death is brought forward. In some instances dementia is symptomatic of underlying physical or other psychiatric illness and treatment of the underlying cause may resolve the dementia (Lishman, 1987). The most common cause of dementia in this country is senile dementia of the Alzheimer type, followed by multi-infarct dementia. Surveys suggest that about 5% of the population over 65 at any one time are impaired by a dementia; the prevalence increases with age, with only 1–2% suffering from the condition in the age bracket 65–74, and 20% or more in the 85+ age bracket (Copeland, 1989). There is evidence that the incidence and prevalence of dementia differ in different places with people from poor inner city areas appearing to be more prone to develop the condition and to survive for a shorter period with it (Copeland *et al*, 1987). There is the possibility that the incidence of dementia is falling in successive generations (Hagnell et al, 1981) and that intellectual capacities are better preserved in successive generations (Berg, 1980).

The morbidity associated with dementia is enormous: patients lose abilities and dignity, and resistance to intercurrent stress and illness is impaired. There is a massively increased likelihood of reliance upon care from others both at home and in institutions. There is an indirect morbidity through the stress upon carers, family members and others (Levin et al, 1989).

Aetiologies

Symptomatic dementias may be produced by a range of alternative pathologies (Lishman, 1987). In older people the possibility of multiple pathology and multiple medication is ever present and may contribute to the development of a dementia syndrome.

Dementia of the Alzheimer type has been demonstrated to have familial genetic origins in some families particularly where the onset is in the pre-senium or early senium (Shalat et al, 1986). The search for environmental factors or factors of lifestyle prejudicing towards the development of Alzheimer's disease has followed a number of trails, none of them giving certain evidence of causation. Possibilities include it being the late sequel to a viral infection or something similar, the direct toxic effect of one or more agents (among these aluminium has been favoured) or an auto-immune process. As outlined above the observation that incidence, survival and prevalence of Alzheimer type dementias differ in different parts of the world, and may differ in different generations, gives encouragement to the prospect of identifying important environmental agents, but for the moment that remains a prospect.

Multi-infarct dementia is associated with male sex and with the occurrence of atherosclerosis which is predicted by the various risk factors which contribute to heart disease, stroke disease, and other atherosclerotic ailments. Hypertension is identified as a certain risk factor for the development of multi-infarct dementia.

Strategies for prevention

Symptomatic dementias. Primary prevention: This looks to the avoidance, early detection and treatment of those physical illnesses or other psychiatric disorders which produce a dementia-type syndrome.

Secondary prevention: This rests on the early identification of cognitive change associated with intercurrent illnesses and with their prescribed treatments, and energetic treatment and reappraisal of the situation, with a view to reducing the cognitive change as far as possible.

Tertiary prevention: Where cognitive change has developed and progressed it still remains possible to arrest further progress. This requires ongoing surveillance and energetic treatment and rehabilitation throughout.

Alzheimer type dementia. Primary prevention: It may be possible in some families to avoid the development of Alzheimer type dementia by genetic counselling. In Huntington's chorea counselling exercises have reduced the incidence of the disorder in some parts of this country and others. The understanding of Alzheimer's disease and the provision of early markers is not so well developed in this condition as in Huntington's chorea, but it remains a very real possibility for the near future.

The unusual forms of Alzheimer type dementia associated with repeated head trauma, particularly from boxing, could clearly be avoided by banning sports in which repeated head trauma occurs.

Secondary prevention: It is not clear that there are any strategies yet available.

Tertiary prevention: Once changes of an Alzheimer type dementia have been identified, progression of the disorder can certainly be influenced by providing a good level of general medical care and appropriate management of the social and personal environment. Thus life expectancy among people with dementia has clearly been increased by the more general availability of good quality care both at home and in institutions (Christie, 1985) and the experience of life within the dementia can similarly be improved by the provision of just such services. It is likely that patients can be enabled to remain at home for longer with the provision of comprehensive support services and adequate back-up from day hospitals and, if needs be, respite care in institutions. Once a person moves into an institution the provision of an appropriate environment near to their home makes life much better than if 'put away' in the squalid conditions which were available in mental hospitals in the 1950s.

An important component of treatment and care involves the treatment of intercurrent psychiatric symptomatology such as anxiety, depression, hallucinations, and paranoid ideation. All these symptoms can be helped by psychotherapeutic approaches, by the provision of a supportive and sympathetic environment and/or by the prescription of appropriate medications.

Multi-infarct dementia. Primary prevention: A number of risk factors are well recognised for the development of atherosclerotic changes in general, and atherosclerosis which may produce heart attacks or stroke disease in particular (Christie, 1985; Welin *et al*, 1987; Smith *et al*, 1989). Energetic pursuit of strategies to reduce these risk factors has been shown to reduce the incidence of coronary artery morbidity and deaths and stroke morbidity (Malmgren *et al*, 1987; Working Group of Coronary Prevention Group and British Heart Foundation, 1991). It is probable that similar strategies reduce the incidence of multi-infarct dementia.

Secondary and tertiary prevention: Once an individual has started to suffer from atherosclerotic brain disease it is more difficult to be sure of the best strategy. It is probable that control of blood pressure within normal limits is helpful (MRC Working Party, 1992). Some people believe that the use of aspirin or similar compounds is justified and helpful (Orme, 1988). Otherwise one is left with the general approaches to good care, good general medical care and appropriate support to the individual on a personal basis in their social context as for Alzheimer's disease outlined above.

Paranoid disorders

Paranoid disorders are less common than either depression or the dementias although paranoid symptoms may occur in the course of mood disorder or dementia. Paranoid personality developments or paraphrenic illnesses, which probably reflect extremes of related dimensions, occur in 1–2% of the elderly population. Most surveys identify more elderly female paranoids than males. There is clearly an association between specific sensory deficits, particularly impairment of hearing and the development of paranoid ideas and auditory hallucinations. Elderly paranoids may remain quite independent and, indeed, cut themselves off from other people almost entirely. They may get into difficulties through their hostility towards neighbours or authorities. Their life expectation is not generally reduced. Problems occur if and when they develop physical illnesses that require extra help.

Aetiology

Lifestyle of independence and suspiciousness often associated with great energy seems to be common among elderly paranoids. The development of physical infirmity, particularly sensory deficits as outlined above, seems to be important.

Strategies for prevention

Primary: Lifestyle is almost certainly impossible to alter but the early detection and treatment of hearing or visual impairment and so forth would seem likely to have potential for reducing the incidence of paranoid states.

Secondary and tertiary: Once identified, paranoid disorders can be effectively treated with neuroleptic medication. This is not without its hazards as unwanted side-effects are more common among elderly people. Whatever is prescribed, it is important that interested and informed professional teams monitor that medication is being taken and that side-effects are being recognised and treated if and when they emerge. It is probably more important than a worthwhile supportive relationship developed between professional carers and the paranoid that they take their medication all the time. Before the availability of community psychiatry and effective neuroleptics many elderly paranoids were admitted to mental hospitals to spend many years there until their deaths. It is relatively unusual for such people to need to be admitted to hospital at all if appropriate regimes are made available, and if they are admitted the time in care may only be short.

Delirium

This is a symptomatic psychosis characterised by the sudden development of confused thinking, disorientation, disordered sleep rhythm and clouding of consciousness. There is a great variability of mood as well as of grasp and there is considerable variability through different parts of the day and night-time, with disturbance being most characteristically at night. Disturbance may include psychomotor changes, hallucinations, particularly in the visual mode and changeable delusional ideas. The development of delirium produces great hazard to the individual who is not capable of providing or protecting for themselves. There is an associated high mortality in excess of uncomplicated similar physical illnesses.

Aetiology

Delirium is caused by underlying physical illness and almost any severe illness may precipitate delirium in a vulnerable person. Elderly people are all deemed vulnerable to delirium and this is particularly so for people suffering from one of the dementias. Medication is often responsible for producing delirious states, the anti-depressants and anti-Parkinsonian agents being particularly common culprits. Of the physical illnesses themselves intercurrent chest infections are probably the most common, although cerebrovascular disease and heart disease are also important (Jolley, 1981).

Strategies for prevention

Primary: The identification of particularly vulnerable individuals, particularly those suffering from dementia, is important. The avoidance of extra stresses and extra illness may be possible, for instance, moving people from one place to another may be sufficient to release confusion and sometimes can be avoided. The prescription of powerful medications which may have side-effects or may interact with other medication, can sometimes be avoided. Early surveillance for the emergence of infections and their energetic and appropriate treatment, if possible at home, may similarly avoid the development of confusional states.

Secondary and tertiary prevention: Once a confusional state is identified it is almost always necessary to manage the patient in hospital unless a great deal of support can be available within the home. Energetic examination, investigation, and treatment of the underlying cause are the most important of activities and will reduce longer term sequelae. In addition appropriate management in a sympathetic, confident, nursing framework reduces distress. Psychotropic medication, particularly the neuroleptics, may play a part in controlling distress, agitation and psychotic thinking. It is important to avoid secondary and tertiary complications such as severe debility, pressure sores, and becoming bedfast. It is most important that family and carers understand that there is the possibility of recovery and that the prospect for delirium is quite different from that for dementia. Recovery from delirium may be complete or it may be followed by a period of sub-acute confusion or persisting dementia. Thus individuals require careful supervision after the acute episode and follow-up. Similarly, having had one episode of delirium clearly identifies that individual as vulnerable to subsequent episodes, and they should be followed very carefully to try and avoid stresses and illness that might precipitate a recurrence.

Other syndromes developing in late life

Outlined above are the most important syndromes in terms of number and severity. Other syndromes may develop and are recognised as perhaps increasingly important. Among these the use and abuse of alcohol is emerging as a particular problem with women who have survived their husbands and become distressed or depressed with the life left to them. The development of anxiety states and phobic states associated with physical disability or with the increase in prevalence of violence towards old people are also worthy of note.

The syndrome of abuse of elderly, or elder abuse, is receiving increasing interest and prominence.

Carers

There is a particular issue of the production of secondary stress and psychiatric disorder among carers of elderly people who develop psychiatric disorders. An enormous number of dependent elderly people are cared for on an informal basis by members of their own family and occasionally unrelated people, and a useful and appropriate literature is being built up on the problems from which they suffer (Levin et al, 1989). It seems clear that the early identification, effective treatment and responsible follow-through of patients with psychiatric disorder in late life will minimise the stress and distress caused to carers. In addition it is often possible with responsible and comprehensive services to enable carers to continue to care for longer than they would otherwise have done, helping them to achieve greater satisfaction with their task.

The occurrence of elder abuse is sometimes associated with exposing carers to too much stress and responsibility because of the unavailability or the insensitivity of services. The personal characteristics of carers as well as their mental health requires careful monitoring and response if the best model of care for elderly people is to be sustained.

Survival into late life with established psychiatric disorders

The concept of 'graduates' has developed to describe those elderly people living out their lives in mental hospitals with major psychotic illnesses, usually schizophrenia or manic depressive psychosis, with onset at an early stage of life. The lifestyle of care in a mental hospital until death, previously available to such chronic psychotics, may not have given them an optimal life. Certainly the availability of asylum care has become less and less in England over the last 10 years and will probably disappear in the near future. This means that elderly people who have experienced a lifetime of mental illness are to be found living with their families or in hostels or, indeed, out of touch with any apparent caring organisation (Campbell, 1991). It behoves us to be aware of their presence and their needs and to make appropriate care available.

Strategies for prevention

Primary: Would require the avoidance of psychiatric disorder in earlier life or its completely effective treatment.

Secondary: All people who have suffered from psychiatric disorder in earlier life which has a chronic progressive or relapsing nature should remain under supervision and active treatment into and through the senium.

Tertiary: Having achieved graduation into late life with an established chronic or relapsing disorder it is important that all appropriate services remain available to individuals. This would probably best be done by maintaining a register of such individuals and being sure that they are kept in touch with services or put in touch with more appropriate services which are available to the elderly. There is the real possibility that people are lost to contact because of the discontinuity between services for the 'general adult population' and the 'elderly population'. This has developed to some extent within the health services and often more particularly so within social services.

It is very likely that social, physical as well as mental health care needs to change as a person gets older, so frequent review of all components of their health is required.

References

BALDWIN, R. & JOLLEY, D. (1986) The prognosis of depression in old age. *British Journal of Psychiatry*, **149**, 574–583.
BARRACLOUGH, B. M., BUNCH, J., NELSON, B., *et al* (1974) One hundred cases of suicide. *British Journal of Psychiatry*, **125**, 355–373.
BENBOW, S. & JOLLEY, D. (1992) A cause for concern – changing fabric of psychogeriatric care. *Psychiatric Bulletin*, **16**, 533–535.
BERG, S. (1980) Psychological functioning in 70 and 75 year old people. *Acta Psychiatrica Scandinavica* **62**, (Suppl. 288).
CAMPBELL, P. G. (1991) Graduates. In *Psychiatry in the Elderly* (eds R. Jacoby & C. Oppenheimer), pp. 779–818. Oxford: Oxford Medical.
CHRISTIE, A. B. (1985) Survival in dementia: a review. In *Recent Advances in Psychogeriatrics* (ed. T. Arie), pp. 33–44. Edinburgh: Churchill Livingstone.
COPELAND, J. R. M. (1989) Epidemiology of the mental disorders of old age. *Current Opinion in Psychiatry*, **2**, 548–551.
——, GURLAND, B. J., DEWEY, M. E., *et al* (1987) Is there more dementia, depression and neurosis in New York? *British Journal of Psychiatry*, **151**, 466–473.
EASTWOOD, R. & CORBIN, S. (1985) Epidemiology of mental disorders in old age. In *Recent Advances in Psychogeriatrics* (ed. T. Arie), pp. 17–32. Edinburgh: Churchill Livingstone.
FAMILY POLICY STUDIES (1991) *An Ageing Population*. Fact Sheet 2. London: Family Policy Studies, 231 Baker St.
FOSTER, E. M., KAY, D. W. K. & BERGMANN, K. (1976) The characteristics of old people receiving and needing domiciliary services. *Age and Ageing*, **5**, 345–355.
HAGNELL, O., LANKE, J., RORSMAN, B., *et al* (1981) Does the incidence age psychosis decrease? *Neuropsychobiology*, **7**, 201–211.
JOLLEY, D. (1981) Acute confusional states in the elderly. In *Acute Geriatric Medicine* (ed. D. Coakley), pp. 175–189. London: Croom Helm.
KAY, D. W. K., BERGMANN, K., FOSTER, E. M., *et al* (1970) Mental illness and hospital usage in the elderly. *Comprehensive Psychiatry*, **11**, 26–35.
LEVIN, E., SINCLAIR, J. & GORBACH, P. (1989) *Families, Services and Confusion in Old Age*. Avebury.
LINDESAY, J. (1991) Anxiety disorders in the elderly. In *Psychiatry in the Elderly* (eds R. Jacoby & C. Oppenheimer), pp. 735–757. Oxford: Oxford Medical.
LISHMAN, W. A. (1987) *Organic Psychiatry*, (2nd Edn). Oxford: Blackwell Scientific.
MALMGREN, R., WARLOW, C., BAMFORD, J., *et al* (1987) Geographical and secular trends in stroke incidence. *Lancet*, **2**, 1196–1200.
MRC WORKING PARTY (1992) Medical Research Council Trial of treatment of hypertension in older adults. *British Medical Journal*, **304**, 405–412.
MURPHY, E. (1982) Social origins of depression in old age. *British Journal of Psychiatry*, **141**, 135–142.
——, SMITH, R. & LINDESAY, J. (1988) Increased mortality rates in late life depression. *British Journal of Psychiatry,* **152**, 347–353.
NAGUIB, M. & LEVY, R. (1991) Paranoid states in the elderly. In *Psychiatry in the Elderly* (eds R. Jacoby & C. Oppenheimer), pp. 758–778. Oxford: Oxford Medical.
ORME, M. (1988) Aspirin all round? *British Medical Journal*, **296**, 307–308.
POST, F. (1982) Functional disorders: treatment and its relationship to causation and outcome. In *Psychiatry of Late Life* (eds R. Levy & F. Post), pp. 197–221. Oxford: Blackwell Scientific.

SHALAT, S. L., SELTZER, B., PIDCOCK, C., *et al* (1986) Case control study of medical and family history and Alzheimer's disease. *American Journal of Epidemiology*, **124**, 540–551.

SMITH, W. C., TUNSTALL-PEDOE, H., CROMBIE, I. K., *et al* (1989) Concomitants of excess coronary deaths – major risk factor and lifestyle – findings from 10 359 men and women. *Scottish Medical Journal*, **34**, 550–555.

WELIN, L., SVARDSUDD, K., WILHELMSEN, L., *et al* (1987) Analysis of risk factors for stroke in a cohort of men born in 1913. *New England Journal of Medicine*, **317**, 521–526.

WORKING GROUP OF CORONARY PREVENTION GROUP AND BRITISH HEART FOUNDATION (1991) An action plan for preventing coronary heart disease in primary care. *British Medical Journal*, **303**, 748–750.

16 Forensic psychiatry

PAMELA J. TAYLOR

Forensic psychiatry is for the problems of people with a recognised mental disease, or suspected mental disease, who also come into contact with the law, or who by virtue of their behaviour or experiences are likely to do so. Most of the work of forensic psychiatry in Britain is concerned with mentally abnormal offenders – whether or not their offending behaviour results in criminal charges and progress through the criminal justice system. The work is weighted towards the provision of clinical assessment and treatment services, but the preparation of reports for the courts and other statutory bodies forms an important part of it too. Some forensic psychiatrists also work extensively with the survivors of criminal assaults or disasters – again both in treatment provision and court reporting. The two patient groups raise different issues, but there is considerable overlap, not least because many offenders have had earlier experience of being victims.

The speciality of forensic psychiatry is, in contrast to that forensic psychiatric work practised as part of general psychiatry, in general, a tertiary referral service. In practice, therefore, prevention work in relation to the mentally abnormal offender inevitably tends to be biased towards the prevention of repetition of unwanted behaviour which has already occurred, to early detection of continuing or extended risk and towards limitation of disability. Although most mentally disordered offenders are between 20 and 50, and most suffer from schizophrenia or a personality disorder, they may be of any age and suffer from any disorder, and so nothing that is a valid option for prevention in other branches of psychiatry can be ignored in forensic psychiatry. There are, however, some special issues too. Much is now known about the antecedents of offending behaviour, which opens possibilities for primary prevention.

Survivors of trauma similarly tend to present as secondary or tertiary referrals, and so direct psychiatric preventive work with them is also generally in secondary prevention fields. Such survivors are most likely to suffer from severe neurotic disorder, perhaps especially anxiety disorders including phobias, or from substance misuse, and they are known to have a high rate of chronic disability and suicide compared with the general population. Only government or social policy can substantially prevent victimisation in, for example, the reduction of accidents, the elimination of negligent practices in production and service industries, and the improvement of social deprivation at both community and family levels. There may be a specific role for psychiatry or psychology in the primary prevention of post-traumatic disorders among people known to be at exceptionally high risk of trauma, for example soldiers or firemen.

Preventing significant trauma and its impact in childhood

The importance of early prevention

Although longitudinal studies have generally failed to show consistent continuities across age bands in such characteristics as intelligence or temperamental traits (Thomas & Chess, 1984), the evidence for continuity of psychiatric disorder (Rutter, 1989; Zeitlyn, 1990; Robins & Price, 1991), of offending behaviours generally (Wolfgang, 1980; Farrington & West, 1990) and of aggression in particular (Loeber & Stouthamer-Loeber, 1986) is considerable. Further, there is evidence that many prenatal events (including youth of the mother, substance use in pregnancy) and perinatal events (including low birth weight, forceps delivery, toxaemia and infant asphyxia) predict later delinquency (Morash & Rucker, 1989; Kandel & Mednick, 1991). In every sense, therefore, the scope for prevention precedes the arrival of the potential delinquent, but it is the themes of the trauma, the impact of trauma and prevention of offending that form the principal focus of this chapter.

It is doubtful whether intervention programmes with established offenders should be accredited solely in terms of their impact on re-offending. Nevertheless, there is evidence, from studies that have included re-offending as an outcome measure, that they have little or no significant impact on secondary prevention strictly in these terms, whether evaluated in relation to young, delinquent populations (Garrett, 1985; Wiesz *et al*, 1990) or adult populations (Gunn *et al*, 1978; Robertson & Gunn, 1987). The apparently greater promise of the Head Start programmes in the USA, aimed at pre-school children, has brought optimism but also cautious commentaries about the dangers of over-generalising. Woodhead (1989) argued that a programme that is successful in one context or at one time may not be reproducible in other settings. Encouraging reports about improved performance and adjustment, or reduction in offending, through programmes targeted in early childhood do, however, persist (Hawkins *et al*, 1991; Tremblay *et al*, 1991).

Targets for prevention

One of the great difficulties in determining the real impact of childhood trauma or the relative aspects of it, is that those children that are traumatised are rarely subject to an isolated trauma in an otherwise well provided lifestyle. Vulnerabilities to traumatic events and vulnerabilities to post-traumatic disorder overlap but they are not identical (Breslau *et al*, 1991). Further, most studies are limited in the degree to which they can examine the issues. Studies which select for pathology or offending, and establish retrospectively a history of childhood abuse or other trauma may overestimate the prevalence and relevance of traumatic careers. Cross-sectional studies are less revealing in terms of causal relationships than prospective, longitudinal studies, of which there are still few. Nevertheless, such studies as those of Harter *et al* (1988) and Mullen *et al* (1988) are with substantial samples of women unselected for adult pathology, and have established beyond reasonable doubt that those with adult psychiatric disorder have a significantly higher history of sexual or physical abuse in childhood than those who do not. Nevertheless, while Mullen's continuing work (Mullen *et al*, 1993) has confirmed that there is a statistically significant relationship not only between abuse and adult psychopathology, but also severity of the abuse and degree of pathology, the overlap between the effects of the abuse and the effects of the matrix of disadvantage was sufficiently great to raise doubts about the real importance of their independence. Dodge *et al* (1990) in a prospective study of four year old children have established that, at least in the short term (one year), experience of physical harm had a statistically significant effect on social information processing patterns and aggressive behaviour that was above and beyond the contribution of other factors in the family environment, such as marital discord or financial hardship, or of other temperamental traits. Not least of the processing defects found was a bias towards attributing hostile intent to others, and to reacting accordingly with a limited repertoire of responses.

In relation to offending *per se*, factors that have consistently, although not invariably, been shown to be associated, include low (rather than subnormal) intelligence (West & Farrington, 1973); hyperactivity or impulsivity-attention-deficit disorder (Loeber, 1987; Farrington *et al*, 1990); family influences, including poor parental supervision, erratic or harsh parental discipline, marital disharmony, parental rejection of the child, family criminality and large family size, particularly of male sibship (McCord, 1979; Robins, 1978; Loeber & Stouthamer-Loeber, 1986). Increasingly, frank abuse in childhood is documented as a key factor. Widom (1991), while cautioning that she was only scratching at the surface of abuse, followed for up to 20 years nearly 800 children against whom abuse and neglect had been substantiated by a juvenile court. Half of them went on to develop well documented problems of various kinds, including early death. Forty-three per cent of the total sample had been arrested for at least one crime. Crime not officially recorded would not have been identified in the study, but was very likely to have occurred in addition. Socio-economic deprivation, poor schools and wider community disorganisation have also been implicated in young offending, both transient and persistent. It is difficult to separate the factors, since people with low socio-economic status tend to live in areas where community provision of services, including schools, are similarly deprived. Nevertheless, a number of studies from all parts of the world have emphasised poverty, parental occupation and educational status and poor housing as key factors associated with recorded offending starting in the teenage years (USA: Hirschi, 1969; Robins, 1978; UK: Douglas *et al*, 1966; West & Farrington, 1973; Kolvin *et al*, 1988; elsewhere in Europe: Janson, 1983; Van Dusen *et al*, 1983). Schools seem similarly to exert an influence, but probably through such factors as high punishment rates and minimal positive reinforcement rather than simple consequences of low financing, such as decayed buildings or the amount of space per child (Rutter *et al*, 1979). Wider community influences would appear to be more in the nature of direct facilitators of criminal acts, rather than moulders of propensities for offending, but peer influences are more complicated. While delinquent acts tend to be committed in groups in the teenage years (Reiss, 1988), adverse peer reaction to such socially disruptive behaviour as aggression and violence tends to isolate the perpetrator and may be a factor in reinforcing disordered conduct, and ultimately offending.

Models of successful prevention

Little is known about the effects of psychosocial intervention in childhood on the effects of specific childhood trauma, including abuse. Terr's (1983) report of work with children who had been kidnapped together in a school bus was discouraging in that all remained highly symptomatic after four years. She has subsequently (Terr, 1991) emphasised a distinction between type 1 trauma reactions, which generally follow a single unanticipated event, and type 2 disorders which follow from prolonged or repeated exposure to trauma, with some overlap between the two. Highlighting psychological features which bode special risk for long-term disorders (repetitive memories, repetitive behaviour, trauma-specific fears and changed attitudes to people, life and the future) she has, as yet, no advances to offer on disorder preventing or limiting techniques.

Work with children who suffer the multiple, more commonplace traumas of inadequate parenting and environmental deprivation, has shown promising results when the intervention is educational and early. Farrington (1985) provides an admirable review of the field, and is clear that one experiment in Michigan, USA, "stands out almost like a shining beacon among a morass of confused and confusing delinquency prevention studies". In both the medium (Schweinhart & Weikart, 1980) and longer term (up to age 18) (Berrueta-Clement et al, 1984), this project, which combined a daily pre-school programme with weekly home visits for three to four year olds, shared advantages in decreasing subsequent school failure, occupational failure and offending. Perhaps because it was a social/education rather than a medical intervention, it is not highly popular with the psychiatric profession (Rutter & Giller, 1983), despite its success. Subsequent American (Hawkins et al, 1991) and Canadian (Tremblay et al, 1991) programmes of a similar kind, targeting parent and teacher training to reduce childhood aggressive behaviour in the early elementary school grades, have proved promising in reducing externally directed aggression in boys and self-destructive behaviour in girls. In contrast to the previously described programme, however, the American effort appeared ineffective with African-American children, while Tremblay and colleagues found that improvement was not invariable in all aspects of the children's lives. While school performances improved in the monitored study, mothers still reported some disruption at home. There is evidence that even at a later stage intervention in the educational scene, particularly by changing schools, can be effective in reducing disordered behaviour (Gold & Mann, 1984; Gottfredson, 1987).

Pitfalls in the prevention of behavioural and emotional problems in childhood

Fiscal limitations dictate that prevention strategies of the kind indicated for psychosocial disorders must be targeted. Although, as outlined, much is now known about identifying high risk groups, it could be argued that this a risky process in itself. The targeting of someone as being at high risk of becoming delinquent or a criminal, or for developing a serious psychiatric disorder is, in fact, a labelling which may not remain a secret and could provoke adverse reaction in others along with the provision of benefits. Mulvey & Phelps (1988) explored in more detail the four areas which create such ethical dilemmas – validity of problem definition, over-identification of cases, informed consent and confidentiality. It is perhaps worth emphasising that many, even of the highest risk children, do not go on to become delinquents, nor to show serious psychiatric disease, and even among those who become delinquent spontaneous remission is not uncommon (Loeber, 1982; Mulvey & Larosa, 1986). Conversely, coyness about potential psychiatric problems is of no benefit. Terr (1981) reported delays in parents seeking help for their children who had been kidnapped on the school bus because a well meaning physician had confidently predicted that only one in twenty-six would develop symptoms. They all did, but no parent wanted to be the first to admit that their child was 'the one'.

Preventing significant trauma and its impact in adults

That 'significant life events' may precipitate psychiatric disease has long been recognised (Birley & Brown, 1970; Paykel, 1974), although the extent to which it is the event *per se* that is associated with the subsequent disorder has been challenged (Fergusson & Horwood, 1987). More recently emphasis has been on the *causation* of disorder by a key event or events, and the concept of post-traumatic stress disorder (PTSD) has emerged (American Psychiatric Association, 1987). Estimates of the prevalence of PTSD alone, even as defined by the rather stringent DSM–III–R criteria that require a trauma 'outside the range of usual human experience', suggest that it is at least as common in the general population as schizophrenia (Helzer *et al*, 1987) and exceptionally common in high risk groups such as Vietnam veterans (Centers for Disease Control Vietnam Experience Study, 1988). Further, co-morbidity in such samples is very high, with 4.5% of the latter group also having depression, nearly 5% anxiety, 14% alcohol misuse or dependency, and the rates of accidental or suicidal deaths being 50–70% higher than expected. There is conflicting evidence over whether the risks of criminal and other violent behaviour are elevated, but it seems likely (Wilson & Zigelbaum, 1983).

At present almost nothing is known about the prevention of disorder or anti-social behaviour in traumatised adults. Lindemann (1944) was clear in his opinion that 'proper psychiatric management of grief reactions may prevent prolonged and serious alteration in the patient's social adjustment as well as potential medical disease'. He was writing of people who had been involved in a major disaster. While this view might have wider application, it has not been subject to adequate testing. Early interventions occur at a time when most people are undergoing a period of maximum change in their symptomatology, and there is still no study that distinguishes between the effects of crisis intervention and natural resolution of symptoms within the first three months of the trauma. There is a suggestion, however, that some kind of intervention may be better than none (Kelly, 1975), and certainly that there is no justification for a hostile medical stance, refusing treatment on the grounds that post-traumatic symptoms are 'imaginary' or 'compensationitis', which will resolve spontaneously on payment of compensation. There are disturbing indications that those perhaps in most need of help – the repeatedly victimised – may be much less likely to accept intervention than the well adjusted suffering a single trauma, and, indeed, in turn the healthy who have not experienced exceptional trauma (Mezey & Taylor, 1988). Nevertheless, increasingly consistent advice from psychiatrists with much experience of working with traumatised people is that *routine enquiry* for a history of trauma and symptoms of PTSD should be part of any psychiatric examination, even though the initial presentation may not obviously indicate it (McFarlane, 1991).

Primary prevention of PTSD, realistically, can only be considered for high risk groups, such as the police, rescue workers or army personnel. There is some work to suggest that the technique of stress inoculation training may be helpful in this regard (Meichenbaum, 1985). Webb (1993) has described potentially important police organisation techniques, while Alexander & Wells (1991) were in the near unique position of being able to compare and contrast pre- and post-disaster ratings for anxiety and depression among police officers attending the Piper Alpha disaster. Selection of those for specific, traumatic tasks – in this case body handling – was seen as one key factor, with organisational and general support factors being others. Psychiatrists or psychologists may contribute by reinforcing recognition of the potential importance of groups. Hoiberg & McCaughey (1984) studied men surviving a naval collision. The initially surprising observation was made that those seriously injured had been significantly less psychologically disabled than the uninjured men. The former, however, had been hospitalised and fortuitously formed a strong peer support group. The uninjured had returned to their respective home communities and had found no such support. Similarly, Weiseth (1989) has commented on the relative importance of community, company and communicational groupings at the time of a disaster. Only the community grouping, which implies living and working together and thus bonds over and above the link of the disaster, conferred any great advantage. Among one small platoon of Norwegian soldiers, for example, half were killed in an avalanche, but among the survivors who stayed together and received some support, some of whom had several high risk factors for PTSD, none developed it. One potentially very vulnerable group is rarely considered in such terms, and that is former psychiatric patients. Lehman & Linn (1984) showed that the risk of becoming a victim of crime was exceptionally high, but did not comment on subsequent reactions, although they did note that the victimised group reported more psychopathology and less life satisfaction than the non-victimised group.

One unfortunate aspect of this field is the creation of, in effect, surrogate victims through media mis-information – about the risks of trauma, its psychological consequences or both. Prevention by informed education of the public might be possible. In the British Crime Survey (Hough & Mayhew, 1983), for example, it was shown that a majority of older women and a minority of older men were to some extent disabled by their fear of crime, in that they avoided going out at night as a result. Their considerable fear of becoming victims and the related behaviour were wholly disproportionate to real risks, which were tiny. Individuals who have actually become victims of a major incident may find that the press or other news agencies become intensely interested in them. The effect of this is virtually unresearched. While some may be helped by the opportunity to tell and retell their story for the widest possible audience, anecdotally many find the persistent pursuit by some sections of the mass media in itself traumatic. In a rather different arena, many people who, as victims of crime, report the crime against them find their subsequent place in the criminal justice system sufficiently traumatic that it compounds their victimisation. It is quite common for women who have been victims of rape to report that their experience under cross examination in court was as bad or even worse than the original rape. At best it vividly recalls the rape and at worst adds a differently brutal dimension. Many victim support schemes try to support and assist in the prevention of further trauma at this stage (Mawby & Gill, 1987).

The mentally abnormal offender

Prevention of offending and re-offending

There continues to be considerable debate over whether offending among people with a mental disorder is more, as, or less likely than among the mentally healthy. The answer depends to a considerable extent on the definition of mental abnormality, the definition of offending and in particular is influenced considerably by whether the criterion for offending is recorded crime or self-reported anti-social behaviour. In relation to recorded crime it has variously been hypothesised that the mentally abnormal are much more likely to be identified as offenders (Robertson, 1989), but also more likely to be diverted to hospital and so not appear on criminal statistics (Lagos et al, 1977). The only community survey of people wholly unselected for mental abnormality or crime did show that those with a mental abnormality, particularly psychosis or substance misuse, were more likely to report having engaged in violence than those not so afflicted (Swanson et al, 1990), but even these findings have been questioned on the grounds that the reported rates of violence among the mentally healthy seem low and the results may have been biased by more frank reporting among the mentally abnormal. Another American study of a community sample, in this case supplemented with known psychiatric samples from the same communities but from a range of data sources, found support for similar conclusions (Link et al, 1992). There is, thus, good epidemiological evidence to suggest that some mental diseases may be more commonly associated with offending, and particularly violent offending, than would be expected by chance, and that when the two occur together one or more clear directions of association may pertain. In relation to schizophrenia, for example, there is considerable evidence for a direct link between the illness and at least some types of offending. Delusions have demonstrably driven violent behaviour in a substantial minority of cases (Taylor, 1985; Link & Stueve, 1994), and in terms of criminal career, violent behaviour, as opposed to other forms of offending, almost invariably follows the onset of a psychotic illness (Taylor, 1993; Wessely et al, 1994). Others too have shown that career patterns of recorded violent offending in men and all criminal offending in women are distinctive among those with a mental disorder (Hodgins, 1992), particularly schizophrenia (Lindqvist & Allebeck, 1990; Coid et al, 1993) compared with those without disorder or the general population. There is also evidence that in many cases the illness is likely to be indirectly associated, through decline in social status and abilities and acquisition of related risk factors for criminal behaviour. In still other cases there may be a common aetiology for both the offending behaviour and the illness (Taylor *et al*, 1992). In a few cases the illness is not established until many years after offending or imprisonment, although this does not necessarily imply that such experiences have caused or even precipitated the illness. There has been less work evaluating this direction of association.

Drug misuse

In some other conditions, the definitions of mental abnormality are often sufficiently entangled with definitions of criminal behaviour – for example anti-social/psychopathic personality disorder – that, to date, the medical debate about cause and effect is rather circular, and the criminology literature, some of which has already been covered, is more helpful (Robins, 1978; Farrington & West, 1990; Robins & Price, 1991; Farrington, 1992). Substance misuse is often reported to be a substantial problem around the commission of a crime, both by victim and offender, whether or not such use or misuse is associated with dependency. This now remains true even when allowance is made for the fact that the use of some drugs is in itself a crime.

Among all drugs of misuse, alcohol has most consistently shown to be associated with violence and homicide (Wolfgang & Strohm, 1956; Zacune & Hensman, 1971; Gillies, 1976). The relationship between alcohol and violence is, however, far from simple, although one review (*Lancet*, 1990) explored initiatives in a number of countries for reducing alcohol-related violence, including drunken driving. Walters (1994) cuts clearly through the conflicting evidence with respect to other drugs. He concludes from his review that the relationship between drug misuse and crime is genuine, meaningful and quantifiable but that the most obvious relationship – crime emanating from the need to sustain the habit or as a direct effect of the substance – is not necessarily the most important. Crime and its consequences may expand drug use opportunities and be as important a pathway. His inclination, however, is to emphasise the similarities in and interaction of drug taking and criminal lifestyles. Both are legally proscribed behaviours. This leads him to some well supported proposals for an informed debate within and between national legislatures about drug legislation. One possibility that must be kept under review as a preventive of pathology and crime is that habit forming drugs other than tobacco and alcohol might be better subject to specific rather than blanket legal limits. Walters, however, is more interested in the similarities of thinking styles, social rituals and social context between criminals and substance misusers. Preventive policies must take all these variables into account if they are to be effective.

Medical supervision

The prevention of offending by people with mental disorder thus has more in common than not with the prevention and treatment of mental disorder, and strategies of primary and secondary prevention for the psychoses, personality disorders and for substance misuse serve particularly well in this field. It is almost unheard of for a mentally abnormal offender either to commit a serious offence or to reach the stage of remand in custody for any offence without being well known to psychiatric services, albeit often not in current, active treatment at the time of their offence (Hafner & Boker 1973/82; Taylor & Gunn, 1984a, b).

To date studies of mentally abnormal offenders leaving prison or hospital have been misleading because they rely almost exclusively on re-offending, re-hospitalisation and mortality rates for indices of progress and are virtually without reference to the conditions of treatment, social support, or general social position prevailing after the patient has left the institution, and in particular around the time of the re-offending. Even on these fairly crude criteria, however, it has been consistently shown that, for a hospitalised offender patient in England and Wales, planned and conditional discharges within the context of a restriction order of the Mental Health Act 1983 have been associated with better outcome than discharge by a Mental Health Review Tribunal or absolute discharge without conditions (Acres, 1975; Tennent & Way, 1984; Bailey & MacCulloch, 1992). Under the Mental Health Act 1983, which applies only to England and Wales, a person convicted in a criminal court may have the sentence set aside and a hospital order imposed instead. A higher Court (Crown Court) may, if it is thought that the individual poses a continuing risk of serious harm to the public, add an order for restrictions on discharge from hospital. It must then be approved by the Secretary of State at the Home Office and in this case is generally attended by conditions, at least for medical and social supervision in the community and continued reporting to the Home Office on the part of the professionals involved. Also under the Mental Health Act 1983, section 117 requires that the designated patient's District Health Authority and local social services authority provide relevant after care services when he or she leaves hospital until they "are satisfied that the person concerned is no longer in need of such services". Although the same moral obligation should apply to voluntary patients, there is no such legal backing for their right to continuing treatment and care.

Anti-social behaviour

The anti-social behaviour of the majority of patients will be of nuisance value rather than a threat to the life or health of others. Extremely dangerous behaviour does, however, occur and, in the wake of the killing of a social worker by a patient, a public enquiry considered measures to prevent further such tragedies (Department of Health and Social Security, 1988). The Royal College of Psychiatrists (1991) has published guidelines to good practice on the discharge of potentially violent patients, but the recommendations of the inquiry following the killing of a member of the general public by a man well known to psychiatric services (Ritchie et al, 1994) have a sobering consistency with these. It is harder to make good practice than good recommendations. Britain is by no means the only country working with such problems. In Denmark, for example, a country with a low national homicide rate, an increase has been recorded between 1959 and 1983 in homicides by people with a mental disorder, mainly substance misuse or psychosis (Gabrielsen et al, 1992). Men with schizophrenia exhibited the single most steep increase during the period of investigation. The authors question the impact of current mental health policies which, in Denmark as in the UK, might as well be described as antagonistic to the provision of hospital beds as promoting of community care. The balance of service provision, with the guarantee of the hospital safety net, almost certainly needs further adjustment if safe community care and treatment for most people is to be safeguarded.

The secondary prevention of violence to others by people with mental disorder has much in common with the secondary prevention of suicide. Once a threat of violence, or an actual violent act has taken place, the most fundamental question is "has the balance of the situation changed since the violent act, and has it changed such as to minimise the risk of further violence?". In relation to externally directed violence, this balance will involve an evaluation of three key elements and their inter-relationship, namely the patient/perpetrator, the victim or potential victim and the environment and circumstances of the patient. Relevant factors in the patient include diagnosis, specific symptoms, motivation for violence, likely compliance with treatment and capacity for taking responsibility for behaviour. The patient's use of alcohol or other drugs, age, gender, size and habitual patterns of response to stress will all need to be taken into consideration. In relation to the potential victim(s), prevention is influenced by whether the victim is a named individual, or could be anyone, and whether it is someone outside the patient's general sphere of activity or intimately involved. The personal characteristics of the victim are also very important – is the victim likely to be provocative, whether knowingly or not, does the victim understand the risks and have strategies for coping? In relation to the environment, some of the crucial variables include availability of weapons or of disinhibiting substances including alcohol and illicit drugs, as well as the presence of stressors which might include unemployment, poor or crowded accommodation or a new, unfamiliar, threatening or constantly changing environment.

Prevention of violence towards professional staff

A fact not often appreciated by the general public is that violence does not necessarily cease because a person is admitted to or confined in prison or hospital. The Health Services Advisory Committee (HSAC) (1987) survey, for example, showed that health service staff are three times more likely to be injured at work than industrial workers, principally because of attacks by violent patients. In psychiatric facilities, equalled only by accident and emergency departments for major incidents, but also by geriatric and general medical units for more minor violent incidents, as many as one in four respondents had suffered injury as a result of attack. Mortality is a real, but tiny risk. The case of a social worker killed by a patient has already been mentioned. In an epidemiological survey of psychiatric in-patients in Sweden over a 10-year period, Ekblom (1970) calculated that the risk of death at the hands of a patient, adjusted for time of exposure, was one in two hundred and fifty million working hours for staff and one in three hundred and fifty million in-patient hours for patients. It is important, however, to prevent both major and minor violence wherever possible, and the HSAC makes a number of important recommendations for the protection of staff. With only minor modifications they remain an extremely sound basis for preventing serious harm.

(a) Attention to the working environment – good lighting, space and good observation lines are particularly important.

(b) Information systems and organisational procedures must be sufficient that staff can be informed of risks and details about patients particularly likely to engage in violence. Effective call and response systems in cases of emergency are essential.

(c) Information, communications and supportive organisational systems apply as strongly to community and domiciliary work as to hospital in-patient work. This will be increasingly important with attempts to manage more and more disturbed patients in the community. Staff should never visit patients without a schedule of their visits being known to a central office or co-ordinator where practical, another team member where not, and occasionally reporting back with progress on the schedule. Emergency call systems should be available as far as possible. All staff must be trained in diversion and calming techniques to increase the chances of diffusing a potential incident, and in basic break away techniques which can help in the event of assault. Risk factors should be calculated before each visit, and solo visits should not be made to an increasingly unstable patient where there has been any hint of violence previously in such circumstances. It follows from this that:

(d) Staffing levels, staff training and experience must be adequate. There is now good evidence that where staff turnover is high, or temporary staffing form a sizeable proportion of the work force, the level of patient violence escalates, at least in acute in-patient units (James *et al*, 1990).

(e) Clear strategies for coping with violence, and staff knowledge of these are essential. An understanding of personal role, command structure and techniques of physical restraint are all important, and such strategies and skills need regular review and maintenance if they are to remain effective in the management of violence.

(f) Support must be available for staff in the aftermath of a violent incident. Their main needs may include medical attention, an opportunity to ventilate or discuss events, time off, or even legal advice on compensation. It is well recorded that some staff fear revealing distress because they are worried about losing control if they admit to it, while others may mistakenly assume that receiving violence is just 'part of the job' and it is not appropriate to do anything which might be construed as complaining about it. It is not easy for a professional person to concede vulnerability – which is an inescapable element of admitting distress or concern – but failure to explore the full impact of violence can not only prevent resolution of possible conflict and thus render the individual staff member potentially less effective in clinical situations, but it can also stop the preventive information coming to light and thus limit the teaching/training value for others of an important episode.

Preventing morbidity and mortality in the mentally disordered offender

A danger that cannot be emphasised too strongly is the risk to the mentally abnormal offender himself. The institutions in which he may be detained may create specific problems which are dealt with below, but in the community he is also at considerable risk. Robertson (1987) followed for 23 years 1347 mentally abnormal offenders defined as such by having been detained in ordinary psychiatric hospitals under hospital orders after conviction for a criminal offence. Nearly one-quarter had died, 25 per cent of these violently, with a coroner's verdict of suicide, accident or open verdict. The rate of suicide among 25–29 year olds was five times that for the general population. Prevention approaches should have more in common than not with those for the seriously disordered who are not offenders. Greater effort may be required, however, for offender patients because of the risk that they are diverted away from health service facilities.

Morbidity and mortality in institutions, particularly prisons

While it is often argued, with much theoretical justification, that prisons are unhealthy and destructive places, there has been remarkably little interest in the extent of the damage that they may cause. Two of the greatest problems for which there is considerable evidence is transmission of infection and suicide.

The origins of the prison medical service lay in preventive medicine. In 1774, as a result of John Howard's investigation into the state of English prisons, Parliament passed an "Act for Preserving the Health of Prisoners in Gaol and Preventing the Gaol Distemper" (Gunn *et al*, 1978). Then, the principal concern was a form of typhus – which threatened to spread beyond the jails into the wider community. All common infectious diseases are likely to pose increased risk of spread in relatively closed communities, but the greatest concerns in prisons have now centred on hepatitis and the AIDS virus. Turnbull *et al* (1991) completed a survey of the extent of risk-increasing behaviour in English prisons, and found that at least 10% of ex-prisoners in their sample of 452 reported sexual activity and illicit drug injection. Farrell & Strang (1991) argued for a number of preventive measures which could be effective both within and without the prisons, including education, ready availability of condoms and training in the sterilisation of injection equipment.

The rate of suicide in English prisons was last estimated to be approximately four times that of the general population (McClure, 1987) and has risen dramatically from 8.6 per hundred thousand receptions between 1972 and 1975 to nearly 16% between 1984 and 1987. It then stabilised, even falling as prisoner numbers fell, but rose sharply again in late 1993. Parasuicide is an even greater problem, but the full extent is not known. The problems that underlie these figures are twofold: first there is a higher rate of psychiatric disease in a prison population – both among prisoners serving custodial sentences (Gunn *et al*, 1991) and those on remand (Taylor & Gunn, 1984*a*); secondly, the stress of imprisonment and the events that lead up to it are considerable for many if not a majority of prisoners. Just a small number of very disordered men and women may find relief in the structured environment. Dooley (1990) confirmed that of 295 coroners' verdict suicides studied, nearly all those occurring in English prisons between 1972 and 1987, a bare majority had followed from a combination of the prison situation and outside pressures, such as relationships breaking. Nearly one-quarter of the total occurred in the context of mental disorder, and 12% apparently as a result of a sense of guilt for the offence. Her Majesty's Chief Inspector of Prisons for England and Wales (1990) further considered the problem and presented recommendations for prevention. Some of the most important are environmental, since almost all deaths are by hanging and the bars in the windows are an important facilitator. There was also much wise advice on the general treatment of inmates, including attention to the day-to-day regime, occupation, communication with people outside prison and opportunities for prison officer/lay counselling. Specific recommendations were also presented for the doctors. The importance of effective screening for mental disease and for suicide potential cannot be too heavily emphasised; all the risk factors applying in other situations such as age, co-morbidity and history of previous suicide attempts are as important in a prison sample as in any other. The importance of the implementation of appropriate observations, treatment and transfer to NHS facilities of the mentally disordered is stressed. More-or-less concurrent advice that people with mental disorder should not be remanded to prison solely for the preparation of psychiatric reports (Home Office Circular 66/90) is, effectively, a very wise piece of prevention advice. Continued failure of its full implementation as much rests with deficits in NHS provision as in identification of the problem, although court diversion schemes offer some prospect of improved practice (Joseph & Potter, 1990).

Research into the risk of psycho-social deterioration in prison, particularly during long-term imprisonment, is very sparse. Some work suggests little overall change (Coker & Martin, 1984), while other work suggests problems like increasing introversion or dependency (Sapsford, 1978) and, particularly where mental abnormality is a feature, it would be expected that some of the elements of institutionalisation would be seen. Almost all the work, however, has been based on cross-sectional studies, and likely to be misleading for that. To date, the best that can be said is that it would appear that educational and occupational programmes, facilitation wherever possible of continuing contacts with family and community of origin, and prisoner contributions to the management of their environment, together with appropriate access to good health services for those with physical or mental disease, are the most important measures with potential for preventing morbidity, assault, riot and death in prisons. Among the most striking examples of the success of such an approach in these terms is the Barlinnie Special Unit in Scotland (Cooke, 1989) and Grendon prison in England (Gunn et al, 1978; Genders & Player, 1989).

Working with patients in the criminal justice system

It has long been understood that people who have mental disorders may have areas of impaired competency. The Confait case was a landmark in changing the rules on police interviewing of suspects after it was revealed that the confessions to murder by three young men with significant learning disabilities were unsafe, and had been the sole basis of criminal conviction (Fisher, 1977).

Procedure for police interviewing of suspected criminals with mental disorder was incorporated into the Police and Criminal Evidence Act 1984 (PACE). Psychiatrists and psychologists may have a small role to play in preventing injustice in the criminal justice system. Gudjonsson & Gunn (1982) have shown that it is possible to apply a scientific approach to the assessment of witness competence, which would otherwise be subject to the risk of crude legal challenge in court, and the dismissal of cases solely on the grounds that the victim or chief witness was mentally disordered. Gudjonsson & MacKeith (1982) have developed assessments of competence in the context of confessions, offering a package which incorporates systematic evaluation of relevant cognitive skills together with the assessment of suggestibility. The Royal Commission on Criminal Justice (1993) considered this among the many other potential avenues for the miscarriage of justice among the healthy and the sick. The principal recommendation of interest here was that when the Police and Criminal Evidence Act 1984 (PACE) is next revised, attention is given to the fact that the relevant section is limited to the 'mentally handicapped', and does not include the 'mentally ill' or other categories of the 'mentally disordered'.

Conclusions

The preventive work of the forensic psychiatrist has much in common with that of psychiatrists working within other specialities, but is particularly sharply focused because of the exceptional risk of serious harm to self or others in a mentally abnormal offender population. Primary prevention depends on liaison with child and adolescent psychiatrists, and in many instances prevention of harm to the children or victims of the primary patient. Secondary prevention covers two main areas – the prevention of offending and re-offending among the psychiatrically disordered and the prevention of further morbidity and mortality among those finding their way into the criminal justice system and the prisons.

References

ACRES, D. I. (1975) The after-care of special hospital patients. (Appendix 3) In *Report of the Committee on Mentally Abnormal Offenders*. London Home Office, DHSS/HMSO: London Cmnd 6244.
ALEXANDER, D. A. & WELLS, A. (1991) Reaction of police officers to body-handling after a major disaster. *British Journal of Psychiatry*, **159**, 547–555.
AMERICAN PSYCHIATRIC ASSOCIATION (1987) *Diagnostic and Statistical Manual of Mental Disorders* (3rd Edn, revised) (DSM–III–R). Washington, DC: APA.
BAILEY, J. & MACCULLOCH, M. (1992) Patterns of reconviction in patients discharged directly to the community from a special hospital: implications for after care. *Journal of Forensic Psychiatry*, **3**, 445–461.
BERRUETA-CLEMENT, J. R., SCHWEINHART, L. J., BARNETT, W. S., et al (1984) *Changed Lives*. Ypsilanti, MI: High/Scope.
BIRLEY, J. L. T. & BROWN, G. W. (1970) Crisis and life change proceeding the onset of relapse of acute schizophrenia: clinical aspects. *British Journal of Psychiatry*, **116**, 327–333.
BRESLAU, N., DAVIS, G. C., ANDRESKI, P., et al (1991) Traumatic events and post-traumatic stress disorder in an urban population of young adults. *Archives of General Psychiatry*, **48**, 216–222.
CENTERS FOR DISEASE CONTROL (1988) Vietnam Experience Study. Health status of Vietnam veterans. *Journal of the American Medical Association*, **259**, 2701–2719.
COID, B., LEWIS, S. W. & REVELY, A. M. (1993) A twin study of psychosis and criminality. *British Journal of Psychiatry*, **162**, 87–92.
COKER, J. B. & MARTIN, J. P. (1985) *Licensed to Live*. Oxford: Blackwell.
COOKE, D. J. (1989) Containing violent prisoners: an analysis of the "Barlinnie Special Unit". *British Journal of Criminology*, **28**, 129–143.
DEPARTMENT OF HEALTH AND SOCIAL SECURITY (1988) *Report of the Committee of Inquiry into the Care and Aftercare of Miss Sharon Campbell*. CM440. London: HMSO.
DODGE, K. A., BATES, J. E. & PETTIT, G. S. (1990) Mechanisms on the cycle of violence. *Science*, **250**, 1678–1683.
DOOLEY, E. (1990) Prison suicide in England and Wales 1972–87. *British Journal of Psychiatry*, **156**, 40–45.
DOUGLAS, J. W. B., ROSS, J. M., HAMMOND, W. A., et al (1966) Delinquency and social class. *British Journal of Criminology*, **6**, 294–302.
EKBLOM, B. (1970) *Acts of Violence by Patients in Mental Hospitals*. Uppsala: Scandinavian University Books; Almquist & Wiksells Boktryckeri AB.
FARRELL, M. & STRANG, J. (1991) Drugs, HIV and prisons. Time to rethink current policy (Editorial). *British Medical Journal*, **302**, 1477–1478.
FARRINGTON, D. (1985) Delinquency prevention in the 1980s. *Journal of Adolescence*, **8**, 3–16.

FARRINGTON, D. P. (1992) Criminal career research: lessons for crime prevention. *Studies on Crime and Crime Prevention*, **1**, 7-29.
FERGUSSON, D. M. & HORWOOD, L. J. (1987) Vulnerability to life events exposure. *Psychological Medicine*, **17**, 739-749.
GABRIELSEN, G., GOTTLIEB, P. & KEMP, P. (1992) Criminal homicide trends in Copenhagen. *Studies on Crime and Crime Prevention*, **1**, 106-114.
GARRETT, C. J. (1985) Effects of residential treatment on adjudicated delinquents: a meta-analysis. *Journal of Research into Crime and Delinquency*, **22**, 287-308.
GENDERS, E. & PLAYER, E. (unpublished). *Grendon: A Study of a Therapeutic Community Within the Prison System*. Report to Home Office (1989).
GILLIES, H. (1976) Homicide in the west of Scotland. *British Journal of Psychiatry*, **128**, 105-127.
GOLD, M. & MANN, D. W. (1984) *Expelled to a Friendlier Place*. Ann Arbor, MI: University of Michigan Press.
GOTTFREDSON, D. C. (1987) Examining the potential of delinquency prevention through alternative education. *Today's Delinquent*, **6**, 87-100.
GUDJONSSON, G. H. & GUNN, J. (1982) The competence and reliability of a witness in a criminal court: a case report. *British Journal of Psychiatry*, **141**, 624-627.
——— & MACKEITH, J. A. C. (1982) False confessions. Psychological effects of interrogation. In *Reconstructing the Past. The Role of Psychologists in Criminal Trials* (eds A. Trankell & A. Nortstedt), Stockholm: Sovers Forlag.
GUNN, J., MADEN, A. & SWINTON, M. (1991) *Mentally Disordered Prisoners*. London: Home Office.
———, ROBERTSON, G., DELL, S., et al (1978) *Psychiatric Aspects of Imprisonment*. London: Academic Press.
HAFNER, H. & BOKER, W. (1973) (English translation by Helen Marshall, 1982) *Crimes of Violence by Mentally Abnormal Offenders*. Cambridge: Cambridge University Press.
HARTER, S., ALEXANDER, P. C. & NEIMEYER, R. A. (1988) Long-term effects of incestuous child abuse in college women: social adjustment, social cognition and family characteristics. *Journal of Consulting and Clinical Psychology*, **56**, 5-8.
HAWKINS, J. D., VON CLEVE, E. & CATALANO, R. F. (1991) Reducing early childhood aggression: results of a primary prevention program. *Journal of the American Academy of Child and Adolescent Psychiatry*, **30**, 208-217.
HEALTH SERVICES ADVISORY COMMITTEE *Violence to Staff in the Health Services*. London: Health and Safety Commission, HMSO.
HELZER, J. E., ROBINS, L. N. & MCEVOY, L. (1987) Post-traumatic stress disorder in the general population. *New England Journal of Medicine*, **318**, 1630-1634.
HER MAJESTY'S CHIEF INSPECTOR OF PRISONS FOR ENGLAND AND WALES (1990) *Report of a Review of Suicide and Self-Harm in Prison Service Establishments in England and Wales*. Cm 1383. London: HMSO.
HIRSCHI, T. (1969) *Cause of Delinquency*. Berkeley, CA: University of California Press.
HODGINS, S. (1992) Mental disorder, intellectual deficiency, and crime. *Archives of General Psychiatry*, **49**, 476-483.
HOIBERG, A. & MCCAUGHEY, B. G. (1984) The traumatic after-effects of collision at sea. *American Journal of Psychiatry*, **141**, 70-73.
HOUGH, M. & MAYHEW, P. (1983) The British Crime Survey: first report. *Home Office Research Study No. 76*. London: HMSO.
JAMES, D. V., FINEBERG, N. A., SHAH, A. K., et al (1990) An increase in violence on an acute psychiatric ward: a study of associated factors. *Brtish Journal of Psychiatry*, **156**, 846-852.
JANSON, C. G. (1983) Delinquency among metropolitan boys: a progress report. In *Prospective Studies of Crime and Delinquency* (eds K. T. Van Dusen & S. A. Mednick), pp. 147-180. Boston: Kluwer-Nijhoff.
KANDEL, E. & MEDNICK, S. A. (1991) Perinatal complications predict violent offending. *Criminology*, **29**, 519-529.
KELLY, R. (1975) The post-traumatic syndrome: an iatrogenic disease. *Forensic Science*, **6**, 17-24.
KOLVIN, I., MILLER, J. F. W., FLEETING, M., et al (1988) Social and parenting factors affecting criminal-offence rates: findings from the Newcastle Thousand Family Study (1947-1980). *British Journal of Psychiatry*, **152**, 80-90.
LAGOS, J. M., PERLMUTTER, K. & SAEXINGER, H. (1977) Fear of the mentally ill: empirical support for the common man's response. *American Journal of Psychiatry*, **134**, 1134-1137.
LANCET (1990) Editorial. Alcohol and violence. *Lancet*, **336**, 1223-1224.
LEHMAN, A. F. & LINN, L. S. (1984) Crimes against discharged mental patients in Board-and Care Homes. *American Journal of Psychiatry*, **141**, 271-274.

LINDEMANN, E. (1944) Symptomatology and management of acute grief. *American Journal of Psychiatry*, **101**, 141-148.

LINDQVIST, P. & ALLEBECK, P. (1990) Schizophrenia and crime. A longitudinal follow-up of 644 schizophrenics in Stockholm. *British Journal of Psychiatry*, **157**, 345-350.

LINK, B. G. & STUEVE, A. (1994) Psychiatric symptoms and the violent/illegal behaviour of mental patients compared to community controls. In *Violence and Mental Disorder: Developments in Risk Assessment* (eds J. Monahan & H. Steadman). Chicago: Chicago University Press.

——, ANDREWS, H. & CULLEN, F. T. (1992) The violent and illegal behaviour of mental patients reconsidered. *American Sociological Review*, **57**, 275-292.

LOEBER, R. (1987) Behavioural precursors and accelerators of delinquency. In *Explaining Criminal Behaviour* (eds W. Buikhuisen & S. A. Mednick), pp. 51-67. Leiden: Brill.

—— & STOUTHAMER-LOEBER, M. (1986) Family factors as correlates and predictors of juvenile conduct problems and delinquency. In *Crime and Justice* Vol. 7 (eds M. Tonry & N. Morris), pp. 29-149. Chicago: University of Chicago Press.

—— & VAN KANMER, E. B. (1990) Long-term criminal outcome of hyperactivity-impulsivity – attention deficit and conduct problems in childhood. In *Straight and Devious Pathways from Childhood to Adulthood*.

MCCLURE, G. M. G. (1987) Suicide in England and Wales, 1975-1984. *British Journal of Psychiatry*, **150**, 309-314.

MCCORD, J. (1979) Some child-rearing antecedents of criminal behaviour in adult men. *Journal of Personality and Social Psychology*, **37**, 1477-1486.

MCFARLANE, A. C. (1991) Victims and survivors. *Current Opinion in Psychiatry*, **4**, 833-836.

MEICHENBAUM, D. (1985) *Stress Inoculation Training*. Oxford: Pergamon Press.

MEZEY, G. C. & TAYLOR, P. J. (1988) Psychological reactions of women who have been raped: a descriptive and comparative study. *British Journal of Psychiatry*, **152**, 330-339.

MORASH, M. & RUCKER, L. (1989) An exploratory study of the connection of mother's age at childbearing to her children's delinquency in four data sets. *Crime and Delinquency*, **35**, 45-93.

MULLEN, P. E., ROMANS-CLARKSON, S. E., WALTON, V. A., *et al* (1988) Impact of sexual and physical abuse on women's mental health. *Lancet*, **1**, 841-845.

——, MARTIN, J. L., ANDERSON, S. E., *et al* (1993) Childhood sexual abuse and mental health in adult life. *British Journal of Psychiatry*, **163**, 721-732.

MULVEY, E. P. & PHELPS, P. (1988) Ethical balances in juvenile justice research and practice. *American Psychologist*, **43**, 65-69.

PAYKEL, E. S. (1974) Life stress and psychiatric disorder applications of the clinical approach. In *Stressful Life Events: Their Nature and Effect* (eds B. S. Dohrerwend & B. P. Dohrerwend). New York: Wiley.

REISS, A. J. (1988) Co-offending and criminal careers. In *Crime and Justice* (eds M. Tonry & N. Morris), pp. 117-170. Chicago: University of Chicago Press.

RITCHIE, J. H., DICK, D. & LINGHAM, R. (1994) *The Report of the Inquiry into the Care and Treatment of Christopher Clunis*. London: HMSO.

ROBERTSON, G. (1987) Mentally abnormal offenders: manner of death. *British Medical Journal*, **295**, 632-634.

—— (1988) Arrest patterns among mentally disordered offenders. *British Journal of Psychiatry*, **153**, 313-316.

—— & GUNN, J. (1987) A ten year follow up of men discharged from Grendon prison. *British Journal of Psychiatry*, **151**, 674-678.

ROBINS, L. N. (1978) Sturdy childhood predictors of adult outcomes: replications from longitudinal studies. In *Stress and Mental Disorder* (eds J. E. Barrett, R. M. Ross & G. L. Klerman), pp. 219-235.

—— & PRICE, R. K. (1991) Adult disorders predicted by childhood conduct problems: results from NIMH Epidemiologic Catchment Area Project. *Psychiatry*, **54**, 116-132.

RUTTER, M. (1989) Pathways from childhood to adult life. *Journal of Child Psychology and Psychiatry*, **30**, 23-51.

——, MAUGHAN, B., MORTIMORE, O., *et al* (1979) *Fifteen Thousand Hours*. London: Opera Books.

—— & GILLER, H. (1983) *Juvenile Delinquency*. Harmondsworth: Penguin.

SAPSFORD, R. J. (1978) Life sentence prisoners: psychological changes during sentence. *British Journal of Criminology*, **18**, 128-145.

SCHWEINHART, L. J. & WEIKART, D. P. (1980) *Young Children Grow Up*. Ypsilanti, MI: High/Scope.

SWANSON, J. W., HOLZER, C. E., GANJU, V. K., *et al* (1990) Violence and psychiatric disorder in the community: evidence from the epidemiologic catchment area surveys. *Hospital and Community Psychiatry*, **41**, 761-770.

TAYLOR, P. J. (1985) Motives for offending among violent and psychotic men. *British Journal of Psychiatry*, **147**, 491–498.
—— (1993) Schizophrenia and crime: distinctive patterns in association. In *Crime and Mental Disorder* (ed. S. Hodgins). Kluwer Academic Publishers.
—— & GUNN, J. (1984a) Violence and psychosis: risk of violence among psychotic men. *British Medical Journal*, **288**.
—— & —— (1984b) Violence and psychosis II. Effect of psychiatric diagnosis on convictions and sentencing of offenders. *British Medical Journal*, **289**, 9–12.
——, MULLEN, P. & WESSELY, S. (1993) Psychosis, violence and crime. In *Forensic Psychiatry: Clinical, Legal and Ethical Issues* (eds J. Gunn & P. J. Taylor). Oxford: Heinemann-Butterworth.
TENNENT, G. & WAY, C. (1984) The English Special Hospital. A 12–17 year follow up study: a comparison of violent and non-violent re-offenders and non-offenders. *Medicine, Science and the Law*, **24**, 81–91.
TERR, L. C. (1981) Psychic trauma in children: observations following the Chowchilla school bus kidnapping. *American Journal of Psychiatry*, **139**, 14–19.
—— (1983) Chowchilla revisited: the effects of psychic trauma four years after a school bus kidnapping. *American Journal of Psychiatry*, **140**, 1543–1550.
—— (1991) Childhood traumas: an outline and overview. *American Journal of Psychiatry*, **148**, 10–20.
THE ROYAL COMMISSION ON CRIMINAL JUSTICE (1993) Report. London: HMSO, Cm 2263.
THOMAS, A. & CHESS, S. (1984) Genesis and evolution of behavioural disorders: from infancy to early adult life. *American Journal of Psychiatry*, **141**, 1–9.
TURNBULL, P. J., DOLAN, F. A. & STIMSON, S. V. (1991)) *Risks and Experiences in Custodial Care*. Horsham: AIDS Education and Research Trust.
VAN DUSEN, K. T., MEDNICK, S. A., GABRIELLI, W. F., *et al* (1983) Social class and crime in an adoption cohort. *Journal of Criminal Law and Criminology*, **74**, 249–269.
WALTERS, G. D. (1994) *Drugs and Crime in Lifestyle Perspective*. Thousand Oaks, CA: Sage.
WEISETH, L. (1989) Individual and organisational response to disaster. Presented to VIII World Congress of Psychiatry, Athens. *Excerpta Medica International Congress Series*, **899**, P706 No. 2743.
WESSELY, S. (1992) The criminal careers of people in one London borough with and without schizophrenia. Presentation to the Winter Workshop on Schizophrenia, Badgastein, Austria, 1 February 1992.
WEST, D. J. (1990) The Cambridge study in delinquent development: a long-term follow-up of all 411 London males. In *Criminality: Personality, Behaviour, Life History* (eds H. J. Kerner & G. Kaiser), pp. 115–138. Berlin: Springer-Verlag.
—— & FARRINGTON, D. P. (1973) *Who Became Delinquent?* London: Heinemann.
WIDOM, C. S. (1991) Avoidance of criminality in abused and neglected children. *Psychiatry*, **54**, 162–174.
WIESZ, J. R., WALTER, B. R., WEISS, B., *et al* (1990) Arrests among emotionally disturbed violent and assaultative individuals following minimal versus lengthy intervention through North Carolina's Willie M Program. *Journal of Consulting and Criminal Psychology*, **58**, 720–728.
WILSON, J. P. & ZIGELBAUM, S. D. (1983) The Vietnam veteran on trial: the relation of post-traumatic stress disorder to criminal behaviour. *Behaviour Science and the Law*, **1**, 69–83.
WOLFGANG, M. E. (1980) Some new findings from the longitudinal study of crime. *Australian Journal of Forensic Sciences*, **13**, 12–29.
—— & STROHM, R. B. (1956) The relationship between alcohol and criminal homicide. *Quarterly Journal of Studies in Alcoholism*, **17**, 411–425.
ZACUNE, J. & HENSMAN, C. (1971) *Drugs, Alcohol and Tobacco in Britain*. London: Heinemann.
ZEITLYN, H. (1990) Current interests in child–adult psychopathological continuities. *Journal of Child Psychology and Psychiatry*, **31**, 671–679.

IV. Prevention in medical settings

17 General hospitals

KEITH LLOYD and SIMON WESSELY

The prevalence of psychiatric disorders among general hospital populations is higher than in community settings, with non-psychotic disorders such as depression, anxiety and somatic symptoms predominating. There is a threefold excess in the risk of psychiatric disorder in those with physical illness compared to those without (Low, 1988; Mayou, 1988; Weyerer, 1990; Lloyd, 1991; Meakin, 1992). Yet, less than 50% of general hospital patients with psychiatric disorders diagnosable according to research criteria will have their disorder diagnosed by the staff looking after them (Maguire *et al*, 1974; Goldberg, 1985; Mayou & Hawton, 1986). Still fewer of those patients in whom psychiatric disorder is recognised will receive specific assessment or treatment for their psychiatric condition (Anon, 1981). This significant pool of untreated psychiatric morbidity among general hospital populations has implications for the organisation of psychiatric services within this setting, and should involve consideration of the nature of that morbidity and the applicability and efficacy of detection, prevention and treatment.

When reviewing the opportunities for preventive strategies the diversity of general hospital psychiatry, its history and development have to be borne in mind. Twenty years ago few hospitals in this country were able to offer a coherent liaison service. In those hospitals where liaison psychiatry was available, interdisciplinary communication was not good. Mezey & Kellett (1971) reported that physicians and surgeons were not over keen to refer patients to psychiatrists for a variety of reasons including the lack of appropriate and readily available services, poor working relationships with psychiatric colleagues and their perception that patients did not like being seen by a psychiatrist. Creed (1991) argued that much has changed over the intervening years with the development of successful policies for dealing with deliberate self-harm patients, and other initiatives raising the profile of liaison psychiatry. However, he contended that there continue to be problems of poor communication between psychiatrists and physicians. On the positive side Creed noted that within general medicine there has been a change of attitude among physicians who now show increasing willingness to recognise the high prevalence of non-organic complaints among medical patients, and there is an increased search for more appropriate management aimed at reducing cost and over investigation. One of the strongest positive influences for change is the availability of a motivated liaison team with appropriate skills (Crisp, 1968; Brown & Cooper, 1987). The prevention and early detection of psychiatric morbidity has an important part to play in this process.

For present purposes, the relevant associations between physical and psychiatric disorders can be summarised thus:

(a) Non-organic psychological consequences of physical disorders
(b) Organic psychiatric disorders
(c) Physical presentations of psychiatric disorders
(d) Psychiatric disorders in specific settings
(e) Emotional and psychiatric problems among patients' relatives
(f) Emotional and psychiatric problems among hospital staff.

Non-organic psychological consequences of physical disorders

Adjustment disorders: epidemiology

Adjustment disorders are the commonest psychological reaction to physical illnesses both acute and chronic (Lloyd, 1991). A period of psychological readjustment following a physical illness or surgery is a normal and early response but it has been suggested that prolonged and maladaptive adjustment reactions are associated with poorer long-term outcome of the physical condition (Hawton, 1981). It is important to note that in general most studies show that the associations of psychological disorders in the physically ill are similar to those in the non-physically ill. Such variables as life events, poor social support, lack of 'mastery', previous psychiatric history have all been implicated. Although the type and severity of the physical illness is indeed relevant, it is not as important a variable as one might expect (Feldman et al, 1987; Turner & Noh, 1988).

Secondary affective disorders: epidemiology and screening

Affective disorders have frequently been shown to be more prevalent among the medically ill than among the general population, even allowing for false positives generated by the use of screening instruments originally developed for use among psychiatric in-patients, most of whom do not have serious concomitant physical illnesses (Feldman et al, 1987). Known associations with affective disorder in general hospital patients include younger age (although there is evidence to suggest that the elderly are at particular risk of depression (Harper et al, 1990)), female sex, lower social class in women, dissatisfaction with living alone, severity of physical illness (in some studies), a previous history of psychiatric illness, and concomitant social problems (reviewed in Mayou & Hawton, 1986). The majority of studies have been cross-sectional in design using screening instruments such as the General Health Questionnaire (GHQ), the Clinical Interview Schedule, Symptom Check list and the Hospital Anxiety and Depression (HAD) scale (Goldberg, 1985). Of these, only the HAD is specifically designed (drawing on clinical experience rather than factor analysis) to detect psychiatric illness among the physically ill (Zigmond & Snaith, 1983). Lewis & Wessely (1990) found that both the HAD and EMG-12 performed well in detecting psychiatric disorder in a dermatology clinic. Its main advantage is its brevity. Reviewing available studies, Mayou & Hawton (1986) found a wide range from 13% to 61% for the prevalence of affective disorder among general hospital in-patients and between 14% and 52% for general hospital out-patients. A key issue is the distinction between an appropriate response to illness and a depressive illness. However, the consensus of such studies suggests that approximately 20 to 30% of new medical out-patients will have a clinically diagnosable affective disorder.

There is evidence to suggest that a proportion of these disorders persisted after discharge especially in those patients with a past psychiatric history (Hawton, 1981; Feldman *et al*, 1987). The relationship of psychiatric co-morbidity to the outcome of a physical disorder is unclear, some workers suggesting that psychiatric disorder slows recovery from physical illness and some suggesting that those patients with the more serious physical illnesses are more likely to be depressed than those with milder conditions (Querido, 1959; Moffic & Paykel, 1975).

Prevention of non-organic disorders

Screening: Proactive targeting of patients at high risk of developing secondary affective disorders could involve either patient selection according to the associations with affective disorder outlined above, or selection of patients suffering from physical conditions known to be associated with a high prevalence of affective disorder. The most effective method of assessing the presence or absence of psychiatric illness is a careful clinical assessment but given the high prevalence of psychiatric disorders and the availability of resources this would be clearly impractical. Nor would it be sufficient to rely on ward staff to detect psychiatric morbidity. Hardman *et al* (1988) found that doctors and nurses identified only 49% of depressed patients on a medical oncology ward. On the other hand they did identify 79% of the patients with clinically significant anxiety detectable by screening with the General Health Questionnaire and standardised psychiatric interview. It is likely that these detection rates by staff were elevated by their knowledge that they were participating in a research project to detect psychiatric morbidity. This raises the important point that when staff are actively seeking psychiatric disorders among their patients they are more likely to find them. Initiatives to train non-psychiatric staff to assess psychiatric disorders have been successful; for example in the management of self-harm (Gardner *et al*, 1978), and have resulted in a drop in demand on psychiatric services.

As regards the method of detection the choice, in practical terms, is between short screening instruments and the brief standardised interview (House, 1988). The disadvantage of administering questionnaires to the elderly and confused or those with confusional states is the patient's ability to complete the test. Meakin (1992) reported that 74% of in-patients were able to complete unspecified pencil and paper tests; in out-patient settings he found higher compliance rates from a review of the literature. Goldberg *et al* (1988) have developed a brief standardised clinical interview which they have used successfully in general practice settings. As yet there are few studies comparing these methods. More is known about screening questionnaires such as the General Health Questionnaire and the Hospital Anxiety and Depression scale (Zigmond & Snaith, 1983). Both have been used successfully with in- and out-patient populations.

Any attempts to screen patients with a view to prevention and treatment would only be successful as part of an integrated assessment and treatment protocol. In the first instance a key issue would be who should administer the instruments. Primary care studies attest to the practicality of nursing staff administering screening instruments to patients prior to their seeing the doctor (Goldberg & Huxley, 1992). Such a move would require cooperation and acceptance of the procedure, a positive attitude to mental illness on the part of staff administering the instrument, and the ability of psychiatric colleagues to offer effective advice and treatment once detection has taken place. Recent research has suggested that the blanket application of psychiatric screening instruments on medical wards followed by brief psychiatric consultation is not cost-effective. Levenson *et al* (1992) confirmed the well known high prevalence of psychiatric disorders on medical wards, and the association between psychiatric morbidity and the use of medical resources. However, they then conducted a randomised controlled trial of brief psychiatric consultation guided by screening. There was no significant difference in psychiatric morbidity, or medical costs, between the groups. It seems that before psychiatric intervention could be shown to be effective, it would be necessary to exclude first those who would get better anyway (with such diagnoses as brief adjustment disorder), and then those with severe medical illness who would not get better even with treatment. Thus psychiatric intervention is most appropriately targeted at high-risk groups, such as those with chronic debilitating illness, medically unexplained symptoms, such as the fatigue and myalgia syndromes, or other conditions with high psychosocial morbidity, such as malignancies or HIV infection.

Organic psychiatric disorders

Secondary to physical illness

Organic mental disorders are associated with many physical illnesses, especially infective and metabolic conditions, diseases of the central nervous system, substance misuse, prescribed drug taking and end organ failure. These are also common in certain environments associated with under or over stimulation, such as intensive care. All become commoner with increasing age (Hodkinson, 1973; Bergman & Eastman, 1974; Lishman, 1987). Overall prevalence estimates among general hospital populations suggest that between one-quarter and one-third of patients have intellectual impairment. By and large these studies did not differentiate between acute, chronic and acute on chronic organic conditions, even though the early identification of acute organic states is crucial because of the need to treat the underlying condition and the high mortality rates associated with acute organic states (Mayou & Hawton, 1986).

Prevention

Wherever possible the prevention of acute confusional states relies on the prompt treatment of the underlying mechanism. This is often the domain of the non-psychiatrist. Primary preventive strategies such as skilled nursing care and a good working relationship and communication skills with the patient are also important. Attention to the physical environment with measures such as providing adequate sensory stimulation and lighting are all important. The psychiatrist is often only involved when the patient's behaviour becomes problematic or when the confusional state has been missed as a cause of changed behaviour or mental state. In those instances where psychotropic medication is considered careful consideration should be given to the choice of drug so as not to worsen the confusional state with inappropriate use of benzodiazepines or aggravate seizures with anti-psychotic medication. Screening instruments for acute and chronic organic disorders include the Mini Mental State (Folstein *et al*, 1975) and the Geriatric Mental State (Copeland *et al*, 1976).

Secondary to alcohol and drug misuse

Male attenders at accident and emergency departments, and in-patients on orthopaedic, surgical and medical wards show a high prevalence of alcohol problems (Holt, 1980; Barrison *et al*, 1982). Many such patients have alcohol-related conditions, but the prevalence of alcohol problems is also high among patients whose current illness is not directly alcohol-related, most studies finding that approximately 20 to 25% of acute hospital admissions are related to alcohol (Lloyd, 1991). Ghodse (1981) estimated that 18.3 per 1000 attendances at accident and emergency departments in London were drug-related.

Prevention

There are several simple screening tests for the detection of problem drinkers which are superior to laboratory tests (*Lancet*, 1980; Wallace, 1986). Johns & Ritson (Chapter 12) have identified the population-based strategies for tackling alcohol-related problems, but in-patient settings offer rich opportunities for the detection of problem drinkers. Again the question is one of how best to employ scant resources. Realistically there is little time in, for example, accident and emergency settings, to screen for alcohol-related problems despite the high prevalence of problem drinkers encountered there. Self-administered screening instruments such as the MAST (Pokorny *et al*, 1972) or CAGE (Mayfield *et al*, 1974) take little time to complete, but are only worthwhile if effective intervention follows.

Screening of in-patients is easier and the same considerations apply as with screening instruments for affective disorders. Detection would need to be followed with appropriate counselling or referral to outside agencies. In a well designed trial Chick *et al* (1985) evaluated the efficacy of brief counselling by a specialist nurse among a group of male medical in-patients with alcohol problems. At 12 month follow-up the counselled group did better than the controlled group on some of the measures used.

Sexual dysfunction

Any physical illness can affect sexual functioning. In a survey of over 1000 male medical out-patients Slag *et al* (1983) found that 34% suffered from impotence. Follow-up investigations indicated that the majority were due to organic causes especially medication. The prevalence of sexual dysfunction is highest among patients with diabetes, renal problems, heart disease and peripheral neurological disorders. Less is known about levels of sexual dysfunction among female patients. Again detection and prevention rely on there being a climate in which patients feel they can express their concerns about sexual dysfunction, and clinicians provide appropriate advice and guidance.

Physical presentations of psychiatric disorders

Somatisation

Somatisation is best understood as a process rather than a disease and is the most common way for psychiatric disorders to present in non-psychiatric settings (see Chapter 18). Certain groups are known to be at particular high risk – those with unexplained somatic symptoms such as irritable bowel, chronic fatigue, facial pain and so on. The range of symptoms is large and somatisation occurs in all medical settings. The primary psychiatric diagnosis in most cases is primary affective disorder, although a significant majority are suffering from somatoform, dissociative or factitious disorders (Slavney & Teitelbaum, 1985). Most patients who somatise receive more medical investigations than are necessary. A proportion are eventually diagnosed as having medical illnesses, but even those may not be sufficient to explain the observed physical and psychological symptoms. The risk of iatrogenic injury is high, as is the risk of prescribed drug misuse, such as benzodiazepines. This is an important area for developing preventive strategies as appropriate detection and intervention have significant cost–benefit implications as well as offering the possibility of improving patients' well being. Strategies for the detection and recognition of somatisation are outlined in Chapter 18 and in Creed *et al* (1992).

Attempted suicide

Deliberate self-harm is discussed in Chapter 8 and will only be mentioned here briefly, although it is of central importance to the development of liaison psychiatry. The size of the problems is indicated from a study which suggested that 11% of admissions to a central London hospital over a four year period during the 1980s were for attempted suicide (Fuller *et al*, 1989). Hawton (Chapter 8) estimated that there are at least 100 000 hospital referrals per year in England and Wales for attempted suicide. The condition represents the commonest reason for acute medical admission in females and comes second only to ischaemic heart disease in men. Completed suicide has been increasing among young males in recent years and this may in time be reflected in referral rates. Secondary and tertiary preventive strategies are reviewed in Chapter 8.

Psychiatric disorders in specific settings and physical illnesses

Obstetrics and gynaecology

About 50% of women experience post-partum blues with symptoms peaking on the fifth day post-partum. There are no indications that this condition can be prevented from occurring, although health education as a part of antenatal care is important to inform women about the condition.

Puerperal depression is more serious and prevalence estimates vary between 3–16%. Onset usually occurs within the first post-partum month, usually between day 3 and day 14. In the majority of women this will be after they return home, and they will often present initially to GPs and health visitors. Education about this condition should be and usually is a feature of antenatal care. However, women with this condition rarely report their symptoms to doctors and a simple scale has been developed which could lead to increased detection and earlier intervention (Cox *et al*, 1987).

The aetiology of puerperal psychosis is unknown. It occurs following 2.6 per 1000 first births and 1.4 per 1000 in later confinements, with symptoms almost always developing within two weeks of delivery (Kendell *et al*, 1981). The main preventive strategy lies in the development of liaison links with the obstetric department to identify mothers at risk, for example those with a past history of psychosis, and to offer prompt and efficient service for those who do develop mental illnesses (Appleby *et al*, 1989).

It is now commonplace to offer brief counselling before termination of pregnancy. This primary preventive strategy has been shown to reduce the likelihood of subsequent psychiatric complications (Greer *et al*, 1976). Psychiatric problems are more common following miscarriage and still birth. A well designed randomised controlled study of prompt bereavement counselling following perinatal deaths, backed up by appropriate obstetric support and advice, demonstrated that intervention was effective in reducing psychiatric complications at six months (Forrest *et al*, 1982).

HIV infection

The prevention of HIV infection is the subject of major public health initiatives. Most HIV services offer well developed counselling services and psychology and psychiatric input, aimed at primary, secondary and tertiary prevention (Miller & Bor, 1988).

Oncology

Much of the psychiatric morbidity associated with cancer, as with other illnesses, goes unrecognised and untreated. Although exact prevalence data are unavailable it is known that mastectomy, chemotherapy and colostomy are associated with substantial psychiatric morbidity. As in other physical illnesses non-psychotic syndromes such as anxiety and depression predominate (Dean, 1987). Rates for psychiatric referral and treatment are higher than are usually found in medical and surgical wards, oncology being an area where physicians increasingly recognise the importance of attending to the patient's psychosocial well being (Maguire *et al*, 1974; Greer, 1985). Many issues pertaining to the prevention of psychiatric disorders associated with serious illnesses apply equally to prevention in association with malignant disorders. There is an increasing body of evidence that in breast cancer a patient's coping style may influence the outcome of the malignancy. Cognitive–behavioural treatments have been designed to optimise patients' coping styles (Moorey & Greer, 1989). This is an area where preventing psychiatric disorders or the modifying psychiatric variables may lead to a decrease in physical morbidity.

Psychological and emotional problems among relatives

The physical illness of a family member can have serious repercussions for other family members which go beyond practical considerations of financial hardship, the burden of caring for a sick relative and uncertainty about prognosis. Following death of the patient, relatives have to cope with bereavement and readjustment. Following myocardial infarction spouses experience similar levels of psychological distress to the patient (Mayou, 1979). During rehabilitation and when looking after a chronically ill, disabled or dying patient the carer often experiences considerable psychological distress (Anderson, 1987). Among the elderly, when one partner is admitted to hospital, the other may not be able to function alone if the sick person was the primary carer for the couple.

The most important preventive strategy involves the provision of adequate and comprehensible information, support and attention given at the appropriate time. Generally psychiatrists are only involved in this process when a relative becomes acutely disturbed. But psychiatrists have an important role to play in educating students and staff in this process (Goldberg & Huxley, 1992), a strategy which could also have useful public relations benefits for the liaison psychiatric team.

Hospital staff

Recent studies among junior hospital doctors (Dudley, 1990) have highlighted something that has been known for a long time: working in hospitals is a stressful experience. Levels of anxiety and depression among doctors are high, and rates of alcohol and drug misuse and self-harm have increased in the medical profession (Rucinski & Cybulska, 1985). Firth-Cozens (1987) reported that over 30% of junior doctors experience significant psychological distress. Rates were even higher among female house officers, 46% of whom were significantly depressed in one study (Firth-Cozens, 1991). Within hospitals certain areas are recognised as being particularly stressful such as intensive care units, oncology, paediatric departments and renal dialysis units. Health professionals are generally poor at seeking help for their own mental health problems. Most hospitals have occupational health departments and in some larger hospitals members of the liaison team are involved in the service provided. Opportunities for primary prevention exist in the provision of support and guidance for staff either formally in groups or by easy access to services. At present little training or teaching is provided for medical students on how to recognise symptoms in themselves and the climate does not exist in which sufferers feel comfortable to admit their symptoms and seek help. There is a national counselling service for sick doctors which performs valuable work in the area of secondary and tertiary prevention (Rawnsley, 1985). Local initiatives depend on the acceptance of the psychiatrist and attention to mental health as a prioritised activity. It would be possible to evaluate this using such measures as rates of sick leave.

Conclusions

Attempted suicide, affective disorders, alcohol-related problems and somatisation are sufficiently common and all have serious or potentially serious consequences to merit their consideration as targets of preventive strategies. Apart from research and service planning needs to detect and estimate the prevalence of these disorders, it is necessary to consider whether specific and sensitive tests exist for these disorders, whether detection and intervention in the natural history of these conditions is possible, whether effective interventions exist, the possibilities for identifying individuals at risk and the cost–benefit and resource implications of preventive strategies (see Chapter 19).

Mayou & Hawton (1991) found that patients with certain physical conditions (such as myocardial infarction, chest pain, diabetes and cancer) were more likely to use psychiatric sessions following medical admissions. One implication of this is that patients with these disorders form a group with special needs who could be targeted for preventive strategies. Together with patients who have alcohol-related disorders, and medically unexplained physical symptoms, these are the three groups who might benefit from better detection of their psychological problems to prevent later psychiatric services utilisation.

The issues of resources, personnel and the status of liaison psychiatry arise. A preliminary target for the prevention of psychiatric disorders in general hospital settings is the establishment of comprehensive liaison services and willingness to collaborate with, educate and be educated by colleagues from medical and surgical disciplines. There are some encouraging signs in this direction which highlight the knock-on effects of establishing effective services. Physicians are becoming more willing to involve psychiatrists in the management of patients (Mayou & Smith, 1986). However, a recent survey of district psychiatric services cited in Creed *et al* (1992) showed that more than 60% had plans to develop a community mental health service, but less than 14% had plans to improve their liaison psychiatry service. The other side of this equation, as Creed (1991) observed, is that adult general psychiatrists should come to regard liaison work as an important part of their clinical work much as child psychiatrists and old age psychiatrists already acknowledge the importance of close collaboration with paediatricians and geriatricians respectively. This will also address the question of available resources – one of the aims of liaison psychiatry should be to help other staff identify and manage psychiatric problems in their patients.

References

ANDERSON, R. (1987) The unremitting burden on carers. *British Medical Journal*, **294**, 73–74.
ANONYMOUS (1981) Psychiatry in the general hospital (Editorial). *British Medical Journal*, **282**, 1256–1257.
APPLEBY, L., FOX, H., SHAW, M., *et al* (1989) The psychiatrist in the obstetric unit: establishing a liaison service. *British Journal of Psychiatry*, **154**, 510–514.
BARRISON, I. G., VIOLA, A., MUMFORD, J., *et al* (1982) Detecting excessive drinking among admissions to a general hospital. *Health Trends*, **14**, 80–83.
BERGMAN, K. & EASTMAN, E. (1974) Psychogeriatric ascertainment and assessment for treatment in an acute medical ward setting. *Age & Aging*, **3**, 174–188.
BROWN, A. & COOPER, A. F. (1987) The impact of liaison psychiatry on patterns of referral in a general hospital. *British Journal of Psychiatry*, **150**, 83–87.
CHICK, J., LLOYD, G. & CROMBIE, E. (1985) Counselling problem drinkers in medical wards: a controlled study. *British Medical Journal*, **290**, 965–967.
COPELAND, J. R. M., KELLEHER, M. J., KELLEHER, J. M., *et al* (1976) A semi-structured clinical interview for the assessment of diagnosis and mental state in the elderly: the geriatric mental state schedule. *Psychological Medicine*, **6**, 439–449.

Cox, J. L., Holden, J. M. & Sagovsky, R. (1987) Detection of post-natal depression: development of the 10 item Edinburgh post-natal depression scale. *British Journal of Psychiatry*, **150**, 782–786.

Creed, F. (1991) Liaison psychiatry for the 21st century: a review. *Journal of the Royal Society of Medicine*, **84**, 414–417.

———, Mayou, R. A. & Hopkins, A. (1992) *Medical Symptoms not Explained by Organic Disease*. London: Gaskell.

Crisp, A. H. (1968) The role of the psychiatrist in the general hospital. *Postgraduate Medical Journal*, **44**, 267–276.

Dean, C. (1987) Psychiatric morbidity following mastectomy. *Journal of Psychosomatic Research*, **31**, 385–392.

Dudley, H. A. F. (1990) Stress in junior doctors (Editorial). *British Medical Journal*, **301**, 75–76.

Feldman, E., Mayou, R., Hawton, K., *et al* (1987) Psychiatric disorder in medical in-patients. *Quarterly Journal of Medicine*, **63**, 405–412.

Firth-Cozens, J. (1987) Emotional distress in junior house officers. *British Medical Journal*, **295**, 533–536.

——— (1991) Science of stress in woman junior house officers. *British Medical Journal*, **301**, 89–91.

Folstein, M. F., Folstein, S. & McHugh, P. R. (1975) Mini Mental State. A practical method for grading the cognitive state of patients for the clinician. *Journal of Psychiatric Research*, **12**, 189–198.

Forrest, G., Standish, E. & Baum, J. (1982) Support after perinatal death: a study of support and counselling after perinatal bereavement. *British Medical Journal*, **285**, 1475–1479.

Fuller, G. N., Rea, A. J., Payne, J. F., *et al* (1989) Parasuicide in central London 1984–1988. *Journal of the Royal Society of Medicine*, **82**, 653–656.

Gardner, R., Hanka, R., Evison, B., *et al* (1978) Consultation liaison scheme for self-poisoned patients in a general hospital. *British Medical Journal*, **11**, 1392–1394.

Ghodse, H. (1981) Drug related problems in London Accident and Emergency departments: a 12 month survey. *Lancet*, **ii**, 859–862.

Goldberg, D. (1985) Identifying psychiatric illness among general medical patients. *British Medical Journal*, **291**, 161–162.

———, Bridges, K., Duncan-Jones, P., *et al* (1988) Detecting anxiety and depression in general medical settings. *British Medical Journal*, **297**, 897–899.

———, Benjamin, S. & Creed, F. (1989) *Psychiatry in Medical Practice*. London: Routledge.

——— & Huxley, P. (1992) *Common Mental Disorders: A Biosocial Model*. London: Routledge.

Greer, H. S., Lal, S., Lewis, S. (1976) Psychosocial consequences of therapeutic abortion. King's termination study III. *British Journal of Psychiatry*, **128**, 74–79.

——— (1985) Cancer: Psychiatric aspects. In *Recent Advances in Clinical Psychiatry* (ed. K. Granville-Grossman). Edinburgh: Churchill Livingstone.

Hardman, A., Maguire, P. & Crowther, D. (1989) The recognition of psychiatric morbidity on a medical oncology ward. *Journal of Psychosomatic Research*, **33**, 235–239.

Harper, R. G., Kotik-Harper, D. & Kirby, H. (1990) Psychometric assessment of depression in an elderly general medical population. *Journal of Nervous and Mental Disease*, **178**, 113–119.

Hawton, K. (1981) The long-term outcome of psychiatric morbidity detected in general medical out-patients. *Journal of Psychosomatic Research*, **25**, 237–243.

Hodkinson, H. M. (1973) Mental impairment in the elderly. *Journal of the Royal College of Physicians*, **7**, 305–317.

Holt, S., Stewart, I. C., Dixon, J. M., *et al* (1980) Alcohol and the emergency service patient. *British Medical Journal*, **281**, 638–640.

House, A. (1988) Mood disorders in the physically ill – problems of definition and measurement. *Journal of Psychosomatic Research*, **32**, 345–353.

Kendell, R. E., Rennie, D., Clarke, J. A., *et al* (1981) The social and obstetric correlates of psychiatric admission in the puerperium. *Psychological Medicine*, **11**, 341–350.

Lancet (1980) Screening test for alcohol (Editorial). *Lancet*, **ii**, 1117–1118.

Levenson, J., Hame, R. & Rossiter, L. (1992) A randomised controlled study of psychiatric consultation guided by screening in general medical in-patients. *American Journal of Psychiatry*, **149**, 631–637.

Lewis, G. & Wessely, S. (1990) A comparison of the General Health Questionnaire and the Hospital Anxiety and Depression Scale. *British Journal of Psychiatry*, **157**, 860–864.

Lishman, W. A. (1987) *Organic Psychiatry* (2nd Edn). Oxford: Blackwell.

Low, C. (1988) Psychiatric clinics in different settings. *British Journal of Psychiatry*, **153**, 243–245.

Lloyd, G. G. (1991) *Textbook of General Hospital Psychiatry*. Edinburgh: Churchill Livingstone.

Maguire, G. P., Julier, D. L., Hawton, K. E., *et al* (1974) Psychiatric morbidity and referral on two general medical wards. *British Medical Journal*, **i**, 268–270.

MAYFIELD, D., MCLEOD, G. & HALL, P. (1974) The CAGE questionnaire: validation of a new alcoholism screening instrument. *American Journal of Psychiatry*, **131**, 1121–1123.

MAYOU, R. A. (1979) The course and determinants of psychological reactions to myocardial infarction. *British Journal of Psychiatry*, **134**, 588–594.

––––– (1988) Psychiatric treatment of somatic symptoms. *Current Opinion in Psychiatry*, **1**, 150–154.

––––– & HAWTON, K. E. (1986) Psychiatric disorder in the general hospital. *British Journal of Psychiatry*, **149**, 173–190.

––––– & SMITH, E. B. O. (1986) Hospital doctors' management of psychological problems. *British Journal of Psychiatry*, **148**, 194–197.

––––– & HAWTON, K. (1991) Use of psychiatric services by patients in a general hospital. *British Medical Journal*, **303**, 1029–1032.

MEAKIN, C. J. (1992) Screening for depression in the medically ill. *British Journal of Psychiatry*, **160**, 212–216.

MEZEY, A. G. & KELLETT, J. M. (1971) Reasons against referral to the psychiatrist. *Postgraduate Medical Journal*, **47**, 315–319.

MILLER, R. & BOR, R. (1988) *Aids: a Guide to Clinical Counselling*. London: Science Press.

MOFFIC, H. S. & PAYKEL, E. S. (1975) Depression in medical in-patients. *British Journal of Psychiatry*, **126**, 346–353.

MOOREY, S. & GREER, S. (1989) *Psychological Therapy for Patient Unit Cancer: a New Approach*. Oxford: Heinmann.

POKORNY, A. D., MILLER, B. A. & KAPLAN, H. B. (1972) The brief MAST: A shortened version of the Michigan alcoholism screening test. *American Journal of Psychiatry*, **129**, 342–345.

QUERIDO, A. (1959) An investigation into the clinical, social and mental factors determining the results of hospital treatment. *British Journal of Preventive and Social Medicine*, **13**, 33–49.

RAWNSLEY, K. (1985) Helping the sick doctor: a new service. *British Medical Journal*, **291**, 922.

RUCINSKI, J. & CYBULSKA, E. (1985) Mentally ill doctors. *British Journal of Hospital Medicine*, **33**, 90–94.

SLAG, M. F., MORLEY, J. E., ELSON, N. K., *et al* (1983) Impotence in male medical out-patients. *Journal of the American Medical Association*, **249**, 1736–1740.

SLAVNEY, P. & TEITELBAUM, M. (1985) Patients with medically unexplained symptoms. *General Hospital Psychiatry*, **7**, 21–25.

TURNER, R. & NOH, S. (1988) Physical disability and depression. *Journal of Health & Social Behaviour*, **29**, 23–37.

WALLACE, P. (1986) Looking for patients at risk because of their drinking. *Journal of the Royal Society of Medicine*, **79**, 129–130.

WEYERER, S. (1990) Relationships between physical and psychological disorders. In *Psychological Disorders in General Medical Settings* (eds N. Satorins, *et al*), pp. 34–46. Bern: Hogrefe & Muber.

ZIGMOND, A. & SNAITH, R. (1983) The hospital anxiety and depression scale. *Acta Psychiatrica Scandinavica*, **67**, 361–370.

18 Somatisation

CHRISTOPHER BASS

Somatisation has been described as "the expression of personal and social distress in an idiom of bodily complaints with medical help-seeking" (Kleinman & Kleinman, 1985). It can be regarded as a basic mechanism which the human species has for responding to stress: we develop pains and discomforts in our bodies. Many definitions of somatisation have been proposed, but the essential features include one or more physical complaints (such as fatigue and gastro-intestinal complaints), and (i) appropriate evaluation uncovers no organic pathology to account for the physical complaints; or (ii) when there is related organic pathology, the physical complaints or resulting social or occupational impairment are grossly in excess of what would be expected from the physical findings.

It is important for psychiatrists to know about somatisation because it is the most common way for psychiatric disorders to present in non-psychiatric settings (Table 18.1). Two studies from primary care and the general hospital respectively illustrate this: (i) one in five patients with new inceptions of illness in primary care satisfies research criteria for somatisation (Goldberg & Bridges, 1988); and (ii) of 94 consecutive referrals to a cardiac clinic with presenting symptoms of chest pain or palpitations, 64% were found to have no heart disease or other serious physical cause for their symptoms (Mayou, 1992).

Somatisation is a process, not a disease entity. One of the most common mechanisms appears to be an affective disorder inducing somatic symptoms, followed by selective perception of bodily symptoms, motivated by fear of disease or other concerns, and a subsequent increase in anxiety with more somatic symptoms forming links in a vicious circle. Somatisation can be acute, sub-acute or chronic, these periods generally being less than four weeks, one to six months, and in excess of six months, respectively.

TABLE 18.1
The prevalence of somatisation in non-psychiatric settings

Setting	Prevalence	Author
Community	4.4%[1]	Escobar *et al*, 1987
Primary care	26–30%	Goldberg & Bridges, 1988; Bhatt *et al*, 1989
Liaison psychiatry service	40%	De Leon *et al*, 1987
Pain clinic	2–53%	Benjamin *et al*, 1988

1. The prevalence of an 'abridged somatisation construct' (at least 4 'unfounded' somatic symptoms for males and 6 for females).

Failure to identify and correctly manage patients with somatic presentations of psychosocial distress can have grave consequences. Chronic somatisation is associated with considerable disability, especially in patients over 40 with a psychiatric diagnosis (Escobar et al, 1987), and with high utilisation of both general medical and mental health resources (Katon et al, 1991). Much of this is a consequence of inappropriate medication, investigations and even surgery (Martin et al, 1977). These harmful and costly secondary effects can all be prevented, and interventions are needed to not only reduce health service and other costs, but also to relieve the non-monetary burden of physical and psychosocial disability on patients and their relatives (Benjamin & Bridges, 1993).

From the point of view of prevention, therefore, the main goal should be to prevent the somatic complaints becoming chronic, i.e. secondary prevention. However, primary prevention also has a role.

Primary prevention

Primary prevention customarily refers to measures which prevent the problem from occurring in the first place. Because somatisation is the presentation of psychosocial distress in terms of physical complaints, primary prevention requires the same effort as primary prevention of anxiety and depression in the population.

The usual course in primary prevention is firstly to identify risk factors and subsequently to initiate measures to eradicate them. Although there is only limited knowledge about risk factors in somatisation, there is some evidence that the psychosocial model proposed by Brown and his colleagues (Brown & Harris, 1989) is relevant and provides a framework for a model of prevention. For example, provoking agents or events, vulnerability or predisposing factors, and protective factors have all been shown to be important in the genesis and maintenance of somatisation (Kellner, 1990).

Primary prevention in children

In primary care investigations indicate a psychological contribution to 17–25% of children's attendances (Garralda & Bailey, 1987). These children tend to present with 'psychosomatic-type symptoms', have relatively high attendance rates in primary and hospital care, and have mothers with health problems.

Inappropriate patterns of invalidism and somatisation in children are associated with a poor prognosis. The great cost and personal distress of chronic disorders in adult life point to the need for primary prevention in children. The potential value is unknown and intervention studies are needed. Benjamin & Eminson (1992) have suggested that these might include public education programmes aimed at both parents and children through the media and in schools. Children who are identified as likely to be at high risk by virtue of their own parents' types of behaviour require special help, the effect of which should be evaluated. Improved training for medical undergraduates and postgraduate students is needed to help them to recognise these problems and their appropriate management.

In recent years factitious illness by proxy (or FIP) has been described in children (Meadow, 1977). The perpetrator is usually the mother and the victim is her child; the parent's aim is to have the child considered seriously ill and subjected to repeated invasive investigations. The typical victims of FIP are children, especially those under five years of age. The iatrogenic damage and unnecessary investigation of these children can be substantial. It is important for both medical and non-medical personnel to be aware of FIP, not only because it can prove very costly. In an American case Schlesinger *et al* (1989) calculated that one admission for their FIP patient cost almost US$9000.

Primary prevention in adults

There is a lot of evidence that life events precipitate a variety of somatising syndromes in predisposed adults (Andrews & House, 1989; Craig & Boardman, 1990). Preventing life events is not plausible, but health promotion strategies may minimise the impact that adverse life events have on the musculo-skeletal and autonomic nervous systems (Linton, 1987). For example, the first development of acute pain may be seen as a warning signal: some people will cope with this signal in appropriate ways, whereas others may complain but nevertheless not deal actively with the problem. Health promotion might teach people how to recognise and cope with such problems while they are still minor. This would involve pain control and problem-solving orientated towards the work place and home. Such an approach might be particularly relevant to individuals at high risk of developing minor musculo-skeletal disorders, such as those engaged in repetitive work involving the hands and back.

Educational programmes in the form of back schools have been studied both as treatment and prevention, but the results have been difficult to evaluate (Linton & Kamwendo, 1986). The same authors used a preventive approach based on work physiology and coping, called the 'relaxation pause'. It is thought that the pauses should interrupt the muscle tension–pain cycle caused by repetitive work routines. Moreover, a use of relaxation could be an important part of pain control and active coping. Linton & Kamwendo (1986) studied the effects of a relaxation–gymnastics programme on neck and shoulder discomfort and found that development of pain and discomfort during the course of the day was affected. However, employees found the frequency of the relaxation gymnastics to be disruptive and there were problems with adherence to the programme in the long term.

Public education

Somatisation is thought to enable people who are unsympathetic to mental disorders to benefit nonetheless when psychologically distressed. It is widespread in Western and other cultures, and the stigma of mental illness is undoubtedly partly responsible. Educating the public about the aetiology of physical symptoms and their relation to stress may therefore have an important contribution. Somatisers will not read leaflets called 'Anxiety' or 'Depression'. The Public Education Committee of the Royal College of Psychiatrists could usefully forge links with organisations such as the British Digestive Foundation and the British Heart Foundation to educate them about the identification and successful psychological management of patients with, respectively, irritable bowel syndrome and non-cardiac pain. The recent joint conference and publication by the Royal College of Physicians and Royal College of Psychiatrists, initiated by the Liaison Psychiatry group, is a step in the right direction (Creed *et al*, 1992).

Many 'somatisers' belong to self-help groups or associations, for example the ME Association. In the last five years psychiatric research has had a substantial effect on the understanding of the pathogenesis and management of this disorder (Jenkins & Mowbray, 1991). There is therefore scope for the Public Education Committee at the Royal College to liaise with and educate these lay organisations about mind–body interactions. The advice that the ME Association gives to its members could and should be influenced by the results of current psychiatric research. This could in turn reduce both lay and medical prejudices about symptoms without disease ('It's all in your mind, it's your fault, pull your socks up' and so forth).

Secondary prevention

Prevention programmes which deal with patients at or after the first health care visit for somatic symptoms may be considered secondary prevention. The major goal of secondary prevention is to prevent the acute disorder from becoming chronic and enduring. This is important because chronic somatisation is associated with both disability and increased use of costly medical resources (Katon *et al*, 1991).

Secondary prevention by non-psychiatrists

Non-psychiatric doctors and nurses have the opportunity to identify these patients through administrative indices such as case note thickness and the number of medical contacts, and not just by some sort of face-to-face interviewing. For example, an audit of certain medical services such as gastroenterology and cardiology might reveal patients with very frequent service contacts, repeated rates of negative investigations, and identification of expensive outliers in the general hospital. Early identification of such patients would lead to improved quality of care and (probably) cost savings.

Most district general hospitals have computerised medical records departments which contain information on both the frequency of patient contacts and the number of specialist departments attended. It is conceivable that 'frequent attenders' could be identified by judicious scrutiny of all patients with, for example, more than 12 visits to hospital departments over a two year period (excluding, of course, those with chronic disorders such as leukaemia and diabetes who may require frequent visits for other reasons). Identification of somatising patients using computerised medical records is underused: there are potential research implications, especially for intervention studies.

Secondary prevention by psychiatrists

In practice, secondary prevention involves targeting interventions in appropriate settings, that is, in primary care and the general hospital. Psychiatrists have an important role to play in implementing these activities. The major thrust of prevention in somatisation should be directed towards three main areas:

(a) helping doctors in non-psychiatric settings to develop skills to identify (and manage) patients with somatisation
(b) once patients have been identified, these doctors need to develop the appropriate skills:
  (i) to inform patients about their negative tests
  (ii) to administer the appropriate treatment, which may or may not involve psychiatric referral
  (iii) to learn how to refer the patient for such a psychiatric or psychological assessment
(c) the development of treatment techniques for relatively homogeneous groups of patients with somatising syndromes at a relatively early stage in the evolution of the disorder, i.e. the first six months (whenever possible).

These skills, discussed in detail in Bass & Sharpe (1993), involve the following:

(a) Be aware of psychosocial problems
(b) Ask some basic screening questions: e.g. how do you feel in your mood?; what do you think is causing the pain?
(c) Perform the minimum number of investigations
(d) Provide unambiguous reassurance when there is no evidence of relevant organic disease
(e) Provide a satisfactory alternative explanation for the pain/symptoms
(f) Withdraw unnecessary medication
(g) Know when to refer for psychiatric/psychological opinion
(h) Know how to expedite such a referral.

These suggestions have implications for the way that psychiatric services are organised. If interventions in somatisation are to be effective, psychiatric services need to be available in the general hospital and in general practice. There has been increasing liaison with general practitioners over the last five years, but there also needs to be a parallel increase in the number of psychiatrists working in general hospitals: there needs to be a recognition by the psychiatric services that both general practice and the general hospital are important pathways to psychiatric care (Gater & Goldberg, 1992). These three areas will now be discussed in more detail.

How can non-psychiatrists develop skills to identify patients with somatisation?

Goldberg and his colleagues have developed a number of techniques aimed at helping patients to see their somatic symptoms in a different way: this process has been called reattribution. They have proposed a three stage model, which is designed to encourage patients to reattribute their symptoms and relate them to psychosocial problems (Goldberg et al, 1989). The various stages of this technique have been incorporated into a videotaped learning package which has been used with vocational trainees in general practice (Goldberg et al, 1989). Other authors, e.g. Craig & Boardman (1990) and Tylee (1991) have also stressed the importance of interview techniques, especially at an early stage of the consultation between the general practitioner and the patient. These skills include appropriate use of open questions, responding to mood cues, and making empathic statements.

The acquisition of these interviewing skills by general practitioners is vital if somatising patients are to be correctly identified and managed. But when should these skills be taught, and by whom? There is a strong case for these skills being taught to medical students during their clinical training, when the negative attitudes to these patients also needs to be addressed. Curriculum committees should be made more aware of this topic, and give it a higher priority. Alternatively, most general practitioner training posts have a psychiatry attachment, and this might be an appropriate time for this teaching to occur.

Educational activities should also be extended to those offering psychological treatment in primary care settings. For example, general practice counsellors and community psychiatric nurses working in primary care often have little experience of assessing or managing these patients.

Management of somatisation by non-psychiatrists after diagnosis

This is critical, because the non-psychiatrist has the opportunity to prevent an acute disorder from being a chronic and potentially costly one. There are a number of separate but inter-related practical skills, all of which can be 'learnt' and which lead to improved management of the somatising patient. These include:

(a) informing the patient about the negative tests and explaining the possible causes of his/her symptoms. This basic skill, which includes exploring the patient's illness beliefs and worries, is not taught routinely in medical schools.
(b) appropriate management of the somatising patient by the non-psychiatrist. This may involve either drug treatment or psychological treatment, or both.
(c) referral for psychiatric treatment. This is a crucial process, which if dealt with adequately will facilitate the acceptance of psychological or psychiatric treatment. As with (a) and (b) above, this is a skill that can be learnt, and should be taught to medical students during their clinical training.

Psychiatrists with liaison psychiatry sessions are ideally placed to teach these skills to both medical students and physicians and surgeons in general hospitals. Alternatively, it may require trainee physicians to work in an appropriate psychiatric unit for a limited time to acquire the requisite skills.

Because there are relatively few liaison psychiatrists, it is important for the training of psychiatrists to be modified so that they can manage somatising patients. Appropriate senior registrar experience in a well developed liaison psychiatry unit is therefore essential if the physician's needs in this area are to be met. The educational and other tasks of senior registrars in liaison psychiatry have recently been described by House & Creed (1993).

Furthermore, undergraduate education must be altered so that psychological and physical disorders are perceived in an integrated way, rather than in separate categories as at present.

Psychological treatment of patients with acute or sub-acute somatising syndromes

In the last ten years there have been numerous studies of patients with relatively homogeneous syndromes, for example irritable bowel syndrome, non-cardiac chest pain, and chronic fatigue syndrome (Bass & Potts, 1992). Cognitive and behavioural techniques have focused on reduction of pain and disability, and the teaching of management techniques that can make sufferers increasingly independent of the medical services.

With the increasing cost and size of this problem (Shaw & Creed, 1991; Bass & Potts, 1992) it is clear that resources need to be focused on those people liable to develop chronic somatoform syndromes (usually chronic pain). This could be achieved if individuals were identified soon after the onset of an acute episode, such as low back pain, non-cardiac chest pain, or facial pain. An appropriate time would be four weeks after a critical negative investigation such as upper gastro-intestinal endoscopy, or a coronary angiogram. This would allow sufficient time to elapse to identify both those patients who recover or who are reassured by the negative tests, as well as those with continuing symptoms who require attention. It is this latter group which should become the focus of interventions in controlled trials, and there should be a mechanism whereby such patients receive early assessment and appropriate management. There is enormous scope for more controlled trials of psychological treatment in this field. Such interventions should prove cost-efficient; efforts to quantify cost savings in studies of this nature should always be attempted (Philips *et al*, 1991).

Finally, there is scope for collaboration between psychiatrists and physicians in this field. Creed (1992) has suggested that algorithms be established for the investigation and management of common circumscribed syndromes such as abdominal pain, chest pain, and back pain. For example, a certain number of investigations to exclude organic disease may be regarded as reasonable, as should the inclusion of a number of questions regarding psychological and social issues. The explanation given to the patient regarding the cause of the symptoms should also be positive, clear and compatible with the patient's previous ideas and beliefs. Such an approach readily lends itself to audit, which could become a routine exercise leading to gradual improvement of the algorithm.

Tertiary prevention

General physicians (or surgeons) and general psychiatrists are often unwilling or unable to take responsibility for 'managing' chronic somatisers with persistent and enduring physical complaints. As a consequence these patients often undergo costly investigations and become dependent on state benefits (Bass & Murphy, 1991). Effective management of patients with chronic somatisation can be achieved by a proactive management plan, which can be implemented by psychiatrists (usually those who are based in general hospitals, where these patients are commonplace). The management involves regular, scheduled out-patient appointments, tapering of unnecessary medication, and 'changing the agenda' to involve discussion of psychosocial stressors rather than somatic complaints and medical procedures. The patient is informed that no further investigations will be carried out and attempts are made to engage the patient in a therapeutic alliance. Such an approach has been found to be cost-effective in the USA (Smith *et al*, 1986), and controlled studies using similar techniques are required in this country.

Shared care

There are opportunities for psychiatrists and general practitioners to carry out 'shared care' of such patients (usually those with somatisation disorder or chronic unexplained pain). This approach, which has been adopted by the author (Bass, 1990, 1992), is described in more detail by Smith (1991). The guidelines below are used for a simple leaflet which is based on research in this field, advising on the management of the heartsink patient, frequent attender or chronic somatiser.

Guidelines for GPs

(a) Try to be proactive rather than reactive. That is, arrange to see the patient at regular, fixed intervals rather than allow him or her to dictate the timing and frequency of visits.

Appointments should take place at approximately the frequency with which the patient has been visiting the doctor, i.e. every two, four, or six weeks. Once this pattern of visits is established, the time between visits can be gradually extended.

(b) During these visits aim to broaden the agenda with the patient. This involves establishing a problem list, eliciting current and relevant psychosocial problems, and allowing the patient to discuss his emotional problems. Try to avoid an 'organ recital' i.e. a long discourse about the many and varied somatic symptoms. Asking the patient to draw up a problem list can be useful. Individual problems can then be addressed in turn.

(c) Reduce unnecessary drugs. Often more than one analgesic or psychotropic drug is being prescribed. Try to negotiate a gradual withdrawal of one drug at a time, for example DF 118, followed by valium. Psychotropic drugs should always be tapered over the course of six to ten weeks.

(d) Treat any co-existing psychiatric disorder such as panic attacks or depression with psychotropic drugs if necessary. Some chronic attenders have these concurrent disorders, which should be treated in the normal way.

(e) Whenever possible try to minimise the contact these patients have with other specialists or practitioners (including alternative practitioners). The reasons for this are:
   (i) the potential for iatrogenic harm is greater if the patients are visiting many doctors (and being told different things by each one)
   (ii) containment is easier if only one (or at most two) practitioners are involved.

(f) Always interview the patient's nearest relative and inform him of the management plan. Your best efforts can be sabotaged by spouses or partners, and so try to co-opt a relative as a therapeutic ally.

(g) Try to reduce your expectation of cure with these patients. The multiple psychosocial and/or medical problems are often chronic and intractable and may be insoluble. Try to aim for containment and damage limitation i.e. limit the iatrogenic damage that may result from doctor-shopping, as well as the damage to your own self-esteem as a doctor. If you encourage the patient (and yourself) to think in terms of coping and not curing, you will feel less frustrated and demoralised.

(h) Don't expect rapid changes. Patients will become less demanding over a matter of months, especially if they feel that their complaints and symptoms are being taken seriously.

(i) If you are in a group practice then inform your partners of your management plan. Share it with them and develop contingency plans for when you are off duty.

(j) Finally, arrange some support for yourself, either from your colleagues or from someone with experience of managing these patients.

References

ANDREWS, H. & HOUSE, A. (1989) Functional dysphonia. In *Life Events and Illness* (eds G. W. Brown & T. Harris), pp. 343–360. London: Unwin Hyman.
BASS, C. (1990) The frequent attender in general practice. *Update*, **40**, 494–501.
—— (1992) Patients with chronic somatization: what can the psychiatrist offer? In *Practical Problems in Clinical Psychiatry* (eds K. Hawton & P. Cowen), pp. 105–117. Oxford: Oxford Medical.
—— & MURPHY, M. (1991) Somatisation disorder in a British teaching hospital. *British Journal of Clinical Practice*, **45**, 237–244.
—— & POTTS, S. (1992) The somatoform disorders. In *Recent Advances in Psychiatry, Vol. 8* (ed. K. Granville-Grossman), pp. 143–163. Edinburgh: Churchill Livingstone.
——, SHARPE, M. & MAYOU, R. (eds) (in press) Management of patients with medically unexplained symptoms in the general hospital. In *Treatment of Patients with Functional Somatic Symptoms*. Oxford: Oxford University Press.
BENJAMIN, S. & BRIDGES, K. (1994) The need for specialised services for chronic somatisers. In *Liaison Psychiatry: Defining Needs and Planning Services* (eds S. Benjamin, A. House & P. Jenkins), pp. 16–23. London: Gaskell.
——, BARNES, D., BERGER, S., et al (1988) The relationship of chronic pain, mental illness and organic disorders. *Pain*, **32**, 185–195.
—— & EMINSON, D. M. (1992) Abnormal illness behaviour: childhood experiences and long-term consequences. *International Review of Psychiatry*, **4**, 55–70.
BHATT, A., TOMENSON, B. & BENJAMIN, S. (1989) Transcultural patterns of somatization in primary care: a preliminary report. *Journal of Psychosomatic Research*, **33**, 671–680.
BROWN, G. W. & HARRIS, J. (1989) *Life Events and Illness* (eds G. W. Brown & T. Harris). London: Unwin Hyman.
CRAIG, T. K. & BOARDMAN, A. P. (1990) Somatization in primary care settings. In *Somatization: Physical Symptoms and Psychological Illness* (ed. C. Bass). Oxford: Blackwell.
CREED, F. (1992) The future of liaison psychiatry in the UK. *International Review of Psychiatry*, **4**, 101–110.
——, MAYOU, R. & HOPKINS, A. (1992) *Medical Symptoms not Explained by Organic Disease*. London: Royal College of Psychiatrists and Royal College of Physicians.
DE LEON, J., SAIZ-RUIZ, J., CHINCHILLA, A., et al (1987) Why do some psychiatric patients somatize? *Acta Psychiatrica Scandinavica*, **76**, 203–209.
ESCOBAR, J. I., GOLDING, J. M., HOUGH, R. L., et al (1987) Somatization in the community: relationship to disability and use of services. *American Journal of Public Health*, **77**, 837–840.
GARRALDA, M. E. & BAILEY, D. (1987) Psychosomatic aspects of children's consultation in primary care. *European Archives of Psychiatry and Neurological Sciences*, **236**, 319–322.
GATER, R. & GOLDBERG, D. (1991) Pathways to psychiatric care in South Manchester. *British Journal of Psychiatry*, **159**, 90–96.
GOLDBERG, D., GASK, L. & O'DOWD, T. (1989) The treatment of somatization: teaching techniques of reattribution. *Journal of Psychosomatic Research*, **33**, 689–695.
—— & BRIDGES, K. (1985) Somatic presentations of psychiatric illness in primary care. *Journal of Psychosomatic Research*, **32**, 137–144.
HOUSE, A. & CREED, F. (1993) Training in liaison psychiatry. Recommendations from the liaison Psychiatry Group Executive Committee. *Psychiatric Bulletin*, **17**, 95–96.
JENKINS, R. & MOWBRAY, J. (1991) *Post-viral Fatigue Syndrome*. Chichester: Wiley.
KATON, W., LIN, E., VON KORFF, M., et al (1991) Somatization: a spectrum of severity. *American Journal of Psychiatry*, **148**, 34–40.
KELLNER, R. (1990) Somatization. Theories and research. *Journal of Nervous and Mental Disease*, **178**, 150–160.
KLEINMAN, A. & KLEINMAN, J. (1985) Somatization: the interconnections in Chinese society among culture, depressive experiences, and the meaning of pain. In *Culture and Depression* (eds A. Kleinman & B. Good). Berkeley: University of California Press.
LINTON, S. J. (1987) Chronic pain: the case for prevention. *Behaviour Research and Therapy*, **25**, 313–317.

—— & KAMWENDO, K. (1986) Relaxation gymnastics as preventative control for neck and shoulder pain: a case study. *Scandinavian Journal of Behaviour Therapy*, **15**, 39–44.

MAYOU, R. A. (1992) Patients' fears of illness: chest pain and palpitations. In *Medical Symptoms not Explained by Organic Disease* (eds F. H. Creed, R. Mayou & A. Hopkins), pp. 25–33. London: Royal College of Psychiatrists and Royal College of Physicians

MARTIN, R. L., ROBERTS, W. V., CLAYTON, P. J., *et al* (1977) Psychiatric illness and non-cancer hysterectomy. *Disease of the Nervous System*, **140**, 974–980.

MEADOW, R. (1977) Munchausen syndrome by proxy: the hinterland of child abuse. *Lancet*, **ii**, 343–345.

PHILIPS, C., GRANT, L. & BERKOWITZ, J. (1991) The prevention of chronic pain and disability: a preliminary investigation. *Behaviour Research and Therapy*, **29**, 443–450.

SCHLESINGER, R. D., DANIEL, D. G., RABIN, P., *et al* (1989). Factitious disorder with physical manifestations: pitfalls of diagnosis and management. *Southern Medical Journal*, **82**, 210–214.

SHAW, J. & CREED, F. (1991) The cost of somatization. *Journal of Psychosomatic Research*, **35**, 307–312.

SMITH, G. R. MONSON, R. A. & RAY, D. C. (1986) Psychiatric consultation in somatization disorder. *New England Journal of Medicine*, **314**, 1407–1413.

SMITH, R. C. (1991) Somatization disorder: defining its role in clinical medicine. *Journal of General Internal Medicine*, **6**, 168–175.

TYLEE, A. (1991) Recognising depression. *Practitioner*, **235**, 669–672.

19 Primary care

KEITH LLOYD and RACHEL JENKINS

The opportunities for primary and secondary prevention in primary care are very great since it is at the level of primary care that recognition of patient risk factors and detection of illness usually occurs (Department of Health, 1989). The general practitioner and primary health care team are the main point of first service contact for the majority of patients. Over 98% of the UK population are registered with an NHS general practitioner. Thus, Shepherd et al (1966) pointed out as long ago as 1966, "the general practitioner by virtue of his provision of primary health care to the population is well placed to monitor psychiatric disorder in the community as a whole and to identify those patients serious enough to warrant treatment". In the 1990s it was recognised that the other members of the primary health care team can also participate in the screening identification prevention and treatment of psychiatric disorder (Goldberg & Huxley, 1992). Given the constraints on team members' time any screening procedures would have to be shown to be of practical value.

The identification and support of those at risk for illness is the key primary preventive strategy. Early detection and prompt treatment of those who are already ill should be priorities for secondary preventive initiatives. Depression has a better prognosis if it is identified by the GP (Johnson & Goldberg, 1976). Screening is therefore a key strategy both in primary prevention (to detect those at increased risk, either by virtue of personal characteristics or of their stressful and unsupported environment) and in secondary prevention (to detect those who are already ill). For example, it has been suggested that 40% of health visitors' clients have evidence of significant emotional disease (Briscoe & Williams, 1985). Identification, using self-rating questionnaires of those at risk could make it easier to target intervention. Outcome studies of social work interventions indicate benefit in selected patients (Corney, 1981). Simple self-report screening instruments such as the General Health Questionnaire (Goldberg et al, 1988) could be handed out by the receptionist so that the GP has a result available when seeing the patient. It has been demonstrated that use of such instruments can significantly improve the detection rates of psychiatric morbidity (Skuse & Williams, 1984; Shapiro et al, 1987).

It is also important to flag up the crucial role of many universal and selective primary prevention strategies which take place in primary care. Specifically health education, immunisation, nutrition, dental hygiene, avoidance of alcohol, family planning, antenatal, perinatal and post-natal care, all of which have important implications for mental health.

Considerations on screening

Primary prevention

Screening can either focus on high risk populations (there tend to be predisposing factors such as loss of mother in childhood or genetic loading) or high risk situations. In practice it is much more difficult to identify high risk populations than high risk situations. In addition the preventive power is greater if one concentrates on the high risk situations, since these are more likely to be followed by mental illness than high risk populations. We need to know the likelihood of illness following a pregnancy with risk factors, the evidence that intervention will avert the occurrence of illness and the cost–benefit analysis of the intervention.

Secondary prevention

Screening seeks to identify the illness with a high degree of accuracy, preferably in early stages of development. Ideally the screening procedure should have a high positive predictive value and a low mis-classification rate. Having detected the condition, it should be possible to reverse, alleviate or modify its impact on a sufferer.

There are various types of screening programmes. Selective screening involves the investigation of identified high risk individuals. This can involve individuals at high risk who develop a single disease and may be single-phasic, such as amniocentesis in elder mothers; or may involve individuals at high risk of developing a number of disorders, and may be multi-phasic such as antenatal investigations in pregnant women. On the other hand, mass screening programmes such as mammography investigate large populations without specific consideration of individual risk factors.

A number of criteria should be considered when setting up a screening programme. These criteria are summarised below and will be considered in turn in relation to the disorders which occur in general practice.

(a) What is the seriousness, consequences and frequency of the condition?
(b) When is detection and intervention possible in the natural history of the condition?
(c) Is there an effective treatment or will detection merely increase the lead time?
(d) Is there a sensitive and specific test?
(e) Is it possible to identify individuals at risk?
(f) What are the cost–benefit analyses and resource implications of the programme?

Psychiatric disorders in general practice

This section will consider prevention of specific mental disorders in general practice as opposed to secondary care settings.

Neurosis

Seriousness, consequences and frequency

Less than 10% of general practice psychiatry is taken up with patients suffering from psychosis (Goldberg & Huxley, 1992). The bulk of psychiatric illness seen in primary care is due to non-psychotic syndromes. It has been estimated that the average GP with a list size of 2000 identifies approximately one in six (300) patients with a neurotic disorder a year (Shepherd et al, 1966; Royal College of General Practitioners, 1973) and there is considerable research evidence that a further one in six i.e. a further 300 patients with a neurotic disorder go undetected by the GP. These groups are known as conspicuous and hidden psychiatric morbidity respectively. The range of symptoms is large but depression is the commonest condition, occurring in over three-quarters of cases, with anxiety and psychosomatic disorders following. GPs tend to over-diagnose anxiety and under-diagnose depression with important therapeutic implications. Therefore both because of the hidden morbidity and frequent faulty diagnosis, screening is potentially extremely important in general practice. Studies have shown that there is considerable overlap in clinical severity between patients seen in primary care and those depressed patients seen in out-patient settings. Many have a good prognosis but a third pursue a chronic course lasting more than 12 months (Mann et al, 1981). There are many important associations with untreated depression such as an increased risk of physical illness (Eastwood & Trevelyan, 1972) an increased risk of suicide and para-suicide, occupational problems such as sickness, absence and accidents (Jenkins, 1992), and problems for children of depressed parents such as cognitive and emotional impairment or neglect and even abuse (Rutter & Madge, 1986).

When is detection and intervention possible?

About 90% of individuals in a community with psychosocial disorders will consult their GP in any given year although not necessarily concurrent with nor indeed complaining of psychological symptoms. Therefore, screening in primary care settings is nearly as rewarding as screening in the community, and is very much easier to do in the GP's surgery than on a house-to-house basis.

Marks et al (1979) studied factors associated with GPs' ability to detect psychiatric morbidity. Doctors who were good at detecting psychological disorder were usually interested in the psychological aspects of disease, conducting interviews in an open-ended and empathic manner and usually having had some training in psychiatry. Patients who presented their psychiatric disorder in somatic terms tended to be missed. Johnson & Goldberg (1976) found that those patients identified by screening and notified to GPs had a better prognosis than those not so identified, particularly if the disorder was severe. Thus screening alone has some therapeutic benefits.

Is there an effective treatment?

The treatment for depression is careful exploration of symptoms and social circumstances followed by support together with antidepressants where necessary (Paykel & Priest, 1992). Antidepressants have been shown to be effective in double-blind studies (Thomson *et al*, 1982). Tyrer *et al* (1988) showed that self-help, cognitive behavioural therapy and tricyclic antidepressants were equally effective in the treatment of non-psychotic disorders. In their study, the self-help option consisted of a relaxation tape, self-help instructions and regular brief sessions with a therapist offering supportive advice. Intervention by nurses who had received a specialist training in behavioural psychotherapy was effective in the management of chronic neurotic disorders in the community. The use of nurse therapists who have more time to devote to such treatments has economic advantages over treatment by a medical practitioner (Goldberg & Huxley, 1992).

The treatment of anxiety is behavioural but tranquillisers are still prescribed in large quantities. They are symptomatic rather than curative drugs and are addictive. In Tyrer's 1980 study they were shown to be less effective than a placebo. Referral to specialist psychiatric help is relatively uncommon: only about 5% of patients with non-psychotic disorders are so referred (Goldberg & Huxley, 1992).

Is there a specific and sensitive test?

There are many screening instruments available for use in general practice settings, the best known being the General Health Questionnaire (GHQ) (Goldberg *et al*, 1988). The purpose of the GHQ is to detect a range of psychiatric disorders – it is not a diagnostic instrument. Well validated and easy to complete and score, it is a pencil and paper self-completion test taking only a few minutes and is widely used as a first stage screening test.

Identificaton of individuals at risk

Risk factors for developing psychological disorders are bereavement, unemployment or difficulties at work, social isolation, marital problems, single parenthood, recent childbirth, caring for a disabled relative, physical or sensory disability, painful or life threatening or otherwise serious physical illness (Goldberg & Huxley, 1992). The elderly are at particular risk of developing affective and other non-psychotic disorders (Blanchard, 1992).

Risk factors for a poor outcome once illness has developed include the severity of the initial psychiatric illness, the presence of significant physical illness and the presence of severe social problems.

Cost–benefit analysis and resource implications

The total direct and indirect costs of depression and anxiety have been estimated at 4.6 billion pounds a year. The routine use of the GHQ in the general practice surgery costs approximately 2p per person (Croft-Jeffreys & Wilkinson, 1989).

Alcohol

Seriousness, consequences and frequency

Only a small proportion of problem drinkers in the community are known to specialised agencies (Edwards *et al*, 1973) (see Chapter 12). It has been estimated that the average practice of 2500 patients contains five known cases of chronic alcoholism and 25 undetected cases (Royal College of General Practitioners, 1973). The Office of Health Economics (1981) has estimated that there are some three million heavy drinkers in England and Wales, 700 000 problem drinkers and 150 000 individuals with alcohol dependence syndrome. The physical, social economic and psychiatric sequelae of problem drinking are well documented (Murray, 1986).

When is detection and intervention possible?

Both are possible at any stage in the natural history of the condition depending upon the patients' willingness to acknowledge the problem and accept intervention.

Is there an effective treatment?

Drug treatment is available for withdrawal symptoms. Alcoholics Anonymous provide a social structure within which individuals can seek peer support. Group psychotherapy is widely employed in clinics. The physical sequelae require treatment in their own right; medication may include Antabuse or similar drugs to discourage alcohol consumption. Murray (1986) in summarising the evidence for the effectiveness of intervention concludes that the key determinants of outcome are the personal and environmental circumstances of the drinker.

Is there a specific and sensitive test?

Several screening instruments exist which have been extensively evaluated such as the MAST and CAGE questionnaires which are simple and quick to apply (Mayfield et al, 1974). There are suggestive haematological and biochemical findings which may be detected on routine blood testing.

Identification of individuals at risk

Extensive epidemiological investigation has been carried out into risk factors for alcohol abuse. These include occupation, family history (both environmental and genetic), past behaviour, cultural factors, personality, gender, and marital status. Recently there has been an increase in alcoholism among young people and especially women. From this work it should be possible to identify those individuals most at risk, although the condition is so all pervasive that the evidence suggests that GPs should have a high index of suspicion for alcohol-related problems among almost all their patients. Wallace (1988) has used self-report health diaries to assist early detection of problem drinkers.

Cost–benefit and resource implications

Alcoholics lost at least two and a half times more time off work than their more sober work mates (Murray, 1986). There are strong associations with marital violence and disharmony, road traffic and industrial accidents and vagrancy. The cost–benefit analysis would depend on the efficacy of treatment interventions.

Most of the screening instruments are easily applicable by general practitioners and are not time consuming.

Childhood and adolescent disorders

Seriousness, consequences and frequency

The Isle of Wight study (Rutter *et al*, 1976) estimated the community prevalence of childhood psychiatric disorder at 6.8%, about two-thirds of which were conduct disorders and about one-third emotional disorders. The prevalence in an Inner London Borough (Rutter *et al*, 1975) has been estimated at approximately twice that of the Isle of Wight. Psychiatric disorder is twice as common in boys as girls. The adult sequelae of childhood psychiatric disorders are the subject of intense interest and research at the present time (Harrington, 1990). It is considered by some that major depression constitutes an increasing public health problem among the young (Klerman, 1988) and the suicide rate has been rising in young men for two decades (Department of Health, 1993). Parasuicide is a major problem among adolescents. Child sexual abuse is still a very contentious issue in terms of frequency (prevalence estimates are being continually adjusted upwards) and its long-term consequences.

When are detection and intervention possible?

Evidence of disturbance is based more on the observations of behaviour made by parents, teachers and others than on the accounts of children themselves.

Is there an effective treatment?

The treatment of childhood psychiatric disorders differs from that of adult disorders in that it often involves other members of the family and the broader network. Psychological treatments are commonly used. Effective treatment strategies have been developed for conditions such as enuresis and encopresis.

Is there a sensitive and specific test?

The Rutter B Scale is a widely used research screening instrument which is completed by teachers. There are a few self-report instruments available for administration to children. Those in use tend to show a high prevalence of emotional symptoms of uncertain significance. There are a few instruments available for screening purposes in a general practice setting. A recent review (Place, 1987) observed that there are few specific instruments for screening adolescents, although the GHQ "proved to be reasonably efficient".

Identification of individuals at risk

Psychiatric disorder in children living in an Inner London Borough (Rutter *et al*, 1975) was associated with family discord, parental psychiatric disorder, large family size, overcrowding and lack of home ownership. Extensive work has been conducted into the identification of children at risk from sexual abuse. Normal child development checks already in use are potential ways of detecting physical and psychological abuse and neglect. Social services are involved in monitoring children at risk.

Cost–benefit and resource implications

The statutory responsibility for monitoring and intervening in child abuse lies with social services departments and has massive financial implications. It is less clear about the cost–benefit and resource implications of screening for other psychiatric disorders.

Schizophrenia

Seriousness, consequences and frequency

The lifetime risk of schizophrenia is in the order of 1%. It is generally assumed that the vast majority of first presentation cases will be detected with relative ease and managed initially by the psychiatric services (Harrison, 1988). The majority of the work in general practice involves the maintenance and monitoring of patients who have already been diagnosed and who are in the poor prognosis group with persistent handicaps and in need of rehabilitation and support. Ten per cent of schizophrenics commit suicide (Jenkins, 1990).

When are detection and intervention possible?

Detection of the first episode is generally not difficult. Subsequent monitoring should focus on the re-emergence of symptoms. To date little emphasis has been placed on the need to monitor for long-term complications of drug treatment such as dystonia and tardive dyskinesia. With the increasing trend towards GP prescribing for long-term patients this will become an increasing area of concern.

Is there an effective treatment?

Drug treatment has been shown to be effective in some groups of patients (Hogarty & Ulrich, 1977). Family intervention and education also have some effect in preventing relapse (Leff *et al*, 1985).

Is there a specific and sensitive instrument?

Relapse is generally assessed on the basis of clinical judgement about the level of symptomatology and social functioning. Sensitive screening instruments such as the PSE are not suited to general practice screening. Extra-pyramidal side-effects can be rated in a number of ways using instruments such as the ADS and TAKE (Holloway, 1988). Assessment of side-effects requires skill and general practitioners may require training in this area. Alternatively this could be carried out by a community psychiatric nurse.

Is it possible to identify individuals at risk?

Genetic risk factors are well documented. Environmental risk factors are less clear. Early intervention strategies aimed at primary prevention have not yet been developed. Anyone taking anti-psychotic medication over time is at risk of developing side-effects.

Cost–benefit and resource implications

The whole process of care in the community has immense resource implications. Screening and intervention in high expressed emotion families could be a cost-effective way of reducing admissions and research is now underway to evaluate the effectiveness of community psychiatric nurses undertaking this work.

Learning difficulties

Seriousness, consequences and frequency

The average general practice list has 10 patients with severe learning difficulties. Between 2 and 3.5% of the population have an IQ of below 70. Severe learning difficulties are associated with intrauterine and perinatal problems, Down's syndrome, inherited abnormalities and congenital malformations (see Chapter 14).

Is early treatment possible?

Prenatal diagnosis is available for Down's syndrome and some other conditions. Early postnatal biochemical checks are available for phenylketonuria (PKU) and hypothyroidism which can be effectively treated.

Are there sensitive and specific tests?

For Down's syndrome, hypothyroidism and biochemical disorders such as PKU, regular antenatal and developmental checks are non-specific screening devices.

Is it possible to identify individuals at risk?

Older mothers are at increased risk of having Down's syndrome babies and can be offered amniocentesis, and blood tests are becoming increasingly available. Genetic counselling is available for inherited conditions.

Cost–benefit and resource implications

Screening programmes for the above conditions already exist. Screening for PKU or congenital hypothyroidism provides an interesting contrast to most other forms of psychiatric screening. Both conditions are very rare and, unlike the neuroses, both have specific aetiologies. Both are readily treatable and therefore it is highly cost-effective to screen for them.

Dementia

Seriousness, consequences and frequency

Only 5% of the elderly are in any form of institutional care and only 14% of those with dementia. It is generally estimated that about 6% of the elderly population suffer from dementia rising to 20% of the over 80s. Community studies show that not all patients with cognitive impairment undergo further significant decline. With an increasing elderly population dementia is going to become more common (Jacoby & Bergman, 1986).

When is detection and intervention possible?

Apart from those patients who are worried about their memories, the vast majority of cases are brought to the attention of the general practitioner by relatives or come to light when some change in the patient's circumstances means that they can no longer function independently. It is particularly difficult to distinguish the effects of mild dementia from the effects of normal ageing or lifelong poor cognitive performance. Williamson *et al* (1964) found that general practitioners were unaware of 87% of the cases of mild to moderate dementia on their lists. Results from a large identification and intervention study among over 75s in East Anglia suggests that although the quality of life of dementia sufferers can be improved by early detection, admission rates are not reduced (O'Connor *et al*, 1991).

Is there an effective treatment?

Alzheimer's disease is not reversible. Its social and psychological accompaniments are amenable to treatment. Underlying physical conditions can also be treated as part of secondary and tertiary prevention. Accompanying toxic confusional states (from infections or drugs) are not uncommon, and are important to treat as they greatly exacerbate problems with cognitive function.

Is there a sensitive and specific test?

Screening instruments are available for the measurement of cognitive state such as the geriatric mental state but as Kay *et al* (1985) observe there is little standardisation of criteria across instruments and centres. Assessments of social functioning and supports are even less standardised. Mostly the GP relies on clinical judgement. Routine measurement of blood pressure and checks for evidence of atherosclerotic disease are of value in the detection of risk factors for atherosclerotic dementia.

Cost–benefit and resource implications

The resource implications of an ageing population are immense. It is not clear how effective earlier intervention in the dementing process will be.

Conclusions

Primary prevention

The general practice setting is the first point of service contact for the vast majority of patients with a psychiatric disorder. The key to successful primary preventive strategies lies with increasing detection in groups who are at risk of developing psychiatric disorders. One of the aims behind the 1990 contract for general practitioners was "to give prevention of illness and health promotion greater emphasis" (Jenkins, 1990). Particular emphasis is given to screening procedures although these are primarily for physical disorders and immunisation procedures. Mention is also given to health checks (Chisholm, 1990). The use of simple screening instruments such as the General Health Questionnaire could form a useful part of health checks for newly registered patients, patients not seen for three years and patients over the age of 75 years. This latter group particularly is known to be at high risk of psychiatric and emotional disorder. As more and more practices establish age/sex registers it will be possible to construct an at risk register to identify groups at particular risk of psychiatric morbidity, for example the sensorally and physically disabled, the bereaved, the socially isolated, the unsupported and the elderly.

Secondary prevention

Early case detection is an important secondary preventive strategy. There is a need to implement and evaluate on-going training packages to assist the members of the primary health care team in the recognition of psychiatric disorders and to evaluate the increasing time spent by psychiatrists in primary health care settings (Goldberg & Huxley, 1992). Health education initiatives for the users are required to raise the profile of mental illness and facilitate sufferers into making positive choices regarding help-seeking behaviour.

Tertiary prevention

As Goldberg & Huxley (1992) state, "another aim of teaching doctors to detect mental disorders is to identify the minority of patients with disorders that are unlikely to restitute without help". They set as examples agoraphobia and chronic schizophrenia. Other disorders often pursuing a chronic course are severe depression, mania and acute schizophrenia. All these disorders can be helped significantly by intervention. The majority of chronic psychiatric morbidity in primary care settings consists of non-psychotic disorders such as depression, anxiety and somatic symptoms and it is in this area that skills packages need to be developed for general practitioners, practice nurses and other members of the primary health care team.

References

BARRACLOUGH, B. M., BUNCH, J., NELSON, B., et al (1974) A hundred cases of suicide: clinical aspects. *British Journal of Psychiatry*, 125, 355–373.
BLANCHARD, M. (1992) The elderly. *International Review of Psychiatry*, 4, 3–4.
BRISCOE, M. & WILLIAMS, P. (1985) Emotional problems in the clients of health visitors. *Health Visitor*, 58, 197–198.
CHISHOLM, J. (1990) Screening in practice: The 1990 contract – its history and content. *British Medical Journal*, 300, 853–856.
CORNEY, R. (1981) Social work effectiveness in the management of depressed women: a clinical trial. *Psychological Medicine*, 11, 417–423.
CROFT-JEFFREYS, C. & WILKINSON, G. (1989) Costs of neurotic disorder in UK general practice: Editorial. *Psychological Medicine*, 19, 551–558.

DEPARTMENT OF HEALTH (1989) *Caring for People, Community Care in the Next Decade and Beyond*, pp. 8–9. London: HMSO.
—— (1993) Health of Men. In *On the State of Public Health*, pp. 99–100. London: HMSO.
EASTWOOD, R. & TREVELYAN, M. H. (1972) Relationship between physical and psychiatric disorder. *Psychological Medicine*, **2**, 363–372.
EDWARDS, G., HAWKER, A., HEASMAN, C., *et al* (1973) Alcoholics known or unknown to agencies: epidemiological study in a London suburb. *British Journal of Psychiatry*, **123**, 169–183.
GOLDBERG, D. (1989) Screening for psychiatric disorder. In *The Scope of Epidemiological Psychiatry* (eds P. Williams & G. Wilkinson). London: Routledge.
——, D., BRIDGES, K., DUNCAN-JONES, P., *et al* (1988) Detecting anxiety and depression in general practice settings. *British Medical Journal*, **297**, 897–899.
—— & HUXLEY, P. (1980) *Mental Illness in the Community: the Pathway to Psychiatric Care*. London: Tavistock.
—— & —— (1992) *Common Mental Disorders. A Biosocial Mould*, pp. 46–48. London: Routledge.
HARRINGTON, R. (1992) The natural history and treatment of child and adolescent affective disorder. *Journal of Child Psychology and Psychiatry*, **33**, 1287–1302.
HARRISON, G., OWENS, D., HOLTON, A., *et al* (1988) A prospective study of severe mental disorder in Afro-Caribbean patients. *Psychological Medicine*, **18**, 643–657.
HOGARTY, G. E. & ULRICH, R. (1977) Temporal effects of drug and placebo in delaying relapse in schizophrenic out-patients. *Archives of Clinical Psychiatry*, **34**, 297–301.
HOLLOWAY, F. (1988) Prescribing for the long term mentally ill. *British Journal of Psychiatry*, **152**, 511–515.
JACOBY, R. & BERGMAN, U. (1986) The psychiatry of old age. In *Essentials of Postgraduate Psychiatry* (eds R. Murray, B. Hill & A. Thorley). London: Grune & Stratton.
JENKINS, R. (1990) Towards a system of outcome indicators for mental health care. *British Journal of Psychiatry*, **157**, 500–514.
—— (1992) Depression and anxiety – an overview of preventive strategies. In *The Prevention of Depression and Anxiety* (eds R. Jenkins & J. Newton). London: HMSO.
JENKINS, S. (1990) Screening and the 1990 contract. *British Medical Journal*, **300**, 825–826.
JOHNSTONE, A. & GOLDBERG, D. (1976) Psychiatric screening in general practice. *Lancet*, **i**, 605–608.
KAY, D. W. K., HENDERSON, A. S., SCOTT, R., *et al* (1985) Dementia and depression among the elderly living in the Hobart area. *Psychological Medicine*, **15**, 771–778.
KLERMAN, G. L. (1988) The current age of youthful melancholia. *British Journal of Psychiatry*, **152**, 4–14.
KUIPERS, L., BIRCHWOOD, M. & MCCREADIE, R. G. (1992) Psychosocial interventions in schizophrenia. A review of empirical studies. *British Journal of Psychiatry*, **160**, 272–275.
LEFF, J. & VAUGHN, C. (1981) The role of maintenance therapy and relative expressed emotion in relapse in schizophrenia: a 2 year follow up. *British Journal of Psychiatry*, **139**, 102–104.
——, KUIPERS, L., BERKOWITZ, R., *et al* (1985) A controlled trial of social intervention in the families of schizophrenic patients: two year follow up. *British Journal of Psychiatry*, **146**, 594–600.
LEWIS, G., PELOSI, A. J. & ARAYA, R., *et al* (1990) Measuring psychiatric disorder in the community. *Psychological Medicine*, **22**, 465–486.
MANN, A. H., JENKINS, R., BEASLEY, E. (1981) The twelve-month outcome of patients with neurotic illness in general practice. *Psychological Medicine*, **11**, 535–550.
MARKS, J., GOLDBERG, D., HILLIER, V. (1979) Determinants of the ability of GPs to detect psychiatric illness. *Psychological Medicine*, **9**, 337–350.
MAYFIELD, D., MILLARD, G. & HALL, D. (1974) The CAGE questionnaire: validation of a new alcoholism screening instrument. *American Journal of Psychiatry*, **131**, 1121–1123.
MURRAY, R. (1986) Alcoholism. In *Essentials of Postgraduate Psychiatry* (eds P. Hill, R. Murray, A. Thorley, *et al*). London: Grune & Stratton.
O'CONNOR, D. W. (1991) Does early intervention reduce the number of people with dementia admitted to institutions for long-term care? *British Medical Journal*, **302**, 871–875.
OFFICE OF HEALTH ECONOMICS (1981) *Alcohol: Reducing the Harm*. London: OHE.
PAYKEL, E. S. & PRIEST, R. G. (1992) Recognition and management of depression in general practice: consensus statement. *British Medical Journal*, **305**, 1198–1202.
PLACE, M. (1987) The relative value of screening instruments in adolescence. *Journal of Adolescence*, **10**, 227–240.
ROYAL COLLEGE OF GENERAL PRACTITIONERS (1973) Present status and future needs of general practice. *Journal of the Royal College of General Practitioners*, Report 16.
RUTTER, M., YULE, B., QUINTON, D., *et al* (1975) Attainment and adjustment in two geographical areas. *British Journal of Psychiatry*, **126**, 520–533.

———, TIZARD, J., YULE, W., et al (1976) Isle of Wight Studies 1964–1974. *Psychological Medicine*, **6**, 313–332.

——— & MADGE, N. (1986) *Cycles of Disadvantage: a Review of Research*, pp. 1–20. London: Heinemann.

SHEPHERD, M., COOPER, B., BROWN, A., et al (1966) *Psychiatric Illness in General Practice*. Oxford: Oxford University Press.

SHAPIRO, S., GERMAN, P., SHINNER, E., et al (1987) An experiment to change detection and management of mental illness in primary care. *Medical Care*, **25**, 327–329.

SKUSE, D. & WILLIAMS, P. (1984) Screening for psychiatric disorder in general practice. *Psychological Medicine*, **14**, 365–378.

THOMPSON, J., RANKIN, H., ASHCROFT, G., et al (1982) The treatment of depression in general practice. *Psychological Medicine*, **12**, 741–751.

TYRER, P., SEIRENIGHT, N., MURPHY, S., et al (1988) The Nottingham study of neurotic disorder. Comparison of clinical and psychological Rx. *Lancet*, **2**, 235–240.

WALLACE, P., CUTLER, S. & HAINES, A. (1988) Randomised controlled trial of general practitioner intervention in patients with excessive alcohol consumption. *British Medical Journal*, **297**, 663–668.

WEINSTEIN, M. & FINBERG, H. (1980) *Clinical Decision Analysis*. Philadelphia: W. B. Saunders.

WILLIAMSON, J., STOHAE, I. H., GRAY, S., et al (1964) Old people at home – unreported needs. *Lancet*, **i**, 1117–1120.

Index

Compiled by JOHN GIBSON

Acts of Parliament (UK)
  Act for Preserving the Health of
    Prisoners in Gaol and Preventing
    Gaol Distemper (1774) 168
  Misuse of Drugs Act (1971) 104
  Mental Health Act (1983) 165
  Police and Criminal Evidence Act
    (1984) 169
  National Health Service Act and
    Community Care Act (1990)
    131, 137
adjustment disorders 178
adolescents, primary care 203–4
adrenocorticotrophic hormone 41
adrenoreceptor blockers 41
ADS 204
affective disorders 53–63
  biological causes 54
  bipolar 53, 54
  causative factors 53–7
  epidemiology 53–4
  genetic factors 54
  personality 54
  prevention 57–63
    primary 57–8
      event centred interventions 58
      genetic counselling 57–8
      parent–child relationships 58
      research 63
    secondary 58–61, 63
      early intervention 60
      event centred intervention 60
      interventions with vulnerable
        families 60
    tertiary prevention 61–2, 63
      prevention of relapse/recurrence
        61–2
      rehabilitation 61
  secondary in medically ill 178–9
  social factors 55–7

  coping repertoire 56–7
  unipolar 53
agoraphobia 94, 207
AIDS 43
  suicide 70
AIDS-related disorders 43
alcohol
  demand reduction 106–8
  advertising 107
  community responses 108
  education 106–7
  drunken driving 164
  foetal alcohol syndrome 126,
    133–4
  general practice care 201–3
  genetics 34
  harm reduction 108
  homicide associated 164
  incidence 202
  intake in pregnancy 126
  legislation 106
  primary care 201–3
  related problems 103–11
  taxation 105–6
  violence associated 164
alliances development 19
alpha-fetoprotein 135
Alzheimer's dementia 40
  aetiology 150
  aluminium in 43
  Apo e4 35
  Down's syndrome associated 34
  genetics 34–5
  head trauma-induced 151
  prevention 150–1
amniocentesis 135
amphetamines 48
Angelmann's syndrome 131
anorexia nervosa 33
  demographic characteristics 97

genetics 34
incidence 96
personality 97
prevention 99–101
twins 97
See also eating disorders
antidepressants 62, 200–1
   after ECT 62
   serotonergic 69
   suicide prevention 69
   tetracyclic 69
anti-Parkinsonian medications 48
antisocial disorders, genetics 34
antisocial/psychopathic personality disorder 164
anxiety disorder 88–94
   anticipatory disorder 92
   early detection 91–2
   factors influencing development 90 (fig.)
   inter-relationship with other neuroses 89
   prevalence 3
   preventable factors 89–90
   prevention prospects 94
   psychosocial stressors 90–1
   secondary anxiety 92–3
      prevention 93
   tertiary prevention 94
apomorphine 41
aspirin 151
atherosclerotic brain disease 151
'at risk' families 28
autism, genetics of 34

Barlie Special Unit, Scotland 169
BEAM (brain electrical activity mapping) 41–2
benzodiazepines 48, 182
Better Services for the Mentally Handicapped (UK, 1971) 131
biological psychiatry 42–3
biotechnology 20
brain damage (kernicterus) 136
breast cancer 183
bulimia 96
   demographic characteristics 97
   family dynamics 98–9
   genetic component 97
   personality 97
   prevention 99–101
   See also eating disorders

CAGE 181, 202
cancer, patient with 185

Caplan, G. 4, 12
carbamazepine 48, 69
causation
   lack of specificity 15
   multifactorial 5
central nervous system 40–2
   disorders of function 40–2
   disorders of structure 42
chest pain 185, 193
child psychiatry 28, 115–27
   control group 119–21
   criteria for good outcome research 119
   effectiveness of therapy 121–3
   genetics 134
   in general practice 203–4
   Isle of Wight study 203
   pre-school intervention 127
   prevention of behavioural/emotional problems 160–1
   primary care 203–4
   primary prevention 18, 115–19
   psychotherapy research future 124
   public health model of prevention 125–7
   risk factors 115–16
   school effect 127
   secondary prevention 117–19
      'at risk' concept 117–18
      early 118–19
      late 119, 124
   seriously disturbed children 122
   sexual abuse 203
cholecystokinin 48
chromosome-21 34–5
chronic fatigue syndrome 182, 193
classification of prevention strategies 14 (table)
Clinical Interview Schedule 178
clonidine 48
clozapine 48
Community Based Rehabilitation 140
Confait case 169
coping response 15
CT scan 42
counselling 91

DART 59
Defeat Depression (R.C.Psych.,R.C.Gen. Pract.) 9, 59
delirium 46, 152–3
Denmark, homicide by people with mental illness 165

dementia 149–51
  Alzheimer's *see* Alzheimer's dementia
  in general practice 205–6
  multi-infarct 40, 150, 151
  prevention 150–1
  primary care 205–6
  symptomatic 150
depression 68–9
  prevalence 3
  elderly patients 148–9
  unipolar, genetics of 33–4
Doll, R., quoted 4
dopamine 40, 41
Down's syndrome 130, 131, 205
  amniocentesis 135
  prevention 132
  primary screening test 135
drug-related problems 103–11
  controls on prescribed drugs 105
  crop control measures 104
  demand reduction 106–8
    advertising 107
    community responses 108
    education 106–7
  harm reduction 110
  HIV risk 110–11
  interception 104
  interdiction 104

eating disorders 96–101
  prevention 99–101
  risk factors 96–9
    constitutional disposition 97
    demographic characteristics 97
    dieting 98
    family dynamics 98–9
    personality 97
    social/cultural influences 97–8
educational activities 9, 19
elder abuse 154
electroencephalography (EEG) 41
EMG-12 78
endorphins 48
environment, shared/non-shared 36
epidemiology 19
evaluation 21–3
expressed emotion 84

facial pain 182
factitious illness by proxy 189–90
foetal alcohol syndrome 126, 133–4
follicle-stimulating hormone 41
forensic psychiatry 157–70
  early prevention 158
  successful prevention models 160
  targets for prevention 158–60
  See also mentally abnormal offender
fragile X syndrome 131–2
  prenatal screening 135

galactosaemia, prenatal screening 136
General Health Questionnaire 178, 179, 198, 201
general hospitals 177–85
  liaison service 185
  prevention of non-organic disorders 179–80
  psychological/emotional problems in relatives 184
  staff 184
genetics 20, 32–8
  current knowledge 33–5
  current research 35–6
  ethics 32–3
  implications for prevention 36–8
  prospects 35–6
Geriatric Mental State 181
'graduates' 154
Grendon Prison 169
growth hormone 41
gynaecology 182–3

Head Start (USA) 177, 126, 158
Health of the Nation (1992) 3
histidinuria 136
HIV 183
  congenital 133
  drug misusers 110–11
  maternal, in developing countries 139
  suicide 70
Homestart 28
homocystinuria 136
Hospital Anxiety and Depression Scale 178, 179
Hunter's syndrome 136
Huntington's disease 35, 37
Hurler's syndrome 131, 136
5-hydroxytryptamine 40
hypothyroidism, congenital, screening for 205

immunocytochemistry 41
'indicated' measures 12–13
information
  modular 36–7
  particular 37
irritable bowel syndrome 182, 193

kernicterus (brain damage) 136

L-dopa 48
learning disorders, primary care 205
Lesch-Nyhan syndrome 131, 136
life event 16–17
lithium 47, 48, 69
    after ECT 62
luteinising hormone 41
lysosomal storage diseases 136

magnetic resonance imaging 42
manic depression, identical twins 33
maple syrup urine disease 136
MAST 181, 202
ME Association 191
mentally abnormal offender 163–7
    morbidity/mortality prevention 167
mental handicap 130–41
    behaviour disorders 138
    biomedical factors 130
    developing countries 139–40
    early intervention 134
    environmental causes 132–4
        drugs 134
        folate deficiency 133
        head injury 134
        hypoglycaemia 134
        infections 133
        ionising radiation 132
        lead poisoning 134
        meningoencephalitis 134
        mercury poisoning 134
        teratogenic drugs 132
        venous sinus thrombosis 134
    family adjustment 138–9
    genetic counselling 131–2
    neonatal screening 136
    prevalence 130
    prevention 140–1
        primary 131–4
        secondary 135–6
        tertiary 136–40
    psychiatric disorder associated 137–8
    'reverse retardation' 139
    socio-cultural factors 130
mental health education 19
Mental Hygiene Movement (US) 89
Mini Mental State 181
Misuse of Drugs Regulations (UK) (1985) 104
multidisciplinary approach 8–10
multifactorial aetiology 12
myocardial infarction 185

national counselling service for sick doctors 184
neurobiology 20

neurofibromatosis, peripheral 131
neuroleptics 47
neuroses 200–1
    genetics 34
    in general practice 200–1
    primary care 200–1
neurotransmission 40–2
'new morbidity' (poor child care, deprivation, abuse, injury) 141
NEWPIN 116–17
nicotine addiction 109–11
noradrenaline 40

obstetrics 182–3
old age psychiatry 148–55
    alcohol use/abuse 153
    anxiety states 153
    carers 154
    delirium 152–3
    dementia see dementia: Alzheimer's disease
    depression 148–9, 178
    elder abuse syndrome 154
    paranoid disorders 151–2
    phobic states 153
    psychiatric disorder survival into late life 154–5
    violence towards old people 153
oncology 183
opiate blocking agents 48
opportunities for prevention 8
organic psychiatric disorder 180–1
    secondary to:
        alcohol abuse 181
        drug abuse 181
        physical illness 180
organisational consultation 19

paracetamol self-poisoning 72–3
perinatal trauma 82
personality disorders, genetics 34
PET 41
phenylketonuria 126, 131
    prenatal diagnosis 136
    screening 205
physical presentation of psychiatric disorders 182
    See also somatisation
positional cloning 33
postpartum blues 182
post-traumatic stress disorder 26, 161–2
    primary prevention 162
Prader-Willi syndrome 131
precipitating factors 15
predisposing factors 15
prevalence of psychiatric disorder 3

primary care 198-207
  primary prevention 199
  screening 199
  secondary prevention 199
prevention, primary 5, 6-7, 12, 13, 206-7
  children 18
  conceptual developments 15-18
  definition 11
  mental health promotion relationship 13-14
  proactive 15
    micro v. macro 16
  reactive 15
  risk factor prevention 15
prevention, secondary 5, 7, 12, 207
  definition 11
prevention, selective 12
prevention, tertiary 5-6, 8, 12, 207
  definition 11
  drug treatment 46-8
prevention, universal 12
prisons
  morbidity/mortality in 167-9
  psychosocial deterioration in 169
professional attitudes 21
propranolol 48
Protocol for Investment in Health Gain (Welsh Office, 1992) 141
PSE 204
psychiatric diagnosis refinement 19
psychiatric disorders and physical illness 182-4
psychiatric disorders in general practice 199-206
  adolescent disorders 203-4
  alcoholism 201-3
  childhood disorders 203-4
  dementia 205-6
  learning difficulties 205
  neuroses 200-1
  schizophrenia 204-5
psychophysiological studies 41
psychosocial stressors 90-1
puerperal depression 183
puerperal psychosis 183

quantitative traits loci 35

relaxation pause 190
research 21-3
rhesus haemolytic disease 136
Royal College of Psychiatrists Special Committee 4-5
rubella, congenital 126, 133
Rutter B scale 203

Samaritans 75
'schizoaffective' psychosis 33
schizophrenia 47, 80-6
  clinical features 80
  CT scan 42
  drug treatment 47-8
  identical twins 33
  in general practice 204-5
  offending associated 163
  outcome 80-1
  peak incidence 80
  primary care 204-5
  primary prevention 81-3
    genetic factors 81
    occurrence of schizophrenic-like psychoses 81-2
    perinatal trauma 82
    social factors in 82-3
    structural brain damage 82
  relapse 47
  secondary prevention 83-4
    drug treatment 83-4
    social treatment 84
  suicide 70
  tertiary prevention 84-6
    social treatment 85-6
  violent behaviour 163
schizophrenic-like psychoses 81-2
serotonin 54
sexual dysfunction 181-2
smoking 43, 105, 109-10
  during pregnancy 133
social factors 25-6
social interventions 26-30
  level 1: the individual 27
  level 2: primary group 27-8
  level 3: social network 28-9
  level 4: culture 29
  level 5: society 29
social phobias 94
social support 17-18
somatisation 182, 188-95
  chronic 189
  prevalence in non-psychiatric settings 188 (table)
  primary prevention 189-91
    adults 190
    children 189-90
    public education 190-1
  psychiatrist-physician collaboration 194
  psychological treatment of acute/subacute syndromes 193-4
  secondary prevention by non-psychiatrists 191
    management after diagnosis 193
    patient identification 192-3

secondary prevention by psychiatrists
    191–4
  tertiary prevention 194
    guidelines for general practitioners
      195–6
    shared care 195
standardised clinical interview 179
substance abuse 8
  schizophrenia-like psychoses 82
  suicide 69
suicide 67–76
  attempted 67, 182
  control of methods used 71–3
  educational measures 73–4
  English prisoners 168
  family problems 71
  general hospital services for
    attempters 75
  limitations of prevention 75–6
  marital breakdown 71
  media prevention 73
  mentally abnormal offender 167
  physical ill-health 70–1
  poverty associated 71
  prevention 68–76
    limitations 75–6
    teenagers 124–5
  psychiatric disorder detection/
    treatment 68
    depression 68–9

schizophrenia 70
  substance abuse 69
schizophrenia associated 70, 81
services for people at risk 74–5
substance abuse associated 69
unemployment associated 71
support systems, natural 18–19
Symptom Check List 178

tacrine 46–7
TAKE 204
targets 20–1, 22 (table)
Tay–Sachs disease 131, 132
  prenatal diagnosis 136
tetrabenazine 46
tobacco 43, 105, 109–10
  See also smoking
tranquillisers 201
tuberose sclerosis 131
tyrosaemia 136

vaccination model 125, 126
ventricular enlargement 42
violence 163, 164, 166–7

Yerkes–Dodson law 88

Zung scale 59